Advance Praise for *Miss Kathi*

"Over multiple decades, Kathi Zellweger had access to North Korea that journalists—and most aid workers—can only dream of. This heartfelt and insightful memoir shows how one extraordinary humanitarian improved countless North Korean lives. A timely reminder that the people should not be punished for the actions of their leaders—and that one person really can make a difference."

Anna Fifield, former Asia editor for *The Washington Post*, author of *The Great Successor: The Divinely Perfect Destiny of Brilliant Comrade Kim Jong Un*

"Kathi Zellweger has an extraordinary story to tell. This book is a gift to the field of North Korea studies, and anyone who wants to get an unbiased, unvarnished, yet compassionate view of life for 'average' Koreans, from the horrific famine of the 1990s to the nuclear saber-rattling of today. Teaming up with the gifted author Mike Chinoy—himself a seasoned North Korea expert—results in a memoir that is as fascinating as it is readable."

John Delury, senior fellow, Asia Society, coauthor of *Wealth and Power: China's Long March to the Twenty-first Century*

"I'm in awe of *Miss Kathi*. This captivating book provides an unvarnished and unrivaled ground-truth account of bluster, heartbreak, and heroics in the world's least understood nation: North Korea."

Eason Jordan, former CNN chief news executive

"*Miss Kathi* provides an unprecedented look inside the real North Korea. Instead of the typical assertions of North

Korea being the *Hermit Kingdom* or the *Impossible State*, it describes the human dimensions of North Korea as seen by Kathi, a humanitarian worker, who through her tireless efforts provided help and hope to a people whose government had failed them."

Siegfried Hecker, former director, Los Alamos National Laboratory, professor emeritus, Stanford University

"Nobody knows North Korea like Kathi Zellweger, and the memoir of this Swiss aid official penetrates this elusive realm like no other. Improbable that a tall, blonde European could become such an insider, but Zellweger resided in Pyongyang for nearly five years and visited at last count seventy-five times, starting during the tragic famine of the 1990s through its baby steps toward economic reform in the 2000s, all taking place under the ominous cloud of the country's nuclear program. Cowritten with Mike Chinoy, no slouch himself when it comes to this country, the book brings out in equal parts the geopolitics, the humanity, and even the humor of life inside North Korea."

Barbara Demick, former *Los Angeles Times* Beijing bureau chief and author of *Nothing to Envy: Ordinary Lives in North Korea* and *Daughters of the Bamboo Grove: From China to America, a True Story of Abduction, Adoption, and Separated Twins*

"The story of Kathi Zellweger's remarkable work in North Korea is comprehensive, practical, and offers invaluable insights for anyone interested in that country. Diplomats and humanitarian professionals returning to the DPRK will find this work a crucial resource. During my own tenure in the DPRK, Kathi served as an essential guide to me and to many of us, demonstrating effective strategies for navigating complex circumstances and consistently supporting efforts to assist the most vulnerable populations in North Korea. A compelling read."

Jerome Sauvage, former UN resident coordinator and United Nations development program representative in the DPRK

"*Miss Kathi* brings to life the side of North Koreans that few outsiders get to see: their resilience, their resourcefulness, and their determination to find humor in the face of food shortages, power outages, and international isolation. *Miss Kathi* is also testament to the patience and persistence of one singular Swiss aid worker who has devoted her life to caring for the orphans, the disabled, and the malnutritional North Koreans that the rest of the world has largely forgotten. This is an important and insightful book about North Korea."

Jean H. Lee, former Pyongyang bureau chief at the Associated Press, presidential chair, East-West Center

MISS KATHI

Saving Lives in North Korea

KATHI ZELLWEGER
MIKE CHINOY

Post Hill
PRESS

A POST HILL PRESS BOOK
ISBN: 979-8-89565-671-6
ISBN (eBook): 979-8-89565-672-3

Miss Kathi:
Saving Lives in North Korea

Cover design by Jim Villaflores

All people, locations, events, and situations are portrayed based on the author's notes and memory. While all of the events described are true, some names and identifying details have been changed to protect the privacy of the people involved.

Post Hill Press
New York • Nashville
posthillpress.com

Published in the United States of America
1 2 3 4 5 6 7 8 9 10

To the people of North Korea

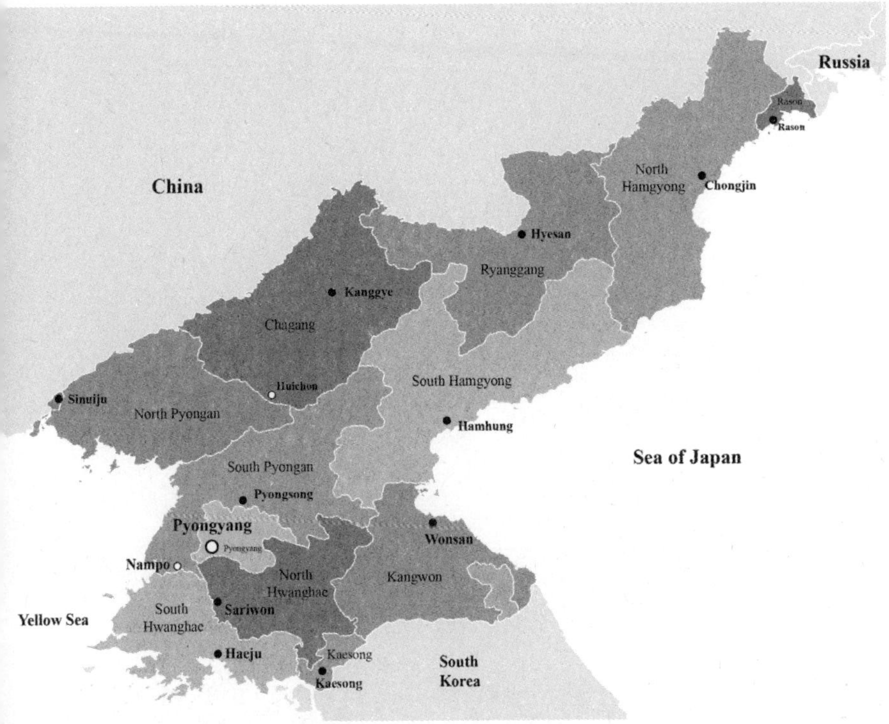

Russia
Rason
Rason
China
North
Hamgyong
Chongjin
Hyesan
Ryanggang
Kanggye
Chagang
South Hamgyong
Huichon
Sinuiju
North Pyongan
Hamhung
Sea of Japan
South Pyongan
Pyongsong
Pyongyang
Wonsan
Pyongyang
Nampo
North
Hwanghae
Kangwon
South
Hwanghae
Sariwon
Yellow Sea
Haeju
Kaesong
Kaesong
South
Korea

Contents

Abbreviations and Organizations

- ACF: Action Contre la Faim—A French global humanitarian organization working to end world hunger.
- ADRA: Adventist Development and Relief Agency—The global humanitarian arm of the Seventh-day Adventist Church.
- APARC: The Walter H. Shorenstein Asia-Pacific Research Center—Stanford University's center for inter-disciplinary scholarship and policy dialogue on Asia issues.
- APMS: Agro-Processing and Marketing Support—An SDC program to assist North Korean agriculture.
- AREP: Agricultural Recovery and Environmental Protection Program—Created by the UNDP to work exclusively on the agricultural sector in North Korea.
- CABI: Center for Agriculture and Bioscience International—International non-profit organization based in Delémont, Switzerland, that applies scientific expertise to solve problems in agriculture and the environment.
- CAFOD: Catholic Fund for Overseas Development—The official aid agency of the Catholic Church in England and Wales and part of Caritas Internationalis.
- Campus für Christus: A major interdenominational Christian organization providing humanitarian aid.
- Caritas-Hong Kong: Part of Caritas Internationalis. Provided the base for operating humanitarian assistance and development programs in North Korea.

- Caritas Internationalis: A confederation of 162 national Catholic relief, development, and social service organisations based at the Vatican and operating in over 200 countries and territories worldwide.
- CASIN: Center for Applied Studies in International Negotiations—A Geneva-based organization focused on training government, business, and civil leaders in governance, diplomacy, and problem-solving.
- CFCB: Canadian Foodgrains Bank—An organization of Canadian Christian churches and church-based agencies working to end global hunger.
- CEU: Central European University—A Budapest-based, Western-oriented university funded by billionaire George Soros.
- CDPF: China Disabled Persons' Federation—China's primary organization for assisting people with disabilities.
- CISAC: Center for International Security and Cooperation—Stanford University's hub for researchers tackling security and international cooperation issues.
- DMZ: The Demilitarized Zone separating North and South Korea since the end of the Korean War.
- DPRK: Democratic People's Republic of Korea—North Korea's official name.
- FALU: Food Aid Liaison Unit—A body set up by a group of NGOs at the Pyongyang office of the UN's World Food Program to help coordinate and monitor aid shipments during the famine.
- FAO: Food and Agriculture Organization—A specialized agency of the UN that leads international efforts to defeat hunger.
- FDRC: Flood Damage Rehabilitation Committee—The body set up by the North Korean government to handle international assistance after the floods of 1995.
- German Agro Action: (Deutsche Welthungerhilfe)—A German NGO working in development cooperation and emergency relief.
- HI: Handicap International—A Belgian-based NGO carrying out occupational and physical therapy training programs in North Korea. Now called Humanity and Inclusion.
- HKMA: Hong Kong Management Association—Hong Kong's leading professional association focusing on business management.

- ICRC: International Committee of the Red Cross—A Geneva-based international humanitarian aid organization.
- IFRC: International Federation of the Red Cross and the Red Crescent Societies – The world's largest humanitarian network.
- ILO: International Labor Organization—UN agency whose mandate is to advance social and economic justice.
- IPM: Integrated Pest Management program—An SDC program to help combat pest infestations in North Korean agriculture.
- JUCHE: A Korean term meaning "self-reliance" and the official ideology of North Korea.
- KCNA: Korean Central News Agency—The state news agency of North Korea.
- KECCA: Korean European Coordination Committee—The unit at the North Korean foreign ministry responsible for liaison with the SDC and other international organizations.
- KFPD: Korean Federation for the Protection of the Disabled—North Korea's main organization for supporting people with disabilities.
- KIC: Kaesong Industrial Complex—A joint venture between North and South Korea employing North Korean labor. Closed in 2016.
- KRCCD: Korean Rehabilitation Center for Children with Disabilities—A North Korean care center in Pyongyang for children with multiple disabilities.
- MCC: Mennonite Central Committee—A relief, development, service, and peace-building agency representing fifteen Mennonite bodies in North America.
- MoLEP: Ministry of Land and Environmental Protection—The North Korean agency which SDC dealt with for its Sloping Land Management program.
- MSF: Médecins Sans Frontières—An international organization providing medical assistance to people affected by conflict or disasters.
- NGO: Non-governmental organization.
- OXFAM: A British-founded confederation of 21 independent NGOs focusing on the alleviation of global poverty.
- PDS: Public Distribution System—North Korea's system for distributing food to the non-farming population.

- POW: Prisoner of War.
- RAC: The Random Access Club—A gathering place for the foreign aid community in Pyongyang. Now closed.
- Save the Children: An international NGO whose goal is to improve the lives of children.
- SDC: Swiss Development Corporation—The Swiss government's agency responsible for international cooperation and humanitarian aid.
- SLM: Sloping Land Management—An SDC program to help cultivate crops in hilly areas.
- TROCAIRE: The official overseas development agency of the Catholic Church in Ireland and part of Caritas Internationalis.
- UIBE: University of International Business and Economics, Beijing.
- UNDP: United Nations Development Program—The UN agency tasked with eliminating poverty and achieving sustainable growth.
- UNESCO: The United Nations Educational, Scientific and Cultural Organization—a specialized UN agency to promote world peace and security through international cooperation in education, arts, science and culture.
- UNICEF: UN agency responsible for providing humanitarian and developmental aid to children.
- UNFPA: United Nations Population Fund—UN agency aimed at improving reproductive and maternal health.
- UNHCR: UN High Commissioner for Refugees—The UN agency that works to aid and protect refugees.
- WFP: World Food Program—A United Nations program that provides food assistance worldwide.
- WHO: World Health Organization—A specialized agency of the UN coordinating international public health responses.

Introduction

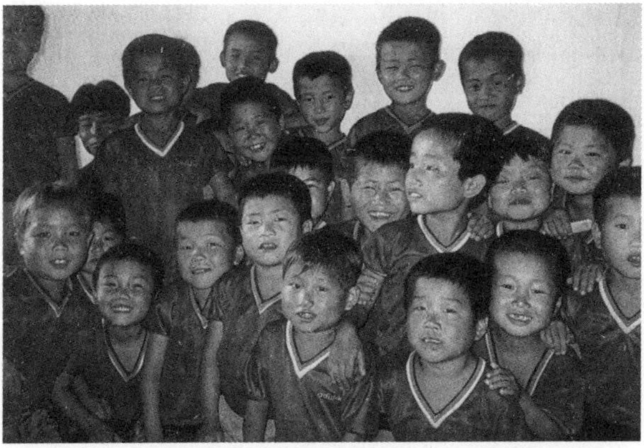

Hardly any signs of difficult times ahead.

Between 1995 and 2019, I made seventy-five trips to North Korea and lived in Pyongyang for five years, working first for Caritas, a Catholic relief, development, and social service organization, then for the Swiss government's development and cooperation arm (SDC), and later running my own nongovernmental organization. My most recent visit to the country was in December 2019, just before its borders were closed because of COVID. To the best of my knowledge, no one else has as long a continuous history of humanitarian engagement with North Korea. This book is an account of my experiences—what I did, saw, thought, and felt as I penetrated deeper and deeper into North Korea's closed society, much of that when the country was suffering one of the worst famines of modern times. It is a story of suffering and tragedy—but also of hope and remarkable resilience under the most difficult of circumstances. I hope my recollections present a picture of ordinary North Koreans different from the one-dimensional clichés that characterize so much of the writing about the country.

In general, books on North Korea can be divided into two types. One consists of high-level accounts of the diplomacy surrounding the North's nuclear and missile programs and the efforts to curb them. The other is based on the accounts of refugees and defectors eager to tell the story of the dreadful suffering that led them, and so many others, to try to leave the country. But the fact is that most North Koreans are neither involved in diplomacy nor seeking to escape, however miserable their situation. Rather, they are simply ordinary people whose lot in life was to be born in North Korea and who are struggling to survive in whatever ways they can. Among them are the most vulnerable—women, children, the poorest, the hungry, and the disabled. It is these people who have been the focus of my work, and who feature most prominently in this book.

My goal is to give the reader a sense of life for such ordinary North Koreans—as well as what it was like to be a humanitarian aid worker operating over so many years in a country as secretive, suspicious of outsiders, and tightly controlled as North Korea. What is it like to arrange a shipment of tons of rice, monitor its delivery, and make sure it reaches those who need it? How does one deal with suspicious government officials? What's involved in arranging lectures on how a modern economy works for midlevel businesspeople coming from a tightly controlled socialist society, or securing permission for them to travel and study abroad? How does one push the limits and encourage individual initiative in a state-run economy? How does one deal with international sanctions that prohibit the import of materials crucial for the running of hospitals or farms? What is life like as a member of Pyongyang's tiny expatriate community, isolated, often under surveillance, and without most of the creature comforts found not only in the West but even in many developing nations? Above all, how does one search for common humanity under such challenging circumstances?

There were many moments over the years when I confronted such intense suffering, especially among the most vulnerable—babies, children, pregnant and nursing mothers, the sick and disabled—that I was overwhelmed with sorrow and despair. Often, it was not easy to carry on. But I was sufficiently moved by what I witnessed that I felt I had no choice but to do what I could do to help. If nothing else, it was a way of reaffirming my own humanity. And watching the many people who did receive food, medicine, and support summon immense courage and determination in their battle to survive against overwhelming odds helped me keep going amidst all the obstacles, setbacks, and frustrations.

The central resource for the writing of this book was the enormous number of written reports I prepared over the years. After every visit, without fail I would write a five-to-ten-page document chronicling every place I went, every institution I visited, virtually every person I met, most of the conversations I had, and my own observations and feelings. In addition, during my five years as the Pyongyang representative of the SDC, in charge of the Swiss government–funded development projects in the country, I wrote detailed monthly or quarterly reports. These were supplemented by letters and journal entries. Altogether, they provided an extensive, detailed contemporary written record of my activities, opinions, and sentiments. I also was able to refer to my enormous collection of photographs taken over more than two decades, as well as dozens of hours of videos I shot, and I provided all the pictures used in this book.

In addition, I spent hundreds of hours in discussions with my friend and collaborator Mike Chinoy, himself an experienced North Korea hand, building on the written record with more insights, memories, and reflections. Mike, a veteran reporter and noted author, spent twenty-four years as a CNN foreign correspondent and made seventeen trips to North Korea, many of them producing groundbreaking journalism. He is the author of five books, including two on the country, *Meltdown: The Inside Story of the North Korean Nuclear Crisis* and *The Last POW*. With access to all my written material, the benefit of our countless conversations, and records of interviews and meetings he conducted with a number of key figures who feature in the book, he then used storytelling skills honed over a lifetime in journalism to write the manuscript, which the two of us carefully reviewed time and time again for clarity, accuracy, and balance.

To avoid burdening the reader with endless footnotes, we have not used any when citing my own reports, letters, or journal entries, which form the backbone of this story. But we have provided footnotes for external sources on which we periodically relied.

Given the sensitivities involved, we have also changed the names of some North Koreans—and a few foreigners—mentioned in the book, as well as a few locations. The North Korean state has a long arm and an even longer memory. So we trust—especially given today's changed political climate, in which Pyongyang is no longer reaching out to the international community in the way it was during many of the years I was traveling there—that the reader will understand why we felt it would be irresponsible not to protect the identities of those who were willing to share their stories, emotions, and feelings, sometimes under the most difficult of circumstances. The names of senior North Korean government officials, diplomats, and other more public figures have not been changed. And a note about my own name: In North Korea, I was invariably called "Miss Kathi" by almost everyone (not least because people found my last name so difficult to pronounce)—which is why it appears in the title of this book.

One other note about names. In Korean, the last name always comes first, and North Korean given names, when rendered in English, are not hyphenated, while those in South Korea are. We have followed this practice throughout the book.

When it comes to North Korea, statistics and other data are notoriously unreliable. Many of the estimates I had to work with were little more than educated guesses. Under these circumstances, we have done our best to provide as accurate a picture as possible, but readers should be aware of the constraints. We of course take responsibility for any errors or inaccuracies in our own accounts.

This is a work of personal history. I was fortunate enough that my engagement with North Korea coincided with crucial moments in the country's development—from the famine of the mid- to late 1990s to cautious experimentation with economic reform, to the limited but real opening to the rest of the world against the backdrop of efforts to negotiate a resolution to the nuclear issue. While our accounts of any of these subjects are hardly definitive, I happened to be on the ground at key moments and was able to witness and experience, perhaps more than most others, how these developments affected both ordinary North Koreans and the country's international interactions. Above all, I was able to gain a sense of the basic human decency I encountered despite the country's repressive political system. It enabled me to see and interact with North Koreans not as brainwashed robots but as unique individuals, each with their own hopes, dreams, and fears. If I can convey some of that to the reader, then I will consider this book a success.

CHAPTER ONE

"Silent Night" in Pyongyang

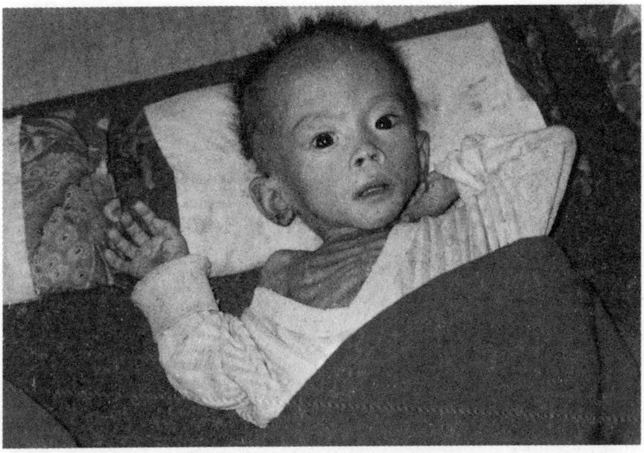

The famine came quickly.

The Kaesong pediatric hospital is a grim stone structure built by Methodist missionaries in 1907. Inside on this day in September 1998 were dozens of kids, weak, emaciated, with stick-like limbs and eyes that haunted me—the hollow, staring eyes of malnourished children. Some of the kids were receiving glucose or water intravenously. What little medical equipment the hospital had was old and outdated. There was no soap or disinfectant. There were no drugs. Although the place was surprisingly clean, the IV drips were attached to unsterilized Fanta or mineral water bottles. The hospital director, his face lined with fatigue, told me several children were dying every month and pleaded for help. I was struck by how quiet it was.

With the harsh Korean winter approaching, I wondered how any of these children would survive.

Kaesong sits just on the northern side of the Korean Demilitarized Zone (DMZ). A millennium ago, it was the capital of the Koryo Dynasty, the kingdom that gave its name to modern-day Korea. In 1998, the city was still full of old buildings with traditional curved, tiled roofs that had escaped destruction during the Korean War. As director of international cooperation for the worldwide Catholic charity Caritas, I witnessed in Kaesong some of the most harrowing consequences of the famine then sweeping North Korea.

That same day, I had also visited an orphanage and nursery in the city. With adults dying, the number of orphans was growing. Flies buzzed around many of the infants, some of whom had jaundice, thrush, or other ailments. At the Full Moon Nursery, a staff member told me there was so little to eat that she and her colleagues had been resorting to "alternative food" made from acorns, which were boiled, dried, crushed, and boiled again. She admitted that many of the children couldn't tolerate what she called acorn jelly, leading to severe digestive problems such as diarrhea, dysentery, and internal bleeding. With the collapse of the government's food distribution system and floods destroying much of the crop, however, there simply wasn't anything else. And the children here were hardly alone. From other places in North Korea had come credible reports of desperate people eating tree bark, sawdust, and grass. One concoction was composed of 80 percent dried fermented grass, 18 percent wheat husks, and 2 percent yeast. A colleague had taken a couple of these small, dark cubes and had them analyzed in a lab abroad. He reported that the substance had no nutritional benefit whatsoever, and the human body was not capable of absorbing it. I looked in the nursery's storeroom. It contained numerous empty jars, plus one bucket of acorns, a bin of maize flour, and one drum of cooking oil supplied by Caritas. Would any of these children be alive by the time of my next visit?

Kaesong is at the southernmost end of North Korea. The previous day, I had witnessed equally distressing scenes in Sinuiju, a city of seven hundred thousand people on the border with China nearly four hundred kilometers to the north and usually off-limits to foreigners. As in Kaesong, my colleague and I had to pass through numerous military and police checkpoints to enter Sinuiju. Along the way, we passed fields that should have been full of rice and maize but that had been devastated by floods and hailstorms. When dusk fell, I could see the lights twinkling in the Chinese city of Dandong across the Yalu River, but with virtually no electricity, Sinuiju was enveloped in gloom.

At Sinuiju Municipal Hospital, I met nine-year-old Kim Chol. Scrawny and still, he lay on a bed. His normally black hair had a reddish color and a straw-like texture—telltale signs of acute malnutrition. In the bed next to him was a five-month-old girl, Yeong Hee. Pale, sickly, and suffering from diarrhea, she had weighed barely four kilos when she was admitted. Her grandmother sat by the bed, coaxing her to sip high-energy milk. I couldn't help thinking it might be too late. Nearby was a fifteen-month-old boy, Chae Il Cheol, his body wasted by malnutrition, also suffering from diarrhea. His mother, a helpless look on her face, watched as the baby received glucose intravenously from a glass test tube covered in gauze. There were no sealed, sterile solutions here. On Il Cheol's drawn, skinny face, the grimaces of pain almost seemed like a smile.

This was not my first trip to North Korea. Since 1995, I had made visits for Caritas. Traveling every few weeks from my base in Hong Kong, I had slowly begun to develop relationships of trust with North Korean officials, with the result that I was being granted more access to more places, many of them usually closed to foreigners, than any other international aid worker. Over those three years, I had also watched the country's slow-motion descent into famine. On my early trips, the children I saw looked OK, and I took many photos of smiling kids. But each time I returned, the adults appeared to have grown thinner and the kids' smiles had faded a little more. I realized it was because the grown-ups were giving their increasingly scant rations to the children. With the passage of time, the kids too began to look emaciated, because their parents no longer had anything to give them.

On this nineteenth trip, in September 1998, the harrowing scenes I witnessed brought home to me the depths of the suffering. As a humanitarian worker, I had learned over the years to compartmentalize my feelings. During my visits to hospitals, nurseries, and orphanages, I focused on objectively assessing the conditions and acquiring as much information as I could. But I was deeply shaken by what I saw. In my spartan hotel each night, I was embarrassed to be served a meal, no matter how simple, knowing that the local people outside had next to nothing. I felt sad and angry. I was well aware of the political controversy that swirled around North Korea, and the idiosyncratic nature of its political system, but the children I saw had done nothing to deserve such a fate. Often, I was swept by a sense of hopelessness. But then, in my gloomiest moments, I also had the sensation that someone was grabbing and shaking me and saying, "Do something now! It can't wait."

And so my resolve to help the weakest and most vulnerable in North Korea, regardless of the politics, only increased. I kept thinking of a slogan I had seen at the Caritas office in Switzerland. "A world where one person suffers less," it declared, "is a better world."

I was born in 1952 in the small Swiss village of Teufen, the fourth of five children. My parents ran a dairy farm, and growing up, my three sisters, one brother, and I all learned to pitch in. While my brother helped my father with the cows, my sisters and I made hay in the summer and cider from the apple and pear trees in autumn. We delivered milk to customers in the village and learned how to make butter from leftover milk.

Most residents of Teufen are Protestants, and a large church dominates the main street. Although my parents were not religious, it was a local tradition that children would go to Sunday school, and we all enthusiastically celebrated religious festivals. While I absorbed Christian values, I did not grow up to be especially religious. From an early age, however, I felt an instinctive sympathy for the underdog, which developed into a commitment that my goal in life should be to help others, especially the poor and downtrodden.

After finishing high school, I did an apprenticeship in agricultural management and studied business administration at a commercial school. After spending eighteen months as an assistant to a team of social workers at a prison near Zurich, I moved to England to learn English and began to volunteer at a senior girls' remand-and-assessment center in the town of Winchester. I had planned to do a degree in social work but was offered a job as a probation officer for young offenders in St. Gallen, a town near Teufen, so I returned home to Switzerland.

When I was a child, my only connection to Hong Kong was that, once every few years, a half-Swiss, half-Japanese schoolmate of my father's would come to see us. He had moved to Hong Kong, married a local woman, and worked there. On one of his visits, he brought a Hong Kong yearbook as a gift. Looking through it, I became fascinated by this distant, seemingly exotic place. So when I saw a newspaper advertisement for a job with the

Caritas charity in Hong Kong, I jumped at the chance. After five years as a probation officer, I wanted a change. Switzerland seemed too small and confining. To my surprise, I was offered the position, and in the summer of 1978, I moved to the part of the world that would shape the rest of my life.

Like so many others, I was entranced and slightly overwhelmed arriving in Hong Kong—Victoria Peak towering over a harbor jammed with boats, the crowded streets pulsating with energy at all hours, the forests of neon signs, the clatter of construction drills. I was struck as well by the contrasts between the city's fabulously wealthy—the Western businessmen and Chinese tycoons with their Rolls-Royces hobnobbing at the Mandarin Hotel and the Hong Kong Club—and the ordinary people squeezed into tiny flats in towering apartment blocks stacked so closely together that parts of Hong Kong were among the most densely populated neighborhoods in the world.

Caritas is a confederation of over 160 Catholic relief, development, and social service organizations operating in more than two hundred countries and territories around the world. Although not a Catholic, I was attracted by its mission statement to help "all people, especially the poorest, the marginalized, and the oppressed, find hope, and come to the fullness of their humanity as part of a global community." In addition to responding to emergencies and supporting development projects, Caritas is also an advocacy network, seeking to have a voice in the public debate and influence policymakers at an international level. It was an exciting place to be.

The office of Caritas–Hong Kong was at 2 Caine Road, named after William Caine, who served briefly as Hong Kong's acting colonial governor in 1859. The building is just a few meters from Government House, the lavish compound with ornate rooms and manicured gardens that had been the official residence for Caine and most of Hong Kong's other British rulers. My immediate boss was Father Francesco Lerda, an Italian priest who had arrived in Hong Kong in 1956. When he joined in the late 1950s, the Caritas office consisted of a handful of staff providing simple social services such as handing out relief material in poor neighborhoods. Lerda was low-key and modest, and spoke such good Cantonese that people who first dealt with him on the phone were flabbergasted to discover he was not a local when they met him. He was also extremely hardworking and very creative, and by the time I arrived, Caritas–Hong Kong had become one of the biggest charities in the territory, and remains so today.

My initial assignment was to help manage a program to assist deprived or disabled children. But by the end of 1978, Hong Kong was facing a new crisis—a huge influx of refugees from Vietnam. Fearful of the new Communist leadership after the end of the Vietnam War, hundreds of thousands sought to flee. They became known as "boat people." With Singapore, Malaysia, and Thailand largely shutting their doors to refugees, Hong Kong, which had declared itself a "port of first refuge," meaning in theory that no one washing up on its shores would be turned away, became the preferred destination for Vietnamese seeking a new life. Soon, thousands were arriving every day. In late December 1978, a Panamanian freighter called the *Huey Fung* sailed into Hong Kong Harbor carrying over 3,000 people. A few weeks later, another dilapidated freighter arrived with over 2,600. Eventually, more than 200,000 Vietnamese would make it to Hong Kong, most of them in small, overcrowded boats.

The refugees were housed in a series of makeshift camps dotted around Hong Kong. Caritas quickly became involved in managing a number of them. Conditions were grim. People slept in three-tiered bunk beds, with only tattered curtains for privacy, waiting, often for years, for their asylum claims to be processed. The camps were initially funded by the Hong Kong government and the United Nations High Commissioner for Refugees, but it soon became clear that more money was urgently needed, and I was given the job of raising funds in Europe to improve conditions for people in the camps. It was an experience that would serve me well fifteen years later, when I faced the challenge of generating international financial support for Caritas operations in North Korea.

I tried to help the refugees in other ways too. When a fire swept through one camp, destroying the meager possessions of many residents, I spent the 1992 Chinese New Year holiday week scouring Hong Kong for blankets, shoes, and other basic supplies. Most stores were closed, but I found one shoe shop open and promptly bought two hundred pairs in different sizes. The bemused shopkeeper shook his head and probably thought I was crazy. I, meanwhile, felt like Imelda Marcos on a shoe-shopping spree. I was also friendly with the concierge at the five-star Mandarin Hotel. At my urging, the hotel donated hundreds of blankets, delivering them to the camp in a catering van normally used to deliver canapés and cakes to high-class social events. It was deeply gratifying to see the smiles on the faces of the shivering, miserable refugees.

I was also involved in helping arrange for a number of refugees classified as problem cases to leave Hong Kong for resettlement in Switzerland. Most had been languishing in the camps for years, rejected for not meeting the strict criteria imposed by nations such as Canada, Australia, and the United States. Some were disabled. Others were one-parent families. After conducting interviews, selecting the candidates, and preparing them for life in the West, I managed to persuade the Swiss authorities to grant visas to hundreds of Vietnamese. I remember telling one man, thirty-four-year-old Nguyen Trong Tan, that he, his wife, daughter, and stepdaughter would be allowed to go to Switzerland. He was so happy, he burst into tears. Altogether, Switzerland accepted almost ten thousand Vietnamese refugees from camps in Hong Kong and elsewhere in Southeast Asia between 1975 and the late 1990s.

The early 1980s also marked the start of the ambitious reform program that over the following decades would profoundly change the landscape of China. Spearheaded by senior leader Deng Xiaoping, the reforms were designed to modernize the country by introducing elements of a market economy without abandoning the Communist Party's monopoly of political power. The people's communes (state-run farms) were disbanded, allowing peasants to farm for themselves, leading to a sharp increase in agricultural productivity. Individuals were permitted to set up small-scale private businesses. And there was a new openness to dealing with foreigners, including welcoming foreign investment and growing interest in tapping foreign expertise. In the following decades, I would watch closely to see if North Korea would adopt similar policies to fix its own economy.

For Caritas, even with its Catholic religious affiliation, the changes in China meant it was now possible to explore setting up projects or supporting existing initiatives in the country. There was certainly a need. After decades in which economic development was ignored in favor of ideological campaigns that had produced massive political upheaval, the People's Republic remained desperately poor. With expertise in education, social services, and health—all areas in which Caritas ran programs in Hong Kong—the organization was well poised to offer help in China. Initially, the Chinese authorities, still feeling their way on collaborating with foreigners, allowed projects only just across the border in neighboring Guangdong Province. But gradually, we were permitted to operate elsewhere, supporting orphanages, old-age homes, medical clinics, and more. Eventually, I was to visit all of China's provinces at a time when few foreigners were allowed to do so.

One of our early projects was to promote literacy among the Salar, a small, predominantly Muslim minority in western China. Descended from Turkic tribes from Central Asia, by the 1980s, the Salar population numbered fewer than one hundred thousand, most of them living in acute poverty. Indeed, on one trip, when I asked to see the notebooks they were using to learn basic reading and writing, I was told the people were too poor to afford such a luxury. Instead, they practiced writing Chinese characters in the sand. On another occasion, we had received a box of bananas from a Chinese project partner in another part of the country, but when we offered the fruit to local children in a village we passed through in Qinghai Province, they didn't know what they were. None of them had ever seen or heard of a banana.

I had a long-standing interest in the plight of disabled people and was excited to help set up China's first residential school for mentally handicapped children in Guangzhou, the capital of Guangdong Province. We brought in Caritas experts to train the local staff there. My work in this area also gave me the opportunity on several occasions to meet with the son of Deng Xiaoping, Deng Pufang, who had become a paraplegic when radical Red Guards threw him out of a building at Peking University during the Cultural Revolution in the 1960s. Deng Pufang had been the driving force behind the establishment of the China Disabled Persons' Federation, of which he was the chairman. As he sat in his wheelchair, I was struck by how open-minded he was, and how eager to get help and funding for training and rehabilitation programs. With his support, Caritas trained the first physio- and occupational therapists in China and created a sponsorship program for four Chinese students to go to Hong Kong for a four-year course in physiotherapy and occupational training.

My role at Caritas-Hong Kong steadily expanded. By the spring of 1993, I was director of international cooperation. That year, I represented the organization at a preparatory meeting in Beijing for the United Nations' Year of the Family initiative. It was here that I met my first North Korean. He was as curious about me as I was about him, peppering me with questions about what Caritas did and my own role. The upshot was an invitation for me to visit North Korea and explore whether there was anything Caritas might do there. I had no way of knowing this would be the first of nearly one hundred trips there, that I would live for five years in Pyongyang, or that North Korea would become the primary focus of my energies for the next quarter century.

In April 1995, I checked in for my first Air Koryo flight to Pyongyang, along with my traveling companions, Park Kyung-Seo, a South Korean who was the executive secretary for Asia at the World Council of Churches, based in Geneva, and a North Korean working at the United Nations Educational, Scientific, and Cultural Organization (UNESCO) office in Beijing. I noticed that virtually all the North Korean passengers were carrying large and beautiful bouquets. I wondered whether, in addition to its other problems, North Korea was suffering from a shortage of flowers. On the Soviet-built aircraft, however, I put the thought aside, as martial music blared and the stewardesses, each wearing a small badge of Kim Il Sung, the North Korean leader who had died the previous July, served a meal of stale bread, tasteless chicken, and dried-up cucumbers. This trip would soon become as familiar to me as taking a local bus.

Two and a half hours later, we landed at a nearly empty Pyongyang airport that was dominated by a huge portrait of Kim Il Sung. I observed that customs gave North Koreans trying to import radios a hard time. Short-wave models were confiscated and destroyed. My traveling companions and I, however, were whisked through the VIP area into three waiting Mercedes—one for each of us. By now, darkness had fallen. The streets were pitch-black. Nevertheless, in some of the apartment buildings we passed, I could see portraits of Kim Il Sung and his son and heir, Kim Jong Il, on the walls, usually illuminated by a single light bulb. The two leaders made their presence felt everywhere.

And then, the mystery of the flowers was resolved. We were driven directly to the giant statue of Kim Il Sung on Mansu Hill, which dominated the skyline of the city. Although it was late, the square in front of the statue was crowded with North Koreans, each carrying a bouquet of flowers, which they reverentially laid at the foot of the twenty-meter-tall statue. Our hosts gave each of us a bouquet, and we did the same. It was a gesture of respect highlighting how worship of the Kim dynasty—the world's most extreme personality cult—appeared to be the central feature of life in North Korea.

We were then taken to a foreign ministry guesthouse on the outskirts of Pyongyang. Our hosts told us we would enjoy the peace and quiet of the countryside, and that we would be safer than in the city. Checking in, we realized we were the only guests.

The Democratic People's Republic of Korea (DPRK), to use its official name, was established following the end of World War Two, when US and Soviet forces entered the country, which had been a Japanese colony since 1905. By prior agreement, two occupation zones were set up: the Soviets in the industrialized North, and the Americans in the agrarian South. In 1948, Kim Il Sung, a Soviet-backed anti-Japanese resistance fighter during the war, became the leader of North Korea. Two years later, he launched a surprise attack across the 38th Parallel, where American and Russian officials had divided the Korean peninsula in 1945. The invasion marked the start of the Korean War, one of the most brutal of the twentieth century; it cost four million lives. Three years of fighting—in which China intervened to oppose United States–led United Nations forces—left the border largely unchanged. The 160 kilometer-long, four kilometer-wide Demilitarized Zone was scarred with barbed wire, dotted with land mines, and guarded by heavily armed troops on both sides. It had been the site of frequent small-scale clashes over the years, each of which raised the specter of renewed hostilities.

At the time of my first visit, North Korea still maintained a million-strong army, much of it deployed just a few hours' striking distance from the South Korean capital of Seoul. Thirty-seven thousand US troops, the latest to serve in a security commitment dating back to the war itself, were stationed in South Korea. And just the year before, in 1994, the two sides had come frighteningly close to war over Pyongyang's effort to develop nuclear weapons, when the Clinton administration seriously considered a preemptive US attack on North Korea's nuclear reactor at Yongbyon, despite the very real risk that it could trigger a broader conflict that could devastate the Korean peninsula. A still-divided Korea remained one of the world's most volatile flash points.

In North Korea, Kim Il Sung created a system based on a unique ideology called *juche*. An extreme form of self-reliance, it was derived from Korea's history as the "hermit kingdom"—the country having long resisted contact with the West—as well as from the bitter experiences of Japanese colonial rule and the devastation of the war. The goal was to make North Korea economically, militarily, and culturally strong enough to counter foreign pressure and influence. Kim achieved some initial economic success. But a combination of socialist inefficiency and mismanagement, limited arable land, and the creation of a large and costly military machine undermined the economy. There were growing reports of factories standing idle and of shortages of food and fuel.

Despite the domestic difficulties and the difficult international climate, my visit appeared to be a small sign that North Korea might be open to at least some limited international engagement. It was not the only such sign. The previous October, just four months after the death of Kim Il Sung, his son and successor, Kim Jong Il, had concluded a deal with the United States called the Agreed Framework, under which Pyongyang agreed to freeze and eventually dismantle its plutonium-based nuclear program in return for pledges of economic aid and a broader improvement in United States–DPRK relations. It seemed like the long-simmering nuclear crisis was on its way to resolution. Moreover, by agreeing to the deal, Kim Jong Il had demonstrated he was in control, confounding the many skeptics who doubted his—and North Korea's—viability after the passing of his father.

On our first full day, we met Chae Ryong Il, the director of the State Education Commission. He presented a glowing picture not only of the educational system but of North Korean society in general—educational opportunities for all children, no drugs, no crime. We were taken to a kindergarten, a primary school, and a middle school. All were spotlessly clean, even sterile, although it was evident that school materials were scarce. In the primary school, there were no exercise books, and several students were sharing tattered textbooks. At all three schools, politics took center stage, from the simple jigsaw puzzles in the kindergarten showing scenes from the Korean War, in which American soldiers were depicted as monster-like figures with long noses, to the revolutionary songs performed in the two other schools. When the teenage girls in the middle school sang about the Great Leader Kim Il Sung, they burst into tears.

Driving around Pyongyang, with its vast boulevards and tall buildings, I was struck by the absence of cars, bicycles, shops, restaurants, advertisements, and markets. The city had little charm, and none of the bustle and crowds one sees in other Asian cities. The citizens walked with expressionless faces, averting their gazes from me. At the Rakwon Department Store, clearly the best in the city (*rakwon* means "paradise"), we found that the only fresh foods were a few battered potatoes and apples. Otherwise, the shelves contained an odd collection of items—cubes of white sugar from Hong Kong, tins of Nestlé Swiss béchamel sauce, and Nestlé chocolate that had expired in September of the previous year. It seemed that people had money, but there was nothing to purchase. As on this and all of my future visits to North Korea, as well as those of virtually every other foreigner, a government guide, sometimes two, acted as escorts everywhere. When I asked about the availability of goods—a pair of shoes, for example—the guide simply said, "To pay for it is not a problem, but we sometimes have to wait a few months for supplies." Further complicating the picture, I would learn later that for most people, it was the work unit that supplied shoes, and many had no idea what a pair would actually cost in a shop.

As a Catholic charity with its headquarters at the Vatican in Rome, Caritas was particularly interested in establishing contact with the church in North Korea. Before World War Two, the northern part of Korea had been a center of Christianity. Indeed, the parents of Kim Il Sung were said to have been devout Christians. Pyongyang had been home to a thriving Christian community, including a large number of American missionaries, some of whom dubbed the city the "Jerusalem of the East." The missionaries had built schools and hospitals. Among those who studied at a mission school in Pyongyang in the 1900s was Ruth Bell. She later married the famous evangelist Billy Graham, who himself visited North Korea, met with Kim Il Sung, and preached at the city's two churches in 1992.

We had asked to visit local churches, and after some stalling and excuses, I was suddenly told I would be able to go to the Catholic church. The Changchun Catholic Church was new, having been built in East Pyongyang in 1988, and was one of three Christian churches in Pyongyang. There had not been a priest in forty-five years, but I was told there were three thousand practicing Catholics, one hundred of whom were at the 10 a.m. prayer service I attended. After the service, I met the leader of the church and two other officials. It was clear that the Catholic Church in the DPRK had virtually no contact with the outside world. The officials talked mostly about reunification, stressing their desire to meet Catholics from the South. For my part, I explained what Caritas did and expressed hope for a future collaboration. I left the church with a strange feeling. The government clearly had little tolerance for religion or independent activities it did not control. I wondered if the whole event had been staged especially for me.

The extreme control that North Korea exercised over foreign visitors was further reinforced when I requested access to a telephone. My guides were nervous. Who was I going to call? What kind of contacts did I have in Pyongyang? Eventually, I was given access to a phone in a locked cabinet and was able to arrange an appointment with Wilhelm Strohe, the charge d'affaires (there was no ambassador) at the German interest section. Strohe was extremely surprised I had been able to reach him. With only five Germans and barely one hundred foreigners altogether living in Pyongyang, he was happy for the company, and eager to talk. He had been in North Korea for two years, he told me, and said access to information in such a controlled society was extremely difficult. With only two international flights a week from Beijing, he and his deputy would often go to the airport just to see if anyone interesting was visiting. He said North Koreans were actively discouraged from having contact with foreigners, and that he felt cut off from North Korean society.

He confirmed from his observations my impression that food was in short supply, that there were clear signs of malnutrition among the population, and that the situation could be moving toward a crisis point. Indeed, barely two months after I would leave Pyongyang, in the early summer of 1995, the DPRK government would swallow its pride and ask two old enemies, Japan and South Korea, for food assistance. Despite political tensions, both countries agreed to provide it—a fact that the regime would publicly confirm to its own people.

The impression that conditions were difficult was underscored when I met the chairman of the State Education Commission. Almost certainly under instructions from his superiors, he asked for help from Caritas in four areas: importing five thousand tons of rice for use in a lunch program for students in parts of the country badly affected by recent hailstorms; $150,000 for the improvement of education for the blind, deaf, and dumb; help in establishing vocational training schools, including bringing foreign experts for consultations and sending North Koreans to receive vocational education in Germany; and purchasing $250,000 worth of paper to produce school textbooks, as the North did not have dollars to purchase paper supplies abroad and, following the fall of the Soviet Union, could no longer barter with Russia.

Although the chairman presented his needs in a low-key manner, I found it striking that a country known for its isolation was now interested in receiving help and collaborating with an international aid organization. I indicated that I was happy to try but did tell him frankly that the last request would be difficult. No donor would find the printing of North Korean propaganda material appealing. Still, we agreed that Caritas–Hong Kong would sign a series of cooperation agreements with the State Education Commission. I suggested as a first step that North Korea send a half dozen people to visit China in coordination with Deng Pufang's China Disabled Persons' Federation. I had been surprised that during my entire visit, I had not seen a single disabled person in public—no one in a wheelchair, with crutches, or even a walking stick. It seemed clear that North Korea preferred to keep disabled people out of sight, and I wondered whether the country even had devices such as wheelchairs and prostheses. Highlighting North Korea's sensitivity about any requests for foreign help, the director asked me to keep all the projects confidential and not to speak with the press. But he did invite me to return later in the year.

As I prepared to leave North Korea, I jotted down some impressions: "People functioning like robots, the reality of brainwashing, the uniformity down to the small details (after a week I could tell the level of the official depending on the cookies served with the tea), the wretched lifestyle, the isolation, even George Orwell's concept of thought-crime. Comparing China to North Korea, China seems like a free country."

But then I thought back to a memorable evening a few days earlier. After dinner, we'd joined our hosts in the entertainment hall of our guesthouse. The room had probably been an air-raid shelter and was now marked by a huge stage with a grand piano. One of our guides produced a guitar and, to my surprise, began singing songs by Franz Schubert in German. I declined a request to yodel. But then we decided to sing a song together. And so, in April 1995, in an underground bunker in Pyongyang, my South Korean colleague, our North Korean guides, and I sang, in German, "Silent Night," the world's most famous Christmas carol, with its message of peace—perhaps a signal that even in a society as rigidly controlled as North Korea, building human connections might be possible.

CHAPTER TWO

Mr. Hugo

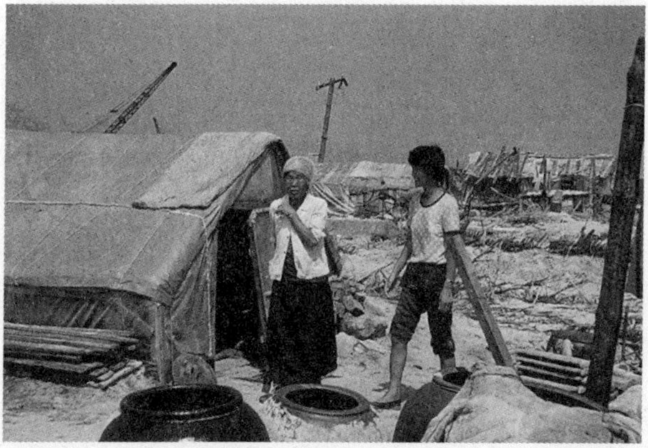

The terrible floods of summer 1995 brought enormous hardship.

A few weeks after I left Pyongyang, the heavens opened, the result of an unusually warm El Niño summer weather pattern. For days on end in July and August 1995, it poured, sometimes 127 millimeters (five inches) an hour. Parts of North Korea were inundated with over 700 millimeters of water in a single day. It was a disaster of biblical proportions, the worst in Korea in the twentieth century, and plunged a nation already suffering from shortages of food, fuel, electricity and much else into a brutal famine.

The terrain of North Korea is rugged and mountainous. Only 15 to 20 percent of the land is suitable for crops, and the growing season is short. To compensate, over the years, the government built elaborate irrigation systems and invested heavily in mechanization and the production of fertilizer. And with the food shortages, people sought to expand arable acreage by cultivating crops on steep hillsides, which often meant clearing heavily forested land. In large-scale cooperative farms, the bigger fields were generally worked by tractors. Crops such as rice and maize were raised on these farms, and then doled out by the state public distribution system (PDS). For the supply of basic foodstuffs such as cereals and vegetable oil, the government used an elaborate scale—the more important the state deemed the work to be, the higher the ration for the person doing that work. Most city dwellers received rations twice a month. In the countryside, farmers got their rations for a full year every autumn after the harvest.

Yet food production remained an issue. In the 1970s and '80s, North Korea had been able to sidestep the problem through its long-standing alignment with the Soviet Union, China, and the socialist bloc, which provided substantial aid and supplies of food and fuel. The latter was especially important, given that the North had no reserves of oil or natural gas. In the early 1990s, however, the Soviet Union disintegrated, and so did the socialist bloc in Eastern Europe, while China accelerated market-style economic reforms. Post-Communist Russia established diplomatic relations with Pyongyang's archrival South Korea in 1991, and China followed suit a year later. Russia soon began to demand payment in hard currency for oil and other products.

China briefly stepped in to supply food and oil at concessionary prices, but by 1994 it too began to reduce what it was willing to provide and also demanded payment in hard currency. The shock to North Korea's economy was enormous, and the impact on agriculture was particularly severe. With few able to afford fuel for pumps, North Korea's irrigation systems largely ceased to operate. Tractors were idled, and fertilizer production, for which petroleum was a key ingredient, fell dramatically, as did the supply of electricity. The state public distribution system came under increasing stress.

And then Mother Nature did her worst, as I saw in grim detail during the eight days I spent in the DPRK in late August and early September 1995. It was still the rainy season when I returned, part of a small group organized at North Korea's request by Hans Roth, the deputy chief of the Swiss embassy in Beijing, and including another Swiss national, Heinrich Gloor, who worked for the humanitarian aid department of the Swiss government. Roth was a good friend and an experienced Asia hand who had studied Chinese in Beijing in the 1970s. He knew that I had visited North Korea earlier in the year and had a background in humanitarian work, so he asked me to join him. At the same time, the North Koreans also invited the United Nations to send personnel to assess the flood damage.

Our hosts were the Ministry of Foreign Affairs and the Flood Damage Rehabilitation Committee (FDRC), an umbrella organization of personnel drawn from various ministries—foreign affairs, agriculture, trade, and internal security—that had been set up to coordinate what would be an unprecedented request for international aid. Our invitation was a small but important step, and the choice of Switzerland was no accident. Switzerland had been a member of the Neutral Nations Supervisory Commission, which monitored the Demilitarized Zone following the end of the Korean War. Switzerland had established diplomatic relations with North Korea in 1974, and its long history of neutral and discreet diplomacy in Korea, as well as elsewhere, evidently appealed to Kim Jong Il. In 1994, Geneva had been the site of the negotiations that resulted in the Agreed Framework deal between the United States and North Korea, which froze Pyongyang's nuclear reactor in return for pledges of economic aid and a promise of better relations with Washington. And for much of the 1980s and '90s, Kim Jong Il's children—including, in the mid-1990s, his eventual heir Kim Jong Un—had studied at schools in Switzerland. If pragmatists in the North Korean government were going to be allowed to take some first cautious steps to open up to the outside world, doing so through Swiss interlocutors made sense.

And it explained why Ri Chol, the North Korean ambassador to Switzerland, returned home to accompany us throughout our trip. A graduate of the Department of French at Pyongyang's University of International Studies, with a receding hairline and black wide-rimmed glasses, Ri was engaging and affable. It was clear he cared deeply about what was going on. As I got to know him better, I found him surprisingly open-minded and willing to deal with foreigners, unusual for such a senior figure in the North Korean system. Posted to the DPRK mission in Geneva in the 1980s and accredited later to the embassy in Berne, he was widely considered to be responsible for relations not only with Switzerland but with much of Western Europe. Some analysts described him as a college classmate of Kim Jong Il's and as the Kim family's personal representative in the region. In the 1980s, he had looked after Kim Jong Il's oldest son, Kim Jong Nam, while he studied in Switzerland, and at the time of our visit, although it was never officially confirmed, he apparently was playing the same role for Kim Jong Un and his younger brother and sister. One of my Swiss colleagues was convinced that Ri was one of the most important figures in the government arguing for greater international outreach. His presence underscored the political importance of our visit.

After a day of intensive and surprisingly candid briefings with multiple ministries and government departments—including the Ministries of Public Health, Agriculture, and Railways; the Grain Administration Service; and the North Korean Meteorological Service—we were taken to survey the worst-hit regions. We set off on a creaky Soviet-built helicopter belonging to the North Korean military to the area near Sinuiju in North Pyongan Province along the border with China. The chopper flight itself was a first. As far as I was aware, no Westerners previously had ever been allowed to travel on a North Korean military aircraft. Although there were only three people in our group, we were given carefully printed boarding passes and sat on seats covered with an ornate lace doily. From Sinuiju, we were then taken to North and South Hwanghae Provinces, the country's breadbasket, where 60 percent of its rice and other types of grain were grown.

The scenes we saw were apocalyptic. Roads, bridges, and railway and communication lines had been swept away. Whole villages had been inundated. Countless homes and schools had been destroyed, along with stocks of food and other daily necessities. I remember being struck by the number of large brown pots used to store kimchi, the spicy fermented cabbage dish that is a staple of the Korean diet, protruding at strange angles in the sand, which now covered so much of the land. I knew that below the surface, whole villages had been buried. There were no chickens, goats, pigs, or other animals to be seen. Most had been drowned in the raging waters.

We saw people housed in makeshift wooden dwellings with roofs made of plastic sheeting or straw. In contrast to just a few months before, the appearance of some children was shocking. I took a photo of one small boy who was naked and covered in dirt, with a protruding belly—a telltale sign of malnutrition. Officials said that diarrhea and other stomach ailments were widespread, and, as the winter approached, measles and acute respiratory infections like pneumonia and whooping cough were likely to increase. Altogether, the North Koreans told us that a quarter of the national harvest—which, given existing economic problems, already would not have been sufficient to feed the population—had been lost. The rice and maize crops were particularly badly affected, with many fields having been flooded for days on end. Over five million people, nearly a quarter of the population, had been affected by the floods. Of North Korea's 209 counties, 145 had sustained damage, estimated in assessment figures the government gave us at some US$15 billion.

The disaster appeared to have produced a remarkable shift in the attitude of some North Korean officials. Instead of the usual practice of restricting access, they did not object to my taking photographs, and allowed me to speak with flood victims and local aid workers. Moreover, unlike on my previous visit, when they had insisted on no publicity, this time they asked me to talk to the international press about the situation when I returned to Hong Kong. These were small but telling additional indications that at least some in the North Korean system were looking for a way to expand international contact and the reception of food aid.

This became even clearer during discussions we had about the provision of aid. It was the first time that North Korea had ever appealed for international assistance. Such a request was a sharp departure from the country's governing philosophy of *juche*, or "self-reliance," and carried the risk that, within the system, it would be seen as an embarrassing loss of face. Indeed, our interlocutors indicated that opposition to reaching out existed, especially within the military. Yet, speaking with unusual frankness, they said the situation was so desperate that there was no other choice, although, to reduce embarrassment and increase political acceptance at home, they framed their requests in terms of relief from natural disasters, rather than deficiencies in the North Korean system. They also made clear their hope that with Switzerland taking the lead in providing aid, other governments would follow.

They told us that food was the first priority, followed by clothing, shoes, medical supplies, paper for schoolbooks, and plastic sheeting for the planting of seedlings for the 1996 crop. Underscoring the self-reliance theme, they stressed they were asking for only the most essential items, which they couldn't produce at home. Our discussions then moved to practical issues of logistics and distribution. It was clear that the North Koreans had no experience in dealing with international aid, especially on such a large scale. Neither, for that matter, had I. The whole experience was a learning process. The most cost-effective option appeared to be to try to acquire needed items in China. To my surprise, however, the North Koreans said that Beijing had imposed an export ban on rice, and urged us to look at Thailand and Vietnam as alternative suppliers. They said they might be able to send vessels to collect the goods, and for air freight, Air Koryo would transport donations free of charge from any destination where the airline operated, but given the country's acute shortage of fuel, we would have to cover that cost.

The three of us produced a report for the Swiss government, and I prepared a separate report for Caritas. The conclusion was the same in both: There was an urgent need for food aid. "The fear that there will be a serious lack of food leading from malnutrition to famine seems justified if nothing is done in the next four months," we wrote to the Swiss authorities. Given the slow-moving Swiss government bureaucracy and internal differences over the whole idea of helping North Korea, Caritas appeared better poised for swift action. "A decision to provide assistance should be viewed from the humanitarian aspect rather than the political one," I argued in my Caritas memo. "Widespread hunger is looming, and without foreign assistance, famine will be inevitable." I urged that we arrange for the first shipments to reach the country by mid-October.

But after returning to Hong Kong, I discovered, as did my two Swiss government colleagues, that the international community was highly skeptical. Given North Korea's dubious reputation, both among governments and more broadly in Western public opinion, many people simply did not want to believe a food crisis existed. Normally reliable donor nations were initially unresponsive. Against this backdrop, I did an interview with CNN at its Hong Kong production studio. It was the first of what, over the years, would be countless media interviews, but at the time, I was terrified. Anchor Patricia Chew calmed me down, saying it would be just a chat where I would show some of my photos. I asked her about the size of the audience, and she replied, "I'm not going to tell you until after the broadcast. It will only make you more nervous." To my surprise, I managed to survive the interview, using the photos I had taken to make the case that, whatever the international politics, the North Korean people needed and deserved humanitarian aid. When we finished, she informed me that millions of people around the world had been watching.

Soon after, Caritas Internationalis launched its first international funding appeal for North Korea, and the organization decided that I should coordinate the relief efforts from my base in Hong Kong. Even before going public, we had already quietly approached a few partner organizations for donations for the school feeding program the North Koreans had asked about during my first trip. Despite the skepticism of many donor organizations and countries, by early October we had received nearly $500,000 from the Caritas chapters in Germany and Switzerland, the German Catholic agency Misereor, and Caritas and other Catholic organizations in South Korea.

The next step was to arrange the rice shipment. I did not have the slightest idea how to do this, so I asked the Caritas offices around Asia for suggestions and advice. My colleagues in Jakarta replied that they had heard of a Swiss man with a trading company in Bangkok who might be able to help, but they did not have his full name. They knew him only as "Mr. Hugo." I set about trying to track him down. Luckily, I knew the assistant to the Swiss ambassador in Bangkok, so I called and told her I was looking for a "Mr. Hugo" who ran a trading company and was based in Thailand. Did she have any ideas? My friend replied, "Yes. His wife happens to work at the embassy."

Ten minutes later, I was on the phone with Mr. Hugo. His company, Bell-Indo Co., Ltd., was a large trading firm, and he had extensive experience shipping rice from Southeast Asia to destinations across the globe. During our long initial conversation, he gave me an instant crash course in the rice trade. He explained about the different kinds of rice—long grain, round, and so on—the different levels of quality, how it was packed, and the numerous certificates required to export it. When he finished, I asked him, "So what is your last name?" to which he replied, "Hörndli"—which in Swiss German means "noodle." So "Mr. Noodle" was to provide the rice. We both broke into laughter.

Two days later, in what with the benefit of hindsight was a breathtakingly naive move, since I barely knew him, I deposited, with the approval of my boss in Hong Kong, $400,000 into his account at the Hongkong and Shanghai Bank. "Mr. Noodle" delivered. Through his contacts in Thailand, he was able to find supplies of rice ready for shipment on short notice. With his help, in just a few weeks, I purchased 1,400 metric tons for Caritas, while also placing an order on behalf of the United Nations' World Food Program (WFP) for 140 metric tons—that agency's first aid shipment to North Korea.

In mid-November, I returned to North Korea to oversee the arrival of the rice shipment and discuss the provision of other relief supplies. This time, I was accompanied by Caritas Secretary General Gerhard Meier, who was based at Caritas Internationalis at the Vatican. I knew him well. He had previously headed the international cooperation department of Caritas

Switzerland and had given me my first Caritas job in Hong Kong. In the two months since my last visit, it was evident that the situation had deteriorated significantly. Because of gasoline shortages, there were even fewer cars on the streets, and I learned that only people with special permission were allowed to drive, but not on Sundays.

All the officials we met spoke openly about food shortages and the need for further belt-tightening. There were a number of times when the lights went off in the middle of meetings because of power cuts. Embarrassed officials would not say a word. Instead, the meeting simply paused, and we all sat in awkward silence until the lights went back on. On a visit to the industrial city of Huichon, I was stuck by how many more undernourished children I saw. The families we visited appeared to have little food in their homes. Many people were coughing or appeared to have colds or respiratory infections. With the harsh Korean winter approaching, I knew things were likely to get worse.

In another sign of how the dire circumstances were forcing a shift in North Korean policy, the UN World Food Program had been given permission to open an office in Pyongyang to coordinate the flow of humanitarian assistance, along with a handful of other agencies. Merete Johansson, a young Swedish officer from WFP Beijing, and a couple of other WFP staffers were helping to coordinate the effort. On November 24, she and I were driven to the port of Nampo, fifty kilometers southwest of Pyongyang, to await the arrival of the M/V *Rabochnya Smerna*, a rusty freighter that had been chartered. The road to Nampo was a concrete two-lane highway along the bank of the Taedong River. It was a cool, clear day. When we arrived, Merete and I sat on a hill overlooking the port and watched the ship sail in.

At the dock, to which we were admitted after stern-faced armed guards carefully inspected our passports, North Korean workmen, assisted by cranes, offloaded hundreds of sacks of rice marked with the Caritas logo and moved them to a nearby warehouse. A satisfied North Korean official turned to us and said, "It's here," suggesting that the mission had been accomplished and that it was now time for us to go. To his consternation, Merete and I replied by saying, "No, we have to count the bags." The North Korean officials looked on in horror, their hands in their pockets to ward off the cold, as Merete and I—two young, blonde, European women—clambered among the sacks, ostentatiously counting.

The process involved piling the sacks in a kind of doughnut with a space in the middle, where Merete stood, shouting out the numbers, which I noted down. Realistically, we knew we weren't going to count every single sack. But this was part of an educational process. Operating in a closed and secretive system, and with no experience in receiving assistance, the North Koreans had no notion of accountability, and of how important that would be for the international community to be willing to provide additional help. Given the relatively lackluster response to Caritas's initial appeal, and the widespread international concern that Pyongyang might divert aid from those most in need to senior government officials or the military, this was a major issue.

As we made our point, we were pleased to see that after their initial skepticism, the North Koreans became more understanding. They even brought a heater to our lunch at a nearby guesthouse. As Merete and I ate, several North Korean officials talked quietly among themselves. Curious, I asked our interpreter what they were talking about. He told us that they were commenting on how stubborn we were, and then he said, "But now we know why you are so stubborn. You are both left-handed, and in the DPRK, left-handed people are generally considered as very stubborn!"

We all laughed. It was a further thawing of the ice.

CHAPTER THREE

Let Them Starve?

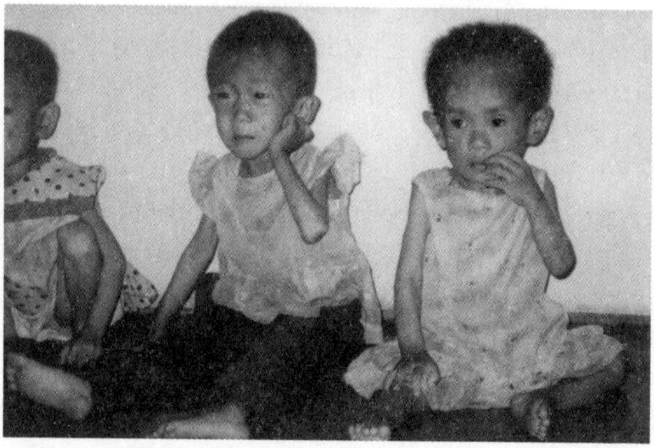

Hungry children and an international community reluctant to help.

In late January 1996, I made the first of what would be five trips to North Korea that year—January, March, May, August/September, and December. As I look back, I see that the experience was like watching a tidal wave form far out in the ocean, grow to terrifying size, and then crash ashore, causing massive death and suffering. The tidal wave was the famine. Like a time-lapse video, on each trip I could see the steadily expanding—and horrifying—impact. The adults looked thinner, the cities at night even darker, the school classrooms emptier, the number of broken-down trucks on the potholed roads greater, the food rations provided by the state smaller.

Even in Pyongyang, I saw people digging up edible roots in the parks and by the roadsides. Elsewhere, I saw a woman picking up individual grains of rice that had fallen from a sack to ensure that nothing was wasted. People told me that parents were giving their food rations to their children, which is why the adults looked increasingly emaciated. During the course of the year, the appearance of children went from simply thin to displaying signs of acute malnutrition. I saw very few pregnant women and was told of low-birthweight babies. While the normal food ration had been 700 grams a day, it had been reduced to 300 grams of uncooked grains by the time of my January 1996 visit. By May 1996, with the autumn harvest of the previous year running out and the new crop still being planted, it was down to 250. Over the summer, in two counties I visited in South Hwanghae Province, the breadbasket of North Korea, it was only 100 grams of cooked rice—barely three ounces. That was less than a fraction of the World Health Organization's recommended daily caloric intake. Indeed, 100 grams of cooked rice contains only 130 calories, while the World Food Program recommends a daily intake of 2,100 calories, including proteins, carbohydrates, and fats. People acknowledged they were reduced to eating edible roots, leaves, and bark from trees. As I noted in a report for Caritas, the whole country was at risk.

The bitter Korean winter accentuated the misery. The frozen ground meant nothing could be grown. The supply of electricity was sporadic at best. By 6:30 p.m., Pyongyang was quiet and dark, with a few dim lights visible in some buildings, although the giant statue of Kim Il Sung on Mansu Hill remained fully illuminated. In my hotel, the dining room was so chilly that I ate while wearing my heavy winter coat. Many buildings had no proper windows. One school was using plastic sheeting, which did little to keep out the cold. With the temperature at minus fifteen degrees Celsius, the floors were covered in ice. I was told that many students were too ill or simply too weak to come to class. A nearby kindergarten, no longer able to provide food for the children, had been shut altogether. I found the school visits to be particularly depressing.

Although the scale was overwhelming, I remained convinced that international food aid could slow—and perhaps, eventually halt—the slide into even greater suffering, although it was already becoming clear to me that such aid could not solve the deeper problems. In some ways, it was like putting a bandage on an uncleaned wound. Long term, assuming North Korea remained open to dealing with outsiders, we would gradually need to shift the focus from relief to rehabilitation and eventually to development, which would require the North Korean government to consider changes to its long-broken economic system. But that was for the future.

By February 1996, the initial 1,400 metric tons of rice I had secured the previous autumn had been distributed and almost used up. I was given access to all the areas where the aid had been sent, and on field trips and during inspections of warehouses, I was able to confirm that the Caritas aid had been signed for and delivered to the schools and vulnerable communities where it was supposed to go. The World Food Program, which now had a permanent presence in Pyongyang, had begun to assist with monitoring, and the workers shared my assessment. Going forward, we agreed to sign a document for each Caritas shipment that would spell out the size of the delivery, where the food would go, who would benefit, and the number of beneficiaries. The Flood Damage Rehabilitation Committee (FDRC) members and I, on behalf of Caritas, would sign each agreement, including a distribution plan. These would form the basis for future monitoring visits.

In March, however, came a new tragedy. I had purchased over 900 metric tons of rice on behalf of Caritas, and WFP had acquired another 5,635 tons in Thailand with the help of the Bangkok-based grain trader Hugo Hörndli. The WFP then chartered a Chinese ship, the M/V *Chengda*. After watching the rice being loaded, Hugo expressed concern to me that the vessel was an "old, rusty lady." His anxiety proved all too accurate when, on March 20, the ship ran into rough weather 370 miles northeast of Hong Kong and sank, with the loss of thirteen of its twenty-two crew members. All the rice was lost as well. It was one of the worst moments of my professional career. The next day, I had to break the news to my North Korean colleagues. I was struck that their initial reaction was not to ask impatiently when the replacement rice would come, but to express concern for the crew. Luckily, the cargo had been insured, and with an emergency infusion of funds from Caritas-Hong Kong, I was able to order another 900 metric tons of rice without even waiting for the payment from the insurance company.

Even as we struggled to arrange for more aid, however, the internal political tensions over Pyongyang's decision to ask for help became glaringly evident. In February 1996, UN and other aid officials were called to a meeting at the North Korean foreign ministry, where officials acknowledged that "internal forces" in the military had not been happy with the decision to request international assistance. Furthermore, one official complained that not much aid had been delivered and that "hostile foreign forces" were exploiting the situation to blacken the DPRK's reputation. He said that under the circumstances, there was no need for the United Nations to make a new international appeal; international agencies could simply complete whatever they were working on now and then leave the country.

Our takeaway from this meeting was that the officials who had advocated requesting aid were under intense internal pressure from the military and internal security agencies, who wanted the foreigners out and who saw soliciting and accepting aid from foreigners as a betrayal of the state's basic ideology. We wondered whether North Korea's brief experiment with openness was already at an end. To my surprise, however, I was taken aside and told that Caritas was not a target, that I was welcome to continue my work and could return at any time. Moreover, it became clear that much of Pyongyang's frustration was the result of the fact that the goal of the United Nations' first international appeal had not been met. It took intensive discussions to explain to the North Koreans that this was very normal. The threat to force all aid agencies to leave gradually subsided, although the deep-rooted suspicion remained.

So too did the lack of international interest in helping North Korea. Although the Canadian Foodgrains Bank, a partnership of fifteen Canadian church-based agencies working to end hunger, had now joined Caritas and the WFP, the amount of money we were able to raise to purchase more food was nowhere close to the 1.04-million-metric-ton shortfall the WFP was projecting. In May 1996, the United Nations issued a new emergency appeal. But the food aid pipeline was now virtually empty. Few nations felt comfortable aiding a regime whose own policies had contributed to the crisis, and which insisted on maintaining large armed forces even as people went hungry. South Korean President Kim Young-sam was particularly vocal on this issue. A conservative who had made no secret of his desire to see North Korea collapse, leading to the reunification of the peninsula under South Korean control, he spoke out repeatedly against providing food aid. Japan, sensitive to Kim's position, also held back, its reluctance to offer food heightened by revelations that several Japanese citizens had been kidnapped by North Korean agents in the 1970s and never returned. For its part, the United States, which did begin to help, sought to use food aid to encourage North Korea to accept a South Korean proposal for four-party talks on an eventual peace agreement that would involve the North, the South, the United States, and China.

Not everyone in South Korea, however, shared Kim Young-sam's hard-line views. One day in the summer of 1996, two South Korean priests arrived at my office in Hong Kong. They said they were part of a group in Seoul called Priests for Justice and were intensely curious about the North. I told them about my experiences, and then one of them pulled out a brown McDonald's bag and placed it on my desk. I looked inside and nearly fainted. The bag was full of hundred-dollar bills. "Here," one of the two men said, "this is something for North Korea." It turned out that to evade Seoul's still-rigid laws on moving funds out of the country—and the South Korean government's hostility toward Pyongyang—the two had asked their parishioners to transfer up to $10,000 each to an account set up in Hong Kong, and had then withdrawn the cash and stuffed it in a bag to deliver to me. I immediately added the roughly $300,000 to our fund to purchase rice to feed children in North Korea.

Like others involved with the aid effort, I too wrestled with the moral dilemma raised by those who argued that providing food was just helping to prop up the North Korean regime. But I was deeply uncomfortable with what I saw as a "let them starve" mentality, which I felt did nothing to feed the hungry and risked heightening tensions in Northeast Asia. My own view was that allowing North Koreans to starve because of distaste for the country's political system was morally wrong. It was not the fault of the children we were trying to feed that they had been born in North Korea. Basic human compassion—trying to alleviate suffering—meant that it was important to proceed, whatever the political pitfalls. In the long run, it was clear to me that North Korea would have to implement some meaningful changes to its economic system, both to weather the famine and to ensure the disaster would not recur. Greater contact with the rest of the world could be an important positive factor. Apart from saving lives now, providing aid was, in my view, a way of engaging the North Koreans on a human level without getting entangled in the nuclear, missile, or other controversial issues. I recognized it would be a slow, uncertain process, and that the results, if any, would be incremental at best. But under the circumstances, I saw no alternative.

In the summer of 1996, a new round of torrential rainstorms and serious floods caused even more devastation. In August, I was taken to particularly hard-hit areas to the east and southwest of Pyongyang, where I saw breached dams, flooded maize and rice fields with crops rotting beneath the water, and other fields covered in silt. At the same time, fuel shortages meant tractors were still sitting idle, and fertilizer and pesticides were still in short supply. I saw entire fields of maize infested with pests. In August, the WFP conducted a flood-damage assessment; it concluded that the grain harvest would be reduced by nearly four hundred thousand metric tons. That autumn, the WFP estimated that the 1996 harvest would be even less than the dramatically reduced one in 1995, leaving a shortfall of over one million metric tons of grain.

By the end of the year, it was clear the country was in a downward spiral. In meetings with officials from the FDRC, they acknowledged that 1997 was going to be a very tough year and spoke openly about the urgent need for food aid as well as agricultural inputs such as seeds, fertilizer, and plastic sheeting. The North Koreans were surprised that I—a Western woman—could talk knowledgeably about farming. I explained that I had grown up on a farm, which left them very impressed.

By now, I felt I was beginning to develop a level of trust with my interlocutors, many of whom I had met on multiple visits, which made it increasingly possible to discuss sensitive topics. This included the need for greater transparency and accountability, allowing international experts to conduct nutritional surveys around the country, and more flexibility in arranging access to different regions. In several meetings, I raised the issue of visiting northern and eastern provinces, such as Ryanggang, Chagang, North and South Hamgyong, and Kangwon, all provinces where it was feared the food situation was particularly grave. No foreign aid personnel had been permitted to go to the first four, and Caritas was at this point the only humanitarian agency permitted to visit Kangwon, where I traveled twice in 1996.

I also encouraged the North Koreans to allow members of the international media to visit and report on the situation. I stressed the importance of press coverage in generating the international sympathy that would pressure donor governments to provide more aid. In these conversations, I felt that the officials I was meeting, some of whom I had been dealing with for more than two years, were showing more flexibility and understanding than before. The question of media access, however, was obviously extremely sensitive, and they made clear to me that any decision to allow foreign reporters to visit would have to be made at a very high level. It was evident that within the country's top leadership, considerable uncertainty and suspicion about engaging with outsiders remained. As I noted in a report to Caritas in early 1997, "The slow step-by-step approach—with the danger of frustrating and deterring donors—will probably continue for the time being."

CHAPTER FOUR

No Access, No Aid

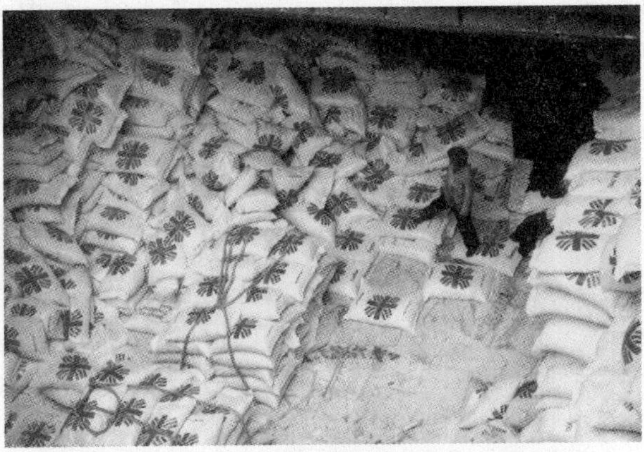

Food aid bags, marked with the Caritas logo, arrived.

In April 1997, the North Korean government staged a huge military parade to mark the sixty-fifth official anniversary of the founding of the Korean People's Army. On a crisp, bright spring morning, tens of thousands of troops goose-stepped through Kim Il Sung Square in the center of Pyongyang, followed by long lines of civilians, each person waving a red plastic flower. Along with the tiny diplomatic corps and a few other foreigners, I was invited to attend. We all had to undergo extensive security checks, and once in the reviewing stand, I realized why. Suddenly, Kim Jong Il appeared on the rostrum. A band played "No Motherland Without You," the rousing song with which the Dear Leader was associated, and which could often be heard blaring from loudspeakers on the streets in Pyongyang and elsewhere.

The military parade offered my first glimpse of North Korea's enigmatic leader. Short, pudgy, with a bouffant hairdo, he did not exactly radiate charisma. Yet the crowds reacted almost hysterically, weeping, clapping, and waving their red flowers as Kim, his face expressionless, soaked up the homage. The message that the carefully choreographed display conveyed, both to North Korea's own people and to the rest of the world, especially adversaries such as the United States and South Korea, was clear: Despite the acute economic crisis, devastating food shortages, and continuing tensions over its missile and nuclear programs, North Korea's political system, and the man who presided over it, remained intact.

In many other countries, famines had led not only to social and economic collapse but to political upheaval. And indeed, by 1997, the US Central Intelligence Agency (CIA) was already predicting that Kim's regime was on the brink of collapse. Yet it never came apart, and I often pondered why this was not the case. It seemed far too simplistic to attribute this simply to sweeping repression. To me, it seemed that several different factors were at play: a deep-rooted Confucian respect for authority; an ability to endure hardship, dating from the half century of Japanese occupation to the upheavals of World War Two, the Communist takeover, and the Korean War; traditional Korean nationalism, which often bordered on xenophobia and was reflected in the national ideology of *juche*—not just the Leninist apparatus of control. The result, I felt, was an absolutist state with some qualities of a religious cult. Whatever the explanation, I had no doubt that the regime would remain intact and that the collapse scenario some were promoting outside the country was wishful thinking. Those of us trying to help had little choice to but to work within the system. That was the reality.

My own experiences during my earlier travels—as well as during the twelve trips I would make in 1997 and 1998, visiting eight of North Korea's nine provinces, from Kangwon on the border with South Korea to Ryanggang in the northeast bordering China—reinforced my conviction that, however acute the suffering, the government's hold over the country remained strong. I never picked up an undercurrent of political dissent, let alone any suggestion that Kim Jong Il was to blame. Indeed, on numerous field trips, I was struck by the resilience and stoicism of a beleaguered people. I watched women uncomplainingly carrying heavy loads on their backs to clear farmland, and men repairing river embankments by hand. Every bit of land seemed to be used for growing food; vegetables were grown on apartment balconies. Crops were even being cultivated on the roof of the Potonggang Hotel, where I would usually stay in Pyongyang. People would speak of an "arduous march." It was a propaganda term used by the government to rally the population, but many of those I met stressed their commitment to overcoming the crisis through courage and determination. As I wrote in a report for Caritas in late 1997, "The people have not given up, and are working hard to solve their problems."

Still, despite the regime's continuing hold on power and the absence of political dissent, the misery of the population was acute—and getting worse. I was well aware that international aid would not on its own be able to solve the country's deep-rooted crisis, but I was more determined than ever to do what I could to help alleviate hunger and save lives. In discussions with colleagues from the WFP and other UN agencies as well from the FDRC, it was becoming clear that the areas I had been most concerned about—Kangwon on the east coast and the three northeastern provinces of South Hamgyong, North Hamgyong, and Ryanggang—did indeed appear to be the worst-hit. Lacking the economic and other benefits provided by proximity to Pyongyang, and with politically sensitive frontiers, mountainous terrain with little arable land, a short growing season, and extreme winter temperatures, the region's nearly seven million people were unquestionably among the most vulnerable.

By mid-1997, my colleagues at the WFP and the FDRC and I identified a half dozen counties in Kangwon as the top priority for the Caritas aid effort. I discovered I was the first international humanitarian worker allowed to visit the province. Initially, getting permission to go anywhere in Kangwon except the provincial capital of Wonsan, a run-down port on the Sea of Japan (or the East Sea, as the Koreans called it), proved difficult. I was told that, for security reasons, some areas of Kangwon close to the border with South Korea would remain off-limits, and indeed, there were a half dozen counties I never managed to visit. Even in areas farther away from the frontier, I could understand the reluctance of local officials to allow me to visit. In a system like North Korea's, they feared being blamed by the central government for the grim conditions in the areas for which they were responsible. But I felt they were out of step with the FDRC members, who had increasingly signaled a willingness to allow me to see the real situation on the ground and were sending that message to the provinces. And over multiple visits, with repeated conversations, constant low-key lobbying, the implied threat of "no access, no aid," plus the fact that Caritas was able to deliver on the assistance it promised, access to other parts of the province slowly expanded.

Thus it was that a few days before the April 25, 1997, military parade, I was taken to two counties in Kangwon. In Ichon County, I visited three families. It was painful to witness their plight. The only meal of the day consisted of rice soup with powdered rice husk. They could not remember the last time they had eaten meat or fish. One local official told me that the daily ration for most people was between 100 and 200 grams—roughly 350 to 700 calories, barely enough to survive—and that food stocks would run out altogether the following month. In another indication of the collapse of the public distribution system, a nearby center had not distributed any food since March 13. When I visited, its warehouse contained only acorns to be crushed, soaked, and powdered.

By this point, the use of alternative foods—bark, grass, roots, seaweed, even sawdust—to make so-called noodles or cakes to stretch what meager rations were available was becoming increasingly common, although it was far from clear that such "food" offered any nutritional benefits. In fact, it likely caused serious intestinal problems for an already weakened population.

At the kindergarten in Ichon County, in northern Kangwon Province, nearly a quarter of the 260 children were absent—too weak or too ill to attend. The youngsters I did see were thin and coughed incessantly. Mrs. Kim, the headmistress, said she had been working at the kindergarten for twenty-three years and had never experienced anything like this. Already, five children had died.

"What is going to happen?" she asked plaintively. Conditions at the kindergarten in Kumchong County, which I also visited, appeared even worse. Many children showed signs of acute malnutrition, such as a distended belly and twig-like limbs. Ten had died. "This is as bad as when the Japanese were here," an official there told me. My interpreter, who had come with me from Pyongyang, struggled to translate my questions—not because he wanted to prevent me from asking them but because he was so shocked by what he was seeing.

I returned to North Korea again in July, September, October, and November. By early autumn 1997, the public distribution system had largely ceased to function, and food rations across much of the country were down to 100 to 150 grams per day, effectively a slow starvation diet. I repeatedly saw people scavenging for seaweed, bark, and herbs, and ragged, emaciated children with watery eyes, runny noses, and deep hacking coughs wandering the streets. The homes I visited not only lacked food, many had no windows, with only plastic sheeting to provide protection from the elements. I wondered how people would survive the bitter North Korean winter.

Moreover, the health sector had virtually collapsed as well. At the County People's Hospital in Anbyon County, in Kangwon, there were no Western medicines, minimal supplies of soap, and only meager stocks of traditional Korean herbal medicine. The supply of electricity and water was erratic at best, and it appeared that many in need of health care were remaining at home to suffer—and perhaps even die—rather than going to hospitals that could not provide for them. One doctor told me that cases of tuberculosis had tripled in recent months. As I wrote in a report for Caritas, "If this hospital is typical, then it is clear that health care in the DPRK is in a critically poor state."

At the Ministry of Health in Pyongyang, officials acknowledged that people were dying because medicines were in short supply. Because of a lack of water and sanitation, other infections were increasing as well. I was told that some 35 percent of North Korean children suffered from diarrhea, while the overall malnutrition rate for children six and under was over 37 percent. That amounted to around eight hundred thousand kids in desperate need of help. In some of my meetings, government officials openly acknowledged their embarrassment and shame at having to ask for international help. Said one, "We have our pride." Yet they became increasingly open in my conversations with them—evidence of the seriousness of the crisis.

By now, the journey to Pyongyang was becoming as familiar to me as a ride on a local bus. I would fly from Hong Kong to Beijing, spend a night or two at the Swissôtel, where the Air Koryo office was located, and then take one of the national carrier's two weekly flights. At the Beijing airport departure lounge, I would run into the same group of old friends and colleagues—UN workers, nongovernmental organization (NGO) staff, foreign diplomats, and the occasional left-wing South Korean. I could always tell the Northerners from the Southerners by their Kim Il Sung and Kim Jong Il badges, and by the flowers they carried—not for their wives, but to place at the statue of Kim Il Sung, which was the obligatory first stop for all travelers.

On the plane, usually a Russian-built Tupolev, named after the great Russian scientist who designed it while in prison for his Catholic beliefs, martial music would blare and lunch boxes with unappetizing snacks would be served. The only in-flight reading material was a glossy propaganda magazine called *Korea Today* and, occasionally, back issues of the *Pyongyang Times*.

At Pyongyang airport, photos of the two Kims looked down from the main building. Customs was slow but usually uneventful, and on the other side, I would find two representatives from the FDRC, my official hosts. We would zoom into town along wide roads that were almost completely free of traffic and spotlessly clean. Closer to the city center, we would pass trams packed to capacity and large numbers of men and women trudging along with packs on their backs.

I usually stayed at the Potonggang Hotel. Built in 1973, the nine-story building stands on the tree-lined banks of the Potonggang River. The Potonggang was considered for many years the nicest hotel in the city. But at this time, I was one of only a handful of guests, which made eating in the huge dining room designed to seat two hundred an eerie experience. From my window, I could see the still-unfinished 105-story Ryugyong Hotel, which towered over the Pyongyang skyline. Construction on the building, intended at the time to be the world's tallest hotel and one of the ten tallest buildings in the world, had begun in 1987 and stopped in the early 1990s because of the country's economic crisis. An empty concrete shell without windows, fittings, or fixtures, it was to me a symbol of so much that had gone wrong in North Korea.

Gaining access to the countryside took careful preparation to avoid running afoul of internal security officials. For each of my trips, I had developed a procedure. A couple of weeks before leaving Hong Kong, I would send a message to my colleagues at the FDRC spelling out the goal of the upcoming visit, where I wanted to go, and who and what I wanted to see. Given the nature of their system, I knew they needed time to make arrangements and secure travel permissions, not only for me and any traveling companions but for the North Koreans accompanying us. After so many visits, I had begun to gain the trust of FDRC officials, which slowly deepened over time. It became increasingly evident that in general, they were making good-faith efforts to accommodate my requests. Often, though, this required them to engage in difficult negotiations with officials in the security apparatus, who were suspicious of allowing any foreigners to go anywhere. Still, more often than not, the FDRC succeeded in securing permission, and I was pleasantly surprised to discover how much access I was beginning to get.

Even more important, my North Korean interlocutors did not appear to be trying to hide from me the extent of the crisis. "We never had this problem before," admitted the director of a nursery in Wonsan. "We are embarrassed. We do not know how to treat these children." Said the chairwoman of a local village council, "I am the mother of the county. I feel bad when I cannot feed everyone." Government officials in Pyongyang expressed concern that food stocks would run out altogether, and it was clear that international aid was probably the only thing keeping millions of people alive.

Despite the growing involvement of other agencies, Caritas remained one of the largest sources of humanitarian assistance. On the day of the huge military parade in April 1997, a ship arrived at the port of Nampo carrying three thousand metric tons of rice and two thousand metric tons of maize. Our other shipments contained multivitamins for children and pregnant and nursing mothers, blankets for children in nurseries and kindergartens, and agricultural inputs such as seeds, fertilizer, pesticides, and plastic sheeting.

As our efforts in North Korea expanded, the Canadian Foodgrains Bank approached Caritas and expressed an interest in collaborating. It became a fruitful partnership. Foodgrains Bank staff accompanied me on my visits, and the organization proved very helpful—not least because of its ability to provide Canadian grain for relief shipments. On the April 1997 trip, Foodgrains Bank colleagues and I raised with the FDRC the idea of using a facility in Nampo to mill the grain as soon as it was offloaded, with the bags of flour to be sent to their intended destinations. The North Koreans agreed, and by summer, the Nampo milling plant was in operation. I made regular inspection visits. The arrangement had many benefits, including that it provided work for some of Nampo's hard-pressed citizens, and it was far less costly to ship large quantities of raw grain than sacks of milled wheat flour to North Korea.

Most important, because we were observing the process from the initial unloading and milling point, we could better monitor where the aid was going. For each shipment, we signed a project agreement with the FDRC, which identified clear locations and beneficiaries and also gave written permission for Caritas to conduct follow-up visits. I was therefore able to trace the transport and distribution of the flour through warehouses and PDS centers, and to check in some homes of villagers where the flour had been made available through the PDS. The flour came in distinctive sacks we had provided, with the Caritas logo on one side and that of the Canadian Foodgrains Bank on the other, and had distributed in small amounts to villagers. Women had to bring their own containers to collect their rations. As the sacks were emptied, the authorities reused them for other storage purposes. I would also make a point of telling local officials when a future shipment would be arriving and how much they could expect, and then point to my Pyongyang-based guide and say, "If you don't get it, here is the person to whom you should complain." It created at least one additional element of accountability.

Yet it remained a challenge to drum up international support for relief supplies for North Korea. Many potential donors were reluctant to be seen as propping up a regime with a reputation for human rights violations and intensifying missile and nuclear programs. Some remained unconvinced that conditions were actually that bad, while others, including Japan, South Korea, and the United States, were linking food aid to North Korean concessions in political talks. Indeed, the World Food Program launched a $99.5 million program for 203,000 metric tons of emergency food aid in the spring of 1997 but by May had received just one-third of the money. It was a climate in which separating humanitarian aid from political considerations was difficult, if not impossible, although I continued to feel strongly that to allow North Koreans to starve because of political differences was morally wrong.

North Korea did not help its cause with its continuing reluctance to issue visas to journalists. I repeatedly urged my counterparts at the FDRC to allow reporters from the international media to cover the famine. I understood their concern that negative news coverage would be seen as a slap in the face for an image-conscious government, but I contended that it would be a small price to pay for generating worldwide sympathy and greater support. Interestingly, the North Koreans appeared to have no problem with my speaking to the foreign press and providing photos and videos, and indeed, I became one of the few regular voices on North Korea with on-the-ground experience in the country.

After my April 1997 visit, I did an interview with the Reuters news agency in Beijing, during which I said, "The overall situation is just going down. It's like a ladder I am climbing down, and I don't know where the bottom rung is. If no major food aid is going in fairly soon, it could deteriorate very, very rapidly." Already there were reports, fueled by North Korean refugee accounts from China, of up to a million deaths and even cases of cannibalism, although I never saw any evidence of the latter in my own travels. For their part, the Chinese never considered the fleeing North Koreans as refugees but rather saw them as illegal migrants, which made it hard for these miserable people get refugee status, let alone be resettled in a third country. Beijing was also reluctant to allow UN High Commissioner for Refugees staff access to the North Korean escapees. Yet talking publicly about the situation remained a delicate balancing act, given Pyongyang's acute sensitivity to anything that could be construed as public criticism that would cause a loss of face. In my case, I felt confident that I had developed enough trust with my North Korean interlocutors that they would not see my accurate descriptions of an increasingly grim situation to be a sign of a deeper anti-regime agenda—something that was not always the case with some staffers at other aid agencies.

This was just one of the challenges as North Korea, despite its reservations, allowed a growing number of international humanitarian aid agencies to base staff in the country as the famine got worse. These included Médecins San Frontières (MSF, aka Doctors Without Borders), Médecins du Monde, German Agro Action, Mercy Corps, World Vision, the International Federation of the Red Cross and Red Crescent Societies, the World Food Program, UNICEF, the UN Development Program, and the European Union's Humanitarian Aid Office (ECHO). Although not allowed to establish a full presence until 2001, the World Health Organization was permitted in 1997 to set up an Emergency and Humanitarian Action office in Pyongyang. From their experiences in places such as Africa and the Middle East, most NGOs were used to humanitarian emergencies characterized by a collapse of local political authority and relative freedom to move around, depending on security or weather or topographical considerations, and to operate where and how they chose. But North Korea was different. The government was profoundly suspicious of, and quick to attribute sinister motives to, outsiders, and was deeply embarrassed at having to ask for international help.

Consequently, as the expat presence grew, so did tensions with the authorities. For many NGOs, the interaction with the FDRC was adversarial from the start. They chafed at the restrictions under which they operated, including an initial ban on sending Korean-speaking staffers; tight controls on travel, with a requirement to apply one week in advance to visit locations outside Pyongyang; and sharp limitations on what was called "random access"—the independent evaluation of conditions on the ground to determine for themselves which parts of the country faced the greatest need.

Above all, there were numerous complaints about the challenge of monitoring aid, which led to widespread speculation—intensified by media coverage—that some assistance was being diverted to feed the North Korean military, security services, and government officials. The issue came up at almost every meeting that aid agencies held in Pyongyang, the concern heightened by the obsessive secrecy of the North Korean system and the thinly disguised hostility on the part of many officials toward the growing foreign presence. The result was frequent confrontations and much bad feeling, with complaints that local authorities were hiding starving children, sprucing up areas to be inspected, and pocketing aid for themselves.

North Korean officials, while expressing gratitude for the assistance, also complained to me that some organizations were more interested in undermining the North Korean system than in helping its people. They repeatedly expressed fears that monitors, especially Americans, might have "alternative agendas," were "interfering in local affairs," or could be spies. To me, though, the reality was much more complex.

As I observed the arrival of aid shipments and traveled the country to inspect deliveries, I remained alert for any signs of diversion. I certainly encountered situations in which the distribution of food and even the conversations were obviously stage-managed. I attributed this both to the secretiveness and regimentation of the North Korean system and to inexperience and fear in dealing with foreigners. And I continually pressed the North Koreans for greater transparency and access. But throughout 1997 and 1998, I felt quite confident that the bulk of the aid Caritas was sending was indeed reaching the intended beneficiaries. Yet the North Koreans were still reluctant to agree to what the aid community felt were crucial steps, especially to allow a nationwide nutritional survey to determine the scale of the hunger and identify the best way to address it.

Watching the situation unfold as the worst of the famine took hold, I came to believe that the attitude of some aid agency personnel—even if they did not have the subversive agenda the North Koreans worried about—was exacerbating the problem. Most aid workers arrived with the best of intentions but knew very little about Korean history, North Korean society, or the unhappy legacy of the Korean War. Not surprisingly, given North Korea's less than stellar international reputation, many were deeply suspicious of their interlocutors and the North Korean system. Used to operating in their own way, they adopted what often seemed to me to be a top-down and sometimes confrontational approach, presenting conditions or making demands, and not displaying an awareness of North Korean culture and sensitivities that might have made their life easier.

The suspicion, distrust, and lack of cultural understanding soured many dealings with the North Koreans. I recall, for example, one NGO aid worker coming back from a family visit during which the housewife had told him, "I have no other food." The worker could see edible things in the home and concluded he was being lied to. He was unaware that when the North Koreans speak of "food," they mean cereals. Other items are just nice little extras. The housewife was not lying but simply expressing a premise of her own culture.

Another time, a foreign woman who had visited a family mockingly recounted to me how a pregnant woman there had said the pregnancy lasted ten months. But ten months in the Korean lunar calendar is nine of our months. Again, it was a case of cultural misunderstanding rather than of someone's trying to pull the wool over an aid worker's eyes.

At Caritas, we debated whether to open our own office in Pyongyang. I felt to do so would be a mistake. Being a foreign resident of North Korea would have meant coping with even more layers of bureaucracy, regulation, and suspicion, not to mention the cost and logistical headaches of arranging accommodations, office space, and the myriad other requirements that would have allowed us to sustain an ongoing presence. To me, having to deal with such matters would have meant diverting time and energy from the need to focus on providing help. Moreover, having by this point established what I felt were positive relationships with North Korean officials, I believed I was just as likely—if not even likelier—to receive meaningful cooperation through visits every couple of months.

The building of relationships took time and enormous patience. Whatever my private feelings about the North Korean system, I made a conscious decision not to be judgmental, to keep an open mind, and to treat the North Koreans with respect. Early on, for instance, I stopped calling those who were escorting me everywhere my "minders." Instead, I used the term "guardian angels" or simply "my colleagues." Aware of the importance of face, I went out of my way to avoid embarrassing North Korean officials. If there was an issue or a problem, whenever possible I would take the person aside later to discuss it. These were small gestures, but they shaped my encounters, and I think those who interacted with me appreciated the fact that I saw them more as colleagues than as adversaries.

As I noted in a report to Caritas, "Accepting the pace of developments the local partners can accept, follow or cope with, is often the source of irritation. Cross-cultural exchange is still new for North Koreans, taking into account that it is less than three years since the North Korean government asked for international assistance. To offer a variety of opportunities to learn about new developments, to look at problems from different perspectives, to grow and transform within a nation and across borders is only valuable if done in a non-threatening manner."

This did not mean that everything always went smoothly. The level of paranoia among North Korean officials remained high. On one trip, a foreign colleague waiting for the rest of our delegation to join him at the dinner table playfully held a pack of cigarettes to his ear, pretending it was a mobile phone. Our North Korean "guardian angels" froze, petrified that this foreigner might have smuggled in a cell phone. When they realized he was only joking, though, we all burst into laughter.

I was occasionally stuck with guides who resisted letting me see what I needed to. On some inspection visits, it was difficult to get straight answers to questions about how much aid had arrived and how it was being distributed. And sometimes, local officials displayed what seemed to me to be appalling insensitivity about the plight of their people. One morning in September 1997, for example, another aid worker and I traveled to Popdong, a mountainous county in Kangwon Province that had been particularly hard-hit. Caritas had initiated several relief projects in Popdong, where we were supplying rice, a corn-soya blend, lentils, and vegetable oil. Although I was repeatedly thanked for the aid, the situation remained grim. I visited the county kindergarten. It had space for over six hundred children, but only a third were there, the rest too weak or ill to attend. It was the same story at the local nursery. But at midday, while hungry children peered through the curtains into the dining room at a local restaurant, county officials served us a huge lunch. I could not eat, because I was so upset that I was unable to swallow. My local hosts were taken aback. But they apparently concluded that I would only behave that way if I were a really powerful VIP. The result was that for the rest of the visit, I was given even greater access.

As frustrating as my experience was, I had some sympathy for the officials and residents in the places I was inspecting. I often thought of how my mother would have reacted in our small Swiss village if a team of unfamiliar Africans or Asians were to have walked into her home at a time of great distress and questioned her in detail about her diet, medical condition, and other personal details. Moreover, in North Korea, not only was I usually the first foreigner that local people had encountered, but I also was asking embarrassing questions while officials from the area looked on as the personnel who had accompanied me from Pyongyang did the translating. No wonder it was awkward. Often during these visits, when no one was watching, I would slip a bar of soap under a piece of furniture, so the family would have a nice surprise after I left. For waitresses in the county restaurants, I would sometimes quietly put lipstick into their hands or apron pockets when saying goodbye. I remember one young girl opening her hand to see what I had given her, and literally jumping up and down with pleasure. It was the least I could do.

In mid-1997, the monitoring effort received a major boost with the creation of the Food Aid Liaison Unit (FALU). Funded by Caritas and a half dozen other NGOs and officially attached to the World Food Program, it was designed to monitor the distribution of food aid and other inputs donated mostly by NGOS, and to serve the needs of international organizations requesting assistance. Its attachment to the WFP magnified its ability to negotiate with the authorities on behalf of the aid agencies, as well as improved coordination among them. Since this involved managing complex relationships and frequent squabbling between NGOs and UN agencies, between NGOs and the North Korean authorities, and between resident and nonresident NGOs, it was a challenging task.

It was headed initially by Erich Weingartner, a Canadian with a long history of church-based humanitarian activism who, in 1986, had arranged the first encounter between North and South Korean Christians at a meeting in Switzerland. He also had worked in conflict zones in Lebanon, El Salvador, the Philippines, and Bosnia. With his keen sense of humor and warm laugh, he immediately became a kindred spirit to me. He was less judgmental about the North Koreans than some other international staff. Like me, he saw our help and expertise as part of a partnership with the

DPRK, not a process to force changes on unwilling subjects. We made numerous trips together.

Still, it remained a struggle to secure the consistent access and transparency that we needed, especially to keep skeptical donors satisfied. Nonetheless, whatever the constraints, the fact that the North Korean government agreed to allow foreign NGOs to station personnel in Pyongyang was, for me, in itself a remarkable development, and by mid-1997, there was a sizable international community in the capital. While I did not formally live there, I was in and out regularly enough to be considered a member. The daily expat existence was a strange one—a routine of often difficult meetings with North Korean officials, often frustrating and tightly controlled trips outside Pyongyang, and constant wrestling with the dilemma of whether we were helping the North Korean people or simply propping up the North Korean regime.

Not all the foreign residents, however, were new arrivals. The Swiss ambassador to China, who was also accredited to North Korea, had told me about an elderly Swiss French woman named Simone Dellamagne, who had lived in Pyongyang since 1983. He urged me to look her up, which I did on one of my early trips. We met first at the coffee shop of the Koryo Hotel, an enormous forty-seven-story twin-tower structure where most foreign visitors stayed. The café was in a dimly lit corner off the lobby and was virtually the only hangout for the tiny foreign community. Later, Simone also invited me to her flat. She was a remarkable woman. Petite, with short white hair, she always dressed elegantly, with bright red lipstick and, in winter, a heavy coat with fur cuffs. She had spent many years as a lawyer for the International Labor Organization (ILO) in Geneva. Although not a member of any Communist party, she had distinctly left-wing politics, and after leaving the ILO, she moved to Beijing in 1981 to work polishing French translations for various Chinese propaganda publications. Two years later, she had taken a similar position in Pyongyang, and had been there ever since.

When we met, she said, "Look, I am old, but here in North Korea, old people are valued, not like in Europe. Gray hair counts in Asian societies. We foreigners are well-treated here. They give you everything." Indeed, later on I visited her flat, in an apartment block where her other foreign colleagues and some North Korean officials lived, and saw that it was spacious, warm, and comfortable, with large, well-worn armchairs. She was paid in US dollars and had a chauffeur-driven Mercedes to take her around. It was the kind of old-world atmosphere where I expected her to put on some classical music, but she instead asked me, "Do you like soft rock?" As the music played loudly in the background, I tried to steer the conversation to what was happening in the country. She stressed that she had "never seen kids with big bellies here in Pyongyang" but acknowledged that even in her position, it was hard to see below the surface.

Simone stayed in Pyongyang until 1999, and after returning to Europe, made numerous visits there. I often wondered how, deep down, she felt about having spent so many years there. But it was clear that her ideological sympathy with North Korea remained intact. When asked, she would say, "One has to risk something in life, and, as the Edith Piaf song goes, '*je ne regrette rien*' (I regret nothing.)" Little did I realize that I would also spend five years living in North Korea.

There were few regrets among the growing numbers of foreign humanitarian workers eagerly arriving in North Korea, but there was abundant frustration, not only in terms of the work but because there was almost nothing to do in one's spare time. A bowling alley, a couple of amusement parks, and the Pyongyang Zoo were literally all that was available. On some earlier visits, I had been taken to what passed for a North Korean version of a disco called the Red Rose. It was a long, dark room with a red rose painted on one wall, and actual dancing took place—although it was always men with men. The society was too conservative for women to go to such places, let alone dance with men in public. A handful of foreigners were allowed to visit the disco, and I have vivid memories of how cold it was inside, to the point that we had to keep our coats on. We also had to bring our own whiskey and music cassettes. Yet even that degree of casual contact was too much for the authorities, and the Red Rose was soon closed.

Soon after his arrival, however, Erich Weingartner and a number of other NGO staffers came up with the idea of creating a place where resident foreigners could hang out without the tension and awkwardness of trying to interact with locals. They procured space in the basement of the building that had been the Bulgarian embassy and was now the office of the WFP, and got some shabby furniture brought in on diplomatic shipments from China, including a large bar as well as a video projector and screen to show movies. A contest was held to find a name, and the bar, which was open only on Friday, Saturday, and Sunday, was quickly christened the Random

Access Club (RAC)—a cynical reflection of the difficulties that aid workers were facing in actually securing random access for their relief work.

The RAC soon became the place to go for aid workers, diplomats, and the occasional visitor, and became so popular that the North Koreans asked about the name. A WFP official responded that "RAC" actually stood for "Relief Agencies Club," and that "Random Access Club" was just a humorous nickname. North Korean contacts told me that the word "random" was particularly hateful, because they had been taught that during the Korean War, the United States conducted random bombing attacks. But to their credit, the North Koreans went along with the joke. The RAC lasted until 2012.

CHAPTER FIVE

"Is This the End of the Great Leader Taking Care of Us?"

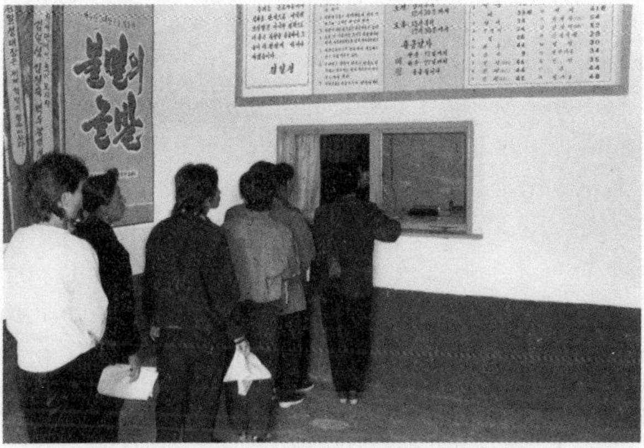

A public distribution center where small groups of women collect their rations.

It was September 1998. I sat on the floor, Korean style, in Mrs. Kim's apartment in Sinuiju, one of North Korea's five largest cities. Located on the banks of the Yalu River just across from the Chinese town of Dandong, Sinuiju had been an important industrial center and a key transit point for trade with China before the North's economy collapsed. Yet even though there was more contact with China in Sinuiju now than in other North Korean cities, it remained shabby and dilapidated, especially in contrast to the bright lights and bustling streets visible on the Chinese side of the Yalu in Dandong. And Sinuiju had not been immune to the devastating impact of the famine. Indeed, earlier in the year, the North Koreans and the WFP had asked Caritas to ship 1,500 metric tons of barley there. As was often the case, providing the aid opened the door for me to visit an area that had previously been off-limits to foreigners. Along with Mary Healy, a nurse and midwife from the Irish NGO Trócaire (Caritas Ireland), which had become one of our most important international partners, I was making my first trip there. Local officials told us that, for many people, our supplies had been crucial in keeping hunger at bay. But the situation remained bleak.

At the Amnokgang Hotel, a large, square building with damp, smelly rooms and balconies whose doors could not be opened, we were virtually the only guests in the cavernous dining hall. The hotel shop offered an eclectic collection of basic necessities, but most striking to me was the jewelry that was also on sale. It was evident that some desperate citizens had pawned their personal valuables to get money to buy food. I bought a pair of earrings inlaid with small red stones. I still have them today. I keep them in a box. They bring back sad memories.

In a dismal gray Stalinist-style building typical of most North Korean cities, sixty-nine-year-old Mrs. Kim shared a tiny flat with her son, daughter-in-law, and six-month-old grandson. The son and his wife both worked in a nearby textile factory. Mrs. Kim and her daughter-in-law kept the apartment spotless. On one wall hung a guitar, which Mrs. Kim's son apparently liked to play. As I entered the room, I was startled to hear the gravel-tinged vocals of American country music legend Kenny Rogers coming from a cassette recorder. It made for an incongruous juxtaposition with the obligatory pictures of Kim Il Sung and Kim Jong Il mounted on another wall. I was tempted to ask about the music, but it occurred to me that the tape and the cassette player likely had come from China, that Mrs. Kim might well not be aware that Rogers was an American, and that the "guardian angels" accompanying us were probably equally ignorant. Inquiring as to why the family had popular music from the United States could have caused trouble for everyone, so I stayed silent. Mary and I just looked at each other with slightly puzzled expressions.

Under other circumstances, owning items such as a guitar and a cassette recorder, or the sewing machines and refrigerators I saw in other urban homes, would, in North Korean terms, have been signs of a decent standard of living. But on this visit, they could not mask the family's grim plight.

"Is this the end of the Great Leader taking care of us?" the daughter-in-law asked plaintively. Her baby was ill. She said she was still breastfeeding and planned to continue to do so as long as possible. She had nothing else to feed her son. Six months had passed since they had received their last rations through the public distribution system. Apart from fourteen kilos of rice and some bean curd delivered to mark North Korea's National Day, they had been subsisting on alternative food plus whatever they could obtain by bartering textiles and other items with relatives who lived in the countryside and were able to grow some food for themselves.

Later that day, Mary and I were taken to meet the family of Mr. Lee, a seventy-one-year-old carpenter. We found him sitting on his living room floor designing some furniture. He was surprised to see two unexpected foreign visitors but was gracious and friendly. Mr. Lee lived with his wife and youngest son. Three older sons were married and lived elsewhere. Like Mrs. Kim, Mr. Lee told us he had last received rations from the PDS in February. He was surviving by making furniture for people in the countryside, which he exchanged for food.

The examples of the Kim and Lee families highlighted two important characteristics of the famine in North Korea. Its epicenter was in urban rather than rural areas. More than two-thirds of the population lived in or near cities and towns. Unlike farmers in the countryside, who had the ability to grow food on small private plots, which the authorities understood were necessary to survive and thus (perhaps grudgingly) tolerated, urban residents, often stuck in large apartment blocks, had no such option. The result was unprecedented hunger in what had been a relatively well-developed modern industrial society. With the collapse of the PDS, which had been the sole source of food, many urban residents, unable to grow anything for themselves, simply wasted away in their homes, starving quietly and out of sight. This was one reason I began to describe the situation as a "hidden famine." In contrast to predominantly rural Somalia or Ethiopia, the worst suffering was not immediately visible. That didn't make it any less real.

For the families we visited in Sinuiju, and many others, bartering was a crucial survival mechanism. What had begun with urban residents trading items of value, either from their homes or what could be stripped from their places of work, for food grown by farmers in private family garden plots became the foundation for the broader development of markets. As I traveled around the country, I would see people by the side of the road selling everything from buns to cigarettes to vegetables to live fish. As time passed, I also started to see little businesses appearing—people mending shoes, sewing, fixing bicycle tires, transporting wood in simple carts. Almost all of those involved appeared to be women, presumably because men were more likely to have fixed jobs or be serving in the military.

The emergence of these markets was a sensitive political issue. As a de facto privatization of an important part of North Korea's economy, they posed not only practical challenges to state control but also an ideological one. Initially, when roadside vendors noticed a foreigner like me approaching, they would quickly cover the plastic buckets containing their products and run away. The government officials accompanying me were visibly uncomfortable as well and would often look in the other direction. But the trend only accelerated with the creation of larger markets, especially in or near urban areas, which took over the role of the largely nonfunctional PDS. Before long, they became not only a source of food but of many other goods, although as they expanded, prices rose as well, and many people remained too poor or too far away to benefit. Indeed, some people told us they were spending up to 80 percent of their salary just to purchase vegetables. The availability of cereals was a particularly sensitive issue. The government jealously guarded its monopoly on distributing items such as rice and maize. Occasionally, these products did make their way to the markets but were usually hidden from the public and sold surreptitiously.

In 2002, in an effort to reform the economy, in conjunction with a broader outreach to Tokyo, Washington, and Europe, Kim Jong Il formally sanctioned the existence of some markets in cities and towns. Before then, however, they operated in a kind of gray area. Foreigners were forbidden from visiting them, which made it hard to determine the precise nature, scale, and impact of the phenomenon, but sometimes on my colleagues' and my travels, we would end up driving right through one, with crowds of people stepping aside to let our vehicle pass. It was yet another of the many paradoxes of North Korea.

I was steadily accumulating more information and insights about the country, as were other humanitarian agencies operating there. But our picture remained frustratingly incomplete. Anecdotal evidence, however interesting, was alone not enough for us to feel confident we had a sufficiently deep understanding of the overall situation. The government's lack of transparency and continuing suspicion added to the challenge. One example of the kind of problems we faced came on a trip I made with four other Caritas members and an official from the Mennonite Church in the United States. The plan was for them to return home while I would stay an extra week. Late in the evening before their departure, an FDRC official came to my hotel room. He was as white as a sheet as he anxiously told me that the security people in a county we had visited had complained that we had photographed military installations, and demanded that I turn over all our film. After a tense conversation, he agreed to take only my film (this was still the pre-iPhone era, when we used actual rolls of film) and to try to convince the security people that nothing of military importance had been photographed. Luckily, I had shot many pictures, so he could tell the security agents he had gotten all the photos from the whole group.

I was not worried about our safety but was concerned that this incident could cause problems for him, as he might face criticism for not watching our delegation more closely. The next morning, however, he had a wide grin on his face when we took the delegation to the airport. The security officials had evidently been reassured. I did not tell my colleagues about the episode; the trip had been challenging enough. But the incident was one example of the difficulty of assembling an accurate idea of the situation in the country.

In an effort to improve conditions for aid work, humanitarian agencies operating in the country, in consultation with the North Koreans, in 1998 came up with a set of nine humanitarian principles to guide our efforts. They included the insistence that aid reach those in the greatest need, that access be granted for monitoring and evaluation, and that assistance would be provided only to areas where access was granted. The principles became a useful tool in determining where aid would be sent, and in negotiating visits. Access remained a challenge, but after the adoption of these principles, we did see some improvement.

For its part, the WFP sought to address this problem by negotiating with the authorities for permission to conduct a comprehensive nationwide nutritional survey. The need for such a survey, which would provide a definitive and internationally credible basis for assessing North Korea's needs, was crucial for sustaining, and hopefully expanding, international engagement and assistance. In my own meetings with North Korean officials, I repeatedly encouraged them to authorize the survey. Moreover, the pressure was acute for more detailed information to provide donors, who deeply distrusted the government in Pyongyang and remained skeptical that the most vulnerable were benefiting from aid.

I encountered that skepticism during a series of trips I made in 1998 to generate more international attention to the crisis and raise funds. During talks, meetings, and media appearances in Geneva, Vienna, Dublin, Seoul, and elsewhere, I made the case that, regardless of the politics, the human needs in North Korea were acute. To emphasize the point, I would show my audience a small plastic bag filled with two hundred to three hundred grams of rice and say, "This is the most that people are getting from the public distribution system. Otherwise, they are on their own—and we have to help." Often, I fielded questions about whether food aid was being diverted to the North Korean military. My usual response was to acknowledge the concern and note that careful planning, signed agreements with the government, detailed distribution plans, and regular monitoring made me confident that, at least in terms of what Caritas was providing, the aid was largely reaching its intended beneficiaries. I was struck by how much more skeptical people were about the diversion issue in North Korea than in other countries. During famines or other food crises elsewhere, there were many instances in which bags of food were simply dropped from planes in the hope that some of it might reach the starving. Yet with North Korea, the pressure for hands-on monitoring was much more pervasive.

Carrying out a nutritional survey, therefore, became an important benchmark for the international aid effort. During the summer of 1998, the North Korean government reluctantly gave its assent for the WFP, UNICEF, and the European Union to work with the DPRK's Institute of Child Nutrition. Given Pyongyang's penchant for secrecy and its sensitivity about the country's international image, the negotiations to secure the agreement had been complex and difficult. The UN agencies stressed that the findings would not be made public until the North Korea government had a chance to go over the data and provide its own comments and input.

In September, as Mary Healy and I were in Sinuiju, fourteen teams, each consisting of one international staffer and four North Koreans—two health workers, an interpreter, and a driver—fanned out across the country to conduct the first-ever random-sample nutritional survey. The project covered 70 percent of the population in eight out of nine provinces and all major cities, and the central government instructed local officials to cooperate. The teams measured the height and weight of approximately 1,800 children between the ages of six months and seven years, and examined them for signs of malnutrition. The international staffers also brought a standardized questionnaire to interview mothers about their experiences regarding other nutrition-related matters, such as food availability and breastfeeding.

My strong impression, shared by most of the humanitarian aid community, was that the survey was extremely well done. Its sobering conclusions, which we learned of at aid agency meetings in Pyongyang, confirmed what those of us working in the field already knew. It found an acute malnutrition rate of 16 percent, the highest in East Asia. The rate was even higher—30 percent—for those between twelve and twenty-four months old, the age when children are weaned from breast milk and are most susceptible to malnutrition that can impair physical and intellectual growth. The teams also found that 62 percent of the children surveyed were suffering from chronic low nutrition or stunting, meaning having a low height for their age. This indicated their having had inadequate food intake for several years. As grim as the data was, the WFP concluded that without international food aid, the situation would have been even more catastrophic.

Although the United Nations in Pyongyang had assured the North Koreans that the data would not immediately be made public, there was intense pressure from skeptical donors, who worried that the North would manipulate the findings, to release the conclusions right away. The pressure got so bad that EU officials threatened to disclose the information themselves if the UN agencies did not do so. The upshot was that the WFP held a press conference in Geneva in mid-November 1998. The presenters accurately noted the data in the survey. But the always sensitive North Koreans were deeply angered by media reports such as that of *The New York Times*, which wrote that the study found the food shortages had "left an entire generation of children physically and mentally impaired,"[1] and by even more sensationalized headlines in the South Korean press.

I was not alone in trying to explain that while I and other humanitarian aid workers could control what we said, we had no control over how headlines or articles were written. It was a classic example of the challenge involved in trying to portray a situation as sufficiently grim for donors to step up with financial support, without slipping into sensationalism or antagonizing the North Korean authorities. But the North Koreans, who were furious as well that the results had been released before they had had time to do their own assessment and put their own spin on the numbers, vowed not to permit another survey like this to be conducted by foreigners.

This was not the only episode that generated tension between the authorities in Pyongyang and humanitarian aid organizations. During the summer of 1998, the French agency Médecins du Monde ended its operations in North Korea, and then, in late September, Médecins Sans Frontières, which had thirteen people on the ground, announced that it too was pulling out. Both organizations claimed they were leaving because the government was preventing them from getting access to those most in need. The departure of MSF, one of the largest and most prominent charities operating in North Korea, sent shock waves through the aid community and beyond. The controversy was heightened because MSF officials coupled their own announcement with a call for all international humanitarian agencies and donor countries to reassess their activities in North Korea as well.

I had encountered many of the MSF workers in Pyongyang and had great respect for their professionalism and commitment. But from the start of its engagement with North Korea, MSF had been faced with conditions quite different from those it was used to when providing medical aid in war zones or in areas where famine or natural disasters had led to a collapse in government infrastructure. In North Korea, the authorities wanted help in securing medical supplies and technical expertise, but as a matter of national pride, they insisted on handling the actual treatment of patients themselves and resisted pressure to allow MSF staff to move more easily around the country. Moreover, in some ways, the whole MSF concept of "without borders" was antithetical to the fundamental way North Korea functioned, maintaining tight controls on internal travel and keeping its external borders largely closed. The tensions were therefore not surprising.

Nevertheless, I and many other humanitarian workers were taken aback by MSF's attempt, in effect, to claim moral superiority over any NGOs who, despite the constraints, chose to stay and continue to operate in North Korea. I knew that even within MSF, the decision to leave had been hotly debated, with many staff on the ground in Pyongyang wanting to remain. This was a frequent topic of discussion among MSF staff and other NGO workers, often over coffee or drinks, and I was occasionally asked for insights about my own experiences dealing with the North Koreans.

Despite the frustrations, I was determined to carry on. I recognized that engaging with foreign NGOs was an utterly new experience for the North

Koreans. Both sides faced a steep, and often bumpy, learning curve. Most of those I dealt with had no idea what humanitarian aid workers did or how they operated, and I had spent countless hours simply trying to explain to my North Korean colleagues the nature of our work. Progress was slow and uneven, but given the scale of the suffering, I felt it would be wrong to walk away. Moreover, I knew that hungry children didn't care about the reason or the politics behind the empty rice bowl. As I wrote in a memo to Caritas headquarters, "Caritas has to continue providing support and stay engaged in North Korea."

Moreover, from my own experience, it was evident that a patient, nonconfrontational approach could produce results. Even as MSF was announcing its withdrawal amid claims that the North Koreans were preventing aid workers from seeing the worst of the famine, I was being given access to some of the grimmest scenes I had yet witnessed. This included visits to an orphanage, a nursery, and a pediatric hospital in Kaesong, near the border with South Korea. Even after I had been witnessing the suffering of ordinary people for three years, they left me deeply shaken.

At the nursery, staff told me that boiled leaves and acorns were mixed with other food, including some provided by Caritas, to make the supplies last longer, even though the children had trouble digesting the meager meals they were given. At the pediatric hospital, all the children I saw were seriously malnourished, and officials told me that fifteen had died. I felt a combination of anger, frustration, sadness, and helplessness. Our mission was to help people and save lives, and I wondered whether, despite all our efforts, we were too late to help those I saw in Kaesong. For once, I felt too distressed to take photographs. And I knew how painfully embarrassing it must have been for local authorities to allow a foreigner to see such appalling conditions. But I was heartened that officials from the Flood Damage Rehabilitation Committee told me they had issued special instructions for the authorities to show me the reality on the ground. One official told me, "The food situation has been bad for some years and will remain like that. Many children are in similar conditions as those in Kaesong. We are running short of food. We cannot overcome the problems alone. We appreciate the aid."

Indeed, by October 1998, when I returned for my twentieth visit, 171 out of a total of 210 counties were accessible to me on a regular basis, although access could fluctuate. Furthermore, on my travels outside Pyongyang, I was able to visit family homes, farms, orphanages, hospitals, nursery schools, and even a chemical factory—visits that, two years earlier, would have been difficult, if not impossible, to arrange. One sign of my increased access was that I was allowed to visit Hamhung, the capital of South Hamgyong Province, one of the worst-hit areas. The city was bleak and desolate, with ugly gray cement buildings and idle factories. Outside the train station, I saw bands of dirty, shabbily dressed children. I wondered if their parents had died in the famine, and who, if anyone, was looking after them.

Traditionally, in hard times, food was given first to the children, then to the men, and the women would have only whatever might be left over. At the places I visited, people spoke openly of the difficulties they faced and the kind of help they needed. Amid all the depressing scenes, I was encouraged by what I saw at the nursery inside the Sinhung chemical factory on the outskirts of Hamhung. I was the first foreigner ever to visit, and officials told me that they had received vegetable oil from Caritas, as well as a corn-soya blend, lentils, wheat flour, maize, and rice. The result was that only five children were reported as being "weak," and the overall nutritional status of the children had begun to improve. It was clear that such targeted food aid was making a difference.

Through my previous travels around the country, I had become aware of an organized system of residential care institutions for children who had lost one or both parents and could not be cared for by other relatives. In my darker moments, I wondered whether the parents' absences were because of the famine or if the parents had gotten into political difficulties and the children were left abandoned. The system had three components: "baby homes" for infants; "orphanages" or "children's centers," where kids of kindergarten age were taken for two years; and "boarding schools" for older children. Most children would stay at a boarding school until the age of seventeen, when they would either join the army or be sent to work at a factory or on a farm. Only a very few were able to pass the entrance exam that would enable them to attend university.

I learned that each province had three or four such large-scale institutions, with a total of around forty for the entire country, looking after approximately ten thousand to twelve thousand children. There were apparently a number of smaller children's homes run by local authorities, but I never got access to them. At my suggestion, Caritas made the entire system a priority target for assistance. Over the next eighteen months beginning in October 1998, visits to these institutions became a regular feature of my travels, to the point that I began to recognize children I had seen at one place who, as they got older, were transferred to another one. I remember in particular a very disabled boy who had been brought to a baby home I visited. No one knew his name or his precise age. He easily could have been left to die, especially considering his disability. But the staff looked after him with particular devotion. Later I saw him, in somewhat better shape, at a children's center. It was heartening to know that he survived, but I would never find out what happened to him as he grew up and moved on.

I found that conditions varied greatly. The North Hwanghae Provincial Baby Home in Hamhung, for example, was a facility designed for 200 infants but caring for over 250. The director said 25 were seriously malnourished and 75 more had milder problems, although additional food aid would put them on the road to recovery. The home did have a garden, where spinach, cucumber, and cabbage had been planted, and had received aid shipments including medicine, clothing, and vitamins. A majority of children at these institutions were stunted—the result of long-term food deprivation, which raised the risk of permanent mental and physical damage. Moreover, the head of the Kaesong Children's Center told me each child had only one set of clothes, despite the sharp differences between the steaming Korean summers and bitterly cold winters. Yet this did not stop the bigger kids from having to go into the mountains to collect roots and herbs to stretch their limited supplies of rice and maize. On the day of my visit to Kaesong, breakfast consisted of noodles made of maize and some cabbage, lunch was bread made of corn flour, and dinner was crushed maize. After visits like these, I would often return to the hotel to discover I could not eat the dinner that was served. I had simply lost my appetite.

At the North Hwanghae Provincial Baby Home and Children's Center, which were housed in the same location, most of the kids I saw also were stunted. The center's headmistress told me their mental development was slower than normal. The psychological and emotional distress among the kids I saw was striking. Many of the babies were rocking uncontrollably back and forth in their cots—a sign of neglect and a lack of stimulation. Indeed, I was told that the Ministry of Education had established a special center to study how best to treat children suffering from such emotional problems. Yet I could see that the staff at these institutions cared deeply for kids who would otherwise slip through the cracks of a society in crisis. In speaking with them, I discovered that they needed almost everything. They asked if I could supply not just food but soap; disinfectant; heaters; underwear; shoes; medicine such as antibiotics, cough medicine, painkillers, and antidiarrheals for the school clinic; and materials such as paper, crayons, toys, and books.

As I repeatedly visited these institutions, I was able to track the delivery of food and other supplies that Caritas had provided. Although at most of the places I visited, the children were shabbily dressed and suffered from skin problems, coughs, or eye infections, I could see that the condition of at least some of them was slowly starting to improve. Some facilities now not only had gardens for growing vegetables but were raising goats, pigs, rabbits, ducks, and dogs. (I could not bring myself to tell the director of Caritas Switzerland, who accompanied me on one trip, that the dogs were for eating.) After the delivery of two shipments of oil, canned fish, and pulses such as beans, lentils, and chickpeas, the headmistress of the Kangwon Provincial Baby Home told me none of the 130 children in her care were now seriously malnourished, although some remained weak.

However precarious the situation in the residential care homes, conditions were even grimmer outside these institutions. Moreover, as kids up to six years of age remained the priority targets for aid deliveries, I saw growing indications that older children were suffering even more. At the pediatric hospital in Wonsan on the east coast, for example, where staff had dealt earlier with extreme malnutrition among young children, doctors told me they were now facing the same problem in adolescents. I met three teenagers there in an advanced stage of malnutrition, suffering from both kwashiorkor, a protein-deficiency condition that causes a swollen, distended belly, and marasmus, or wasting, in which a starved body eats its own muscle tissue. It was evident to me that children in this age group would be the next to suffer the effects of extreme hunger if we were not able to expand the delivery of food to include them.

In its 1999 appeal, Caritas sought to raise $5,925,000 for its North Korea programs. Unfortunately, "donor fatigue" kept us from raising even half that amount. Continuing political tensions on the Korean peninsula did not make our job any easier. Four-party talks in Geneva between the North, the South, the United States, and China, first proposed by the Clinton administration in 1997, had produced few concrete results. Meanwhile, because of opposition in the US Congress, funding for the fuel supplies promised to Pyongyang under the 1994 Agreed Framework deal began to dry up, while Pyongyang remained convinced that Washington's real goal remained the collapse of Kim Jong Il's regime. Then, despite the election of longtime opposition leader Kim Dae-jung, a proponent of engaging the North, as president of South Korea in August 1998, the North launched its first multistage rocket in a failed attempt to place a satellite into orbit. It flew over Japan, deeply alarming the Japanese government, before landing in the Pacific Ocean, and fueled speculation about the North's ability to strike US troops in Japan.

With Pyongyang still widely seen as a pariah state, advocating for expanded humanitarian relief became an increasingly daunting challenge. But I persisted. As I noted in a memo to Duncan MacLaren, the secretary general of Caritas Internationalis, in mid-1999, "The suffering goes on. We encourage members of the Caritas family not to forget the plight of the North Korean people. Help is desperately needed if we want to save lives and reduce suffering."

CHAPTER SIX

"My Heart Will Go On"

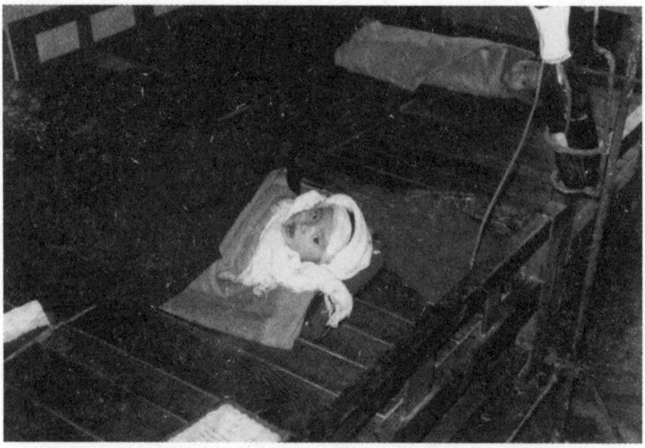

Medical supplies were in extremely short supply, with some hospitals using beer bottles as drips.

In August 1999, on my twenty-fourth trip, I spent three weeks on the road in North Korea. I traveled over 3,600 kilometers, mostly by jeep, visiting six provinces and dozens of institutions and individuals that were receiving Caritas aid—nurseries, children's centers, boarding schools, hospitals, distribution centers, and families. It was my longest continuous stay in the country, and as I drove from Kaesong near the Demilitarized Zone with South Korea to Ryanggang on the Chinese border in the far northeast, it provided a remarkable opportunity to observe daily life at one of the darkest times in the country's history.

On the roads, there was hardly any traffic. Broken-down vehicles dramatically outnumbered those that were operating. I was struck by the number of people in tattered clothes that were on the move, very likely in search of food. Many looked unwell, with protruding bones, loose-fitting skin, and frozen facial expressions. Everyone seemed to be carrying something—food or firewood, a heavy rucksack, bundles in both hands, loads balanced precariously on their heads. A few had pushcarts. Most of those trudging along seemed tired, often sitting, squatting, or even lying down on the roadside. Some women dressed in rags were nursing babies in the shade. The sense of profound exhaustion reflected a society that had been stretched to the limit by the ordeal of the past few years.

Yet, as I had seen previously, I also detected a kind of stoicism that accompanied the fatigue, a sense that these people used to hardship were not giving up but were still struggling to find a way to survive. I often wondered how they managed to summon the will to carry on, but I saw it in those searching the fields for edible herbs or small animals to catch; in a group of skinny kids hacking maize cobs, probably for alternative food; and in those working to repair roads, bridges, irrigation systems, and other parts of the infrastructure by hand, with no machinery and only the simplest of tools. I spoke with one elderly lady who was gathering leaves in the middle of a field. Referring to the suffering she had experienced during the Korean War, she told me, "I am glad I still know what is edible."

Perhaps fittingly, the soundtrack for my effort to make sense of what I was seeing on this trip turned out to be "My Heart Will Go On," sung by Celine Dion in the 1997 hit movie *Titanic*. The song also briefly became the object of a test of wills with my North Korean driver and guide. It was the only music cassette they had—how they acquired it, I had no idea and did not ask—and as we drove across the country, they played it over and over again. My travel companion worked at the FALU office with Erich Weingartner, and the tune began to drive us somewhat crazy. After intense discussions that almost felt like negotiations over a food shipment, they agreed to "ration" the song to three times a day—once in the morning, once in the afternoon, and once in the evening. But as sick as I was of the song, I came to feel that its sentiments reflected an important element of what I was seeing in North Korea—a refusal, despite everything, to give up.

Yet the scale of the challenge was evident everywhere I visited, and no more so than in Ryanggang, a dry, mountainous province in the northeast that was among the areas worst hit by the famine. It had been largely off-limits to humanitarian workers, but after Caritas arranged the delivery of 128 metric tons of lentils and green peas for nurseries, kindergartens, and residential childcare institutions, I was given permission to make a second visit. During a briefing in the provincial capital of Hyesan, the head of the local Flood Damage Rehabilitation Committee acknowledged that since the start of the summer, despite international aid, 20 percent of all families in the province, which had a population of 580,000, had been forced to survive on alternative food for ten days every month. Moreover, projections for the next harvest were dismal, due first to a drought and then to excessive rain, compounded by a lack of fertilizer. Visiting nearby Pochon County, I was told that only alternative food made of potato peels, milled stalks of maize and barley, and edible herbs was available, although a shipment of peas from Caritas had just arrived and promised to ease the situation somewhat. At the Pochon County hospital, doctors said that because of the poor diet, stomach problems had increased significantly. When I was visiting a local family, the mother, Mrs. Lee, told me she wanted to continue breastfeeding her two-year-old son, Jong Suk, but was having problems because the alternative food she was eating consistently gave her diarrhea.

Compounding the misery was the fact that the North Korean medical system, which until the famine had provided the public with better health care than in pre-Communist times, had now virtually collapsed. In 1998 and 1999, I visited more than two dozen hospitals and clinics. Although I was impressed by the cleanliness of most facilities and the commitment of the staff, all of them were desperately short of medicine and supplies such as sterilization equipment (access to clean water was a huge problem), stethoscopes, syringes, and operating tables. Doctors said they were often forced to perform operations without using anesthesia. I was told the most common problems were diarrhea and other stomach disorders, made worse by the consumption of so much alternative food, as well as respiratory diseases and multiple ailments caused by malnutrition. At one hospital in Wonsan, I saw five-year-old Cheng Sang. He was nearly ninety centimeters (three feet) tall but weighed just eleven kilos. A sixteen-year-old girl, Hwang Mi, weighed only twenty-two kilos. One elderly doctor said he could not remember such hard times since the Korean War.

One key goal on this and other trips was to keep track of the aid that Caritas was providing. By 1999, Caritas began to deliver simple medical kits to help alleviate some of the acute shortages in hospitals and clinics. The kits were designed in consultation with the Ministry of Health, the

FDRC, and the World Health Organization (WHO); the latter had set up an emergency and humanitarian action office in 1997. Hugo Hörndli, the Bangkok-based trader who had helped me procure the earliest Caritas grain shipments, sourced the kits in China. Each contained basic supplies: a stethoscope, a thermometer, scissors, a reflex hammer, tweezers, cotton balls, bandages, swabs, and so on.

In Ryanggang, the kits were intended for *ri* (village) clinics. We started the project with one hundred kits to test if working in the province was possible. The idea was that if things went well, all *ri* clinics would get kits. But after visiting several clinics, I felt something wasn't right. As I looked in the kits, I saw that some of the items were missing. Given the ongoing doubts about diversion and the lack of transparency, my traveling companion and I were immediately suspicious.

Monitoring was still a sensitive issue, since both donors and aid workers needed reassurance that the help was going to those most in need. With the passage of time and the development of relations of trust, the process had become somewhat easier, but it was still potentially problematic. Could some things have been sold on the black market or appropriated by the military? I pushed for answers. At times it was awkward, because, especially in a place like Ryanggang, where so few foreigners visited, people were uncomfortable dealing with strangers, unfamiliar with concepts like distribution plans or follow-up inspections, and were definitely not used to probing questions, especially from a European woman.

Moreover, they operated in a culture in which information was closely guarded, and the idea of volunteering it to anyone, let alone an outsider, was almost unthinkable. But the local officials did eventually provide an explanation. In North Korea, they told me, they did not feel it was fair for one clinic to get a full kit while others got nothing. As a result, they had taken the Caritas kits apart and shared the contents among several more villages.

"In our system," they said, "everybody has to get something." It was a kind of "sharing in poverty" concept that, to me, risked being counterproductive, since a kit without all of its components would not afford the same benefits to doctors or patients. But it explained the missing items. And it underscored as well the very different perspectives of the North Koreans and those of us coming from outside. It was another point on my continuing learning curve as I sought to understand the country.

Similar problems arose during inspection visits to hospitals. Distribution plans for food aid normally were based on what we were told was the number of beds in each facility. But in many hospitals, I noticed there were far fewer patients than beds. So where had the food gone? Again, suspicions arose. Were the North Koreans inflating the numbers when the distribution plans were drawn up just to get more? These questions also led to several awkward exchanges, but, as in the case of the medical kits, the ultimate answer seemed plausible to me. I was told that doctors could never be sure how many patients they would have at any given time. The number depended not only on the health of those seeking treatment but on whether a hard-pressed facility had the resources to look after them. If not, people would stay home, no matter how sick they were.

Moreover, I learned that hospitals were responsible for feeding not only their patients but their staff as well, and that doctors in North Korea do house calls, with each doctor being responsible for a certain number of families. Although no one had previously mentioned these things to me, they explained why I had arrived at a hospital on more than one occasion and been told that a number of doctors and nurses were not there, as well as where the food went. There was no "cheating." It was just another way of managing an acutely difficult situation.

Reports that bags with the Caritas or WFP logo had been seen in places where no deliveries had been made also fueled concern about diversion of aid. In several cases, Caritas chapters from different parts of the world had made their own donations directly to the FDRC without a distribution or monitoring plan and with no target group, so it was not surprising that bags from these shipments ended up in unexpected places.

Also, from my own experience, I knew that the North Koreans saved and reused almost everything. In fact, they asked us to provide jute bags rather than plastic ones, as they lasted longer. This included bags in which grain or other supplies originally had been shipped. When I inquired more closely, I found that it was usually the case that bags turning up in unexpected places were used ones, not new, and were storing something different from what was originally inside them. The suspicion of diversion was understandable, but this was yet one more instance in which something that initially appeared questionable turned out to have an entirely reasonable explanation.

There were other instances. I often would bring small tins of Camembert cheese on my trips—as a Swiss, I liked my cheese. I discovered that the empty tins often were used as ashtrays. And five-liter cans of oil donated by the United States were frequently turned into buckets. The women would poke a hole in each side and carry the can with a rope, blissfully unaware that it had an American flag, almost never seen in North Korea, on the outside.

These were hardly the only examples of North Korea's ability to make use of items that would be discarded in the West. At the Ryanggang Boarding School, where 170 children were being cared for, I was startled to notice an old black Swiss-made rotary telephone on the desk of an official. Years earlier, such phones had been declared obsolete by the Swiss government and replaced by newer touch-tone models. But I learned that Ri Chol, the North Korean ambassador to Switzerland, with whom I had become friendly, had paid next to nothing to acquire thousands of the old phones, and the technology that went with them, from Switzerland. I saw them not only in Ryanggang but on desks in many places I visited around the country. Every time I saw one, I smiled.

Ryanggang was also the location of one of the most beautiful—and, to the Koreans, sacred—natural wonders: Mount Paektu. In 1999, on August 15—the day Japan surrendered to end World War Two in 1945, and which both North and South Koreans celebrate as the end of Japanese colonial rule—I had an opportunity to visit the mountain, even though the county in which it is located was closed to international aid. A still-active volcano with an enormous lake at its center, caused by an eruption in AD 946 that was one of the five biggest in the world in the past five thousand years, Paektu is the tallest mountain on the Korean peninsula. In Korean mythology, it was the birthplace of Tangun, the founder of the first Korean kingdom, who was said to be the son of a god and a bear who was transformed into a woman. It is also central to the legend of the Kim dynasty—the place where Kim Il Sung established a base to fight the Japanese, and where Kim Jong Il is supposed to have been born, his birth heralded by a double rainbow. North Korean propaganda describes the younger Kim as a "great man of the Mount Paektu type," a status that was later extended to Kim Jong Un after he succeeded Kim Jong Il in late 2011.

Thickly forested and home to wild boar, deer, and even Korean tigers, Mount Paektu is spectacularly beautiful. On the peak, we met a group of soldiers. Despite the fearsome reputation of the Korean People's Army (KPA), they were extremely friendly, and we all posed for photos before clambering down a set of steep stairs to the lake, where I waded into the frigid water. We had a most enjoyable picnic in the forest before ending up at a nearby hotel for the night. My North Korean companions were extremely happy to have had the opportunity to visit Mount Paektu. That evening, the lights in the hotel kept flickering on and off because of the erratic electricity supply. By now, I had become so used to conditions in North Korea that I barely noticed.

However bad the situation, it is clear with the benefit of hindsight that by 1999, the famine had actually peaked. Indeed, as I continued my travels, the picture I saw also contained some small signs of hope. On the way back from Ryanggang, we stopped in Tanchon, a city in South Hamgyong Province. At the pediatric ward of a local hospital, all nine patients were severely malnourished, suffering from diarrhea and kwashiorkor. But doctors also told us that conditions were slowly improving, the number of pregnant and nursing women had increased, and the number of births was up as well.

I also heard these things at other locations. UNICEF had recently added a new initiative that was dubbed "safe motherhood," which involved providing delivery room equipment for county and *ri* hospitals, as they were not adequately equipped to handle pregnancies and births. It was particularly satisfying to see such help having immediate and practical positive consequences. And we continued to send food targeting pregnant and nursing mothers. In Kosan County, in Kangwon Province, I visited the Kim family, which consisted of parents, grandparents, and a five-month-old boy. The mother told us she had received extra food from aid shipments—maize, wheat, a corn-soya blend, peas, and cooking oil—during her pregnancy. Her son weighed 2.85 kilograms when he was born. She was breastfeeding, and he was growing well. However, she had shared with other family members the extra food that had been allocated to her, a reality that I also encountered elsewhere.

For all the frustrations the aid effort had faced, enough food was now arriving to make a real difference, something that both North Korean officials and other international aid workers acknowledged. In 1999, over one million metric tons of food was delivered, the largest amount for any single year. Caritas was providing mainly peas, lentils, a corn-soya blend, milk powder, and cooking oil, while other international organizations were delivering grains such as rice, wheat, and maize. Despite concerns about monitoring and diversion, my experiences convinced me that the vast bulk of the aid was reaching the most vulnerable sectors of the population. Moreover, despite the gloomy prospects for Ryanggang, a study by the United Nations' Food and Agriculture Organization (FAO) that summer predicted a slightly better harvest for the country as a whole.

On my own travels, I saw not only that large fields of rice and maize now existed but that potatoes, sweet potatoes, millet, sorghum, and vegetables had been planted. Indeed, every available piece of land was being farmed, including hillsides and mountainsides, although that raised the prospect of serious soil erosion and environmental damage—an issue I would get more deeply involved with in the coming years. Although the FAO was warning of a shortfall of between six hundred thousand and one million metric tons of grain, it appeared that the end of the emergency phase of the crisis was nearing. Fewer people were dying. Although chronic malnutrition was now the lot of large segments of the population, more were getting help. Slowly, the situation was starting to stabilize.

It was an appropriate moment to take stock of the previous four years. The suffering had been enormous. Although North Korea officially acknowledged a death toll of only 225,000, outside estimates were much higher, with some claims that it exceeded two million. Even now, it remains difficult to know for sure. With the benefit of all the data and studies that have been conducted since those days, the best guess is that between six hundred thousand and a million people died—representing close to 5 percent of North Korea's pre-crisis population. Many survivors would be stunted and scarred for life. A comparison with South Korea underscored the scale of the damage. Although North and South Korean children are the same race, studies later made clear that as a result of the famine, North Korean children were roughly seven centimeters (three inches) shorter than their South Korean counterparts and up to three kilograms lighter. Overall, in 1999, life expectancy in the North (sixty-one years) was approximately fourteen years shorter than in the South.

Although still dismal, there was no question the picture would have been much, much worse without international aid. Yet among a number of international agencies, the frustration was so acute that in late 1999, two more of them followed the 1998 example of MSF and left North Korea. One was the British-founded charity Oxfam, which had been running an emergency water and sanitation program in Pyongyang and three other provinces. In December 1999, Oxfam halted the program and withdrew its five staffers, claiming the government was preventing them from confirming that their assistance was reaching those for whom it was intended.

At the same time, the French-based agency Action Against Hunger (Action Contre la Faim, or ACF) also pulled out. A key point of contention was the refusal of the government to allow ACF to set up soup kitchens for the legions of homeless children now roaming the streets in many North Korean cities and town. I had seen these gangs of kids myself and understood the need, but for reasons both of national pride and social control, the authorities would not permit foreigners to engage in such a visible activity highlighting the failings of the system.

By now, Caritas had provided over $20 million in aid, almost all in kind, to North Korea and, in my view, saved countless lives, mostly of children and pregnant and nursing mothers. Nonetheless, the withdrawal of the two NGOs triggered renewed debate and pressure within the organization about whether we too should consider ending our efforts. In January 2000, I distributed an organization-wide memo making the argument for staying. I wrote, "To accept the difficult working environment in the DPRK, a tightly controlled and often secretive country, poses a challenge to aid agencies. But withdrawing now, and closing the door, would be morally wrong and deprive people of aid. It would also present much greater difficulties if attempts were made to re-open it in the future, once the established relationships and the trust that goes with it has ceased. Only engagement, dialogue, mutual exchange, and patient negotiations may bring solutions to the many problems North Korea is facing."

I held this view not only because my own experiences had demonstrated that it was possible, despite the obstacles, to get help to those most in need, but because going forward, to improve North Korea's chances of fully emerging from this crisis and avoiding a future famine, it would be crucial for Caritas and other humanitarian organizations to shift from providing purely emergency aid to assisting in rehabilitation and development. Interestingly, FDRC and other government officials began to make the same point.

We were still continuing to deliver food and other aid for hospitals and residential child care centers and expanding the provision of medical kits. To help people living in unheated institutions and homes survive the bitter North Korean winter, we also had started to supply padded jackets and shoes for farmers, and warm clothing, shoes, and blankets for nurseries, orphanages, and other childcare institutions. My sense was that the North Koreans were becoming increasingly receptive to new approaches. Because of my long engagement, it became evident I was probably the foreign humanitarian worker they trusted most, putting me in a unique position to raise new ideas with them. One was to help revive North Korean agriculture, including arranging for the delivery of plastic sheeting for use in farming, as well as for fertilizer, seeds (including 150 metric tons of spinach seeds), tractor tires, and, in a few cases, small trucks.

Perhaps most intriguing, in my conversations with the FDRC and other officials, there was growing interest in "capacity building"—helping North Koreans acquire the skills necessary for a broader recovery of the economy. For the first time, this included a willingness on the North Korean government's part to send personnel abroad beyond the socialist bloc for training and study. As one FDRC official explained the government's thinking to me, "We are members of the UN. We are searching for good collaboration with other member states."

One interesting example involved Switzerland and fish farming. Ambassador Ri Chol had established links with a man named Thomas Wettstein, whose family ran a fish farm near Berne, Switzerland. The family agreed to host North Koreans for training, and to send an expert to Pyongyang to provide technical advice. The expert duly arrived, and so did five hundred thousand donated rainbow trout eggs and two hundred thousand river trout eggs. The expert was shocked by what he saw and said the North Korean fishing industry program was one hundred years out of date, producing only a tenth of the output of Swiss fish farms. The North Koreans then sent two fish farmers and one interpreter to Switzerland to work and learn on the Wettstein farm.

When I went home to Switzerland to see my family, I visited the fish farm and found all three North Koreans wearing knee-high rubber boots and vigorously scrubbing a large fishpond. After witnessing this, when the initial Swiss government funding for the program ran out, I convinced Caritas to step in and support the project. It was a modest initiative, but when I had lunch with Ambassador Ri in Berne, he made clear how important the project was for him. It was also a sign that North Korea was increasingly open to international engagement.

Around the same time, the North Koreans agreed to send a delegation of agricultural experts to Canada at the invitation of the Canadian Foodgrains Bank. Traveling across the country, exchanging views with Canadian farmers, they returned full of ideas, especially in terms of potato seed production and storage; the use of fertilizers, pesticides, and farm machinery; and the possibility of introducing canola, a type of crop derived from rapeseed, to produce cooking oil. Roberto Christen, a Peruvian agronomist at the UN Development Program office in Pyongyang, had extensive dealings with the delegation after their trip. He made the interesting observation that the new knowledge and techniques the North Koreans had acquired made them more influential in shaping policies at home.

Another initiative was much more sensitive—so much so that we had to keep it confidential at the time. I was able to convince the Central European University (CEU) in Budapest, Hungary, where an old friend was vice president for external relations, to offer full scholarships to North Korean officials involved in trade and economic affairs to study for periods ranging from three months to a full academic year. CEU had been founded by the Hungarian American financier George Soros in 1991, following the collapse of communism in the Soviet Union. Its goal was to help the transition from dictatorship to democracy, initially in Eastern Europe but then more broadly, by training scholars, academics, politicians, and civil society leaders in the workings of an open society.

Under these circumstances, I was frankly surprised that the North Korean authorities agreed to send anyone. It was never clear whether they were fully aware of Soros's background, or whether this simply appealed to them as an opportunity to have their people receive much-needed training. In any case, once Caritas agreed to cover travel, visas, insurance, and other costs, thirty-five people were sent to study in Budapest, while forty-six more attended CEU-run training courses in Pyongyang over a period of several years, with the first group going in the late 1990s.The participants came from a variety of organizations and ministries, including the Committee for the Promotion of International Trade, the Korea International Trade Arbitration Committee, and the Chamber of Commerce. All of them were required to demonstrate English proficiency by passing the Test of English as a Foreign Language (TOEFL); they also had to pass an exam in basic economics administered by CEU staffers who came to Pyongyang.

The process was not entirely smooth. Once the eight members to attend the first course had been selected, the North Korean foreign ministry insisted on adding additional people who clearly were not technocrats but minders. Initially, CEU said no, but when the North Koreans threatened to withdraw from the project altogether, the CEU backed down, and at least one minder then accompanied every group. Since he had no other expertise, my friend at the university and I jokingly dubbed the minder the "goulash cook." But eventually, I realized the importance of such guides, because they had the most influence back home.

Another problem emerged when the South Korean embassy in Budapest learned of their presence. The South Koreans were desperate to contact the North Koreans, and even sent diplomats to the CEU campus to find them. The North Koreans, of course, were under strict instructions to avoid all contact with their archenemies. Had any contact taken place, the North Koreans could have gotten into serious trouble at home. When CEU officials learned of the situation, they banned the South Koreans from entering the university grounds.

The first group was all men, but going forward, I insisted that women also be included, and subsequent groups usually had at least two women. Their studies focused on economics and trade, with all the participants taking courses in business English, basic law, and economics. But there was a deeper educational purpose as well—to expose them to life in a Western society emerging from communism. Even with the restrictions and complications, for me, the program was a small but valuable part of a broader process of opening closed minds that I believed was central to engagement with North Korea. As one North Korean participant said, "My stay in Budapest showed me how the real world works."

Meanwhile, the evidence continued to mount of a growing recognition within the North Korean leadership that, given the devastation of the famine, some kind of change was necessary to ensure the regime's survival. In May 2000, Kim Jong Il traveled secretly to Beijing. After the visit, China's official *People's Daily* newspaper quoted him as praising Beijing's policies of reform and opening the door to the outside world, which had sparked a dramatic economic transformation in the People's Republic of China. That same spring, North Korea opened diplomatic relations with Italy and Australia. In the next year, ties were established with the United Kingdom, Germany, the Netherlands, Belgium, and the Philippines.

Even more dramatic, in June 2000, Kim Jong Il hosted South Korean President Kim Dae-jung for an unprecedented summit in Pyongyang. It was the first time that talks had ever been held between the leaders of the two Koreas. The summit produced an agreement that included allowing visits between families separated by the Korean War, creating a series of steps to encourage trade and investment, toning down harsh propaganda on both sides, and, most memorably, the two Korean teams marching together under an Olympic flag at the opening ceremony of the 2000 Olympics in Sydney, Australia. When I visited Pyongyang in July 2000, officials I met all spoke of how the summit was an important step in easing the North's international isolation.

Four months later came an even more remarkable breakthrough: a visit to Pyongyang by US Secretary of State Madeleine Albright. She and Kim discussed a possible freeze on the North's missile program and a broader rapprochement with the United States. Kim asked her to convey an invitation for President Bill Clinton, in the final months of his second term, to visit Pyongyang. For North Korea, a presidential visit would symbolize an end to its pariah status and an affirmation of its international legitimacy.

It was a remarkable change from the political climate that existed when I had first visited North Korea five years earlier. There was no question that the impact of the famine was a key factor in North Korea's decision to seek greater international contact. But I was convinced that the humanitarian aid effort also had played an important role. As I wrote in a memo to Caritas following a trip soon after the Albright visit, "Aid not only eases human suffering. It also brings about changes in attitude and approaches."

The challenge now was to build on the momentum of these dramatic developments, in the hope of both further improving the lives of ordinary North Korea people and helping the country emerge further from its long-standing international isolation.

CHAPTER SEVEN

Holy Peas

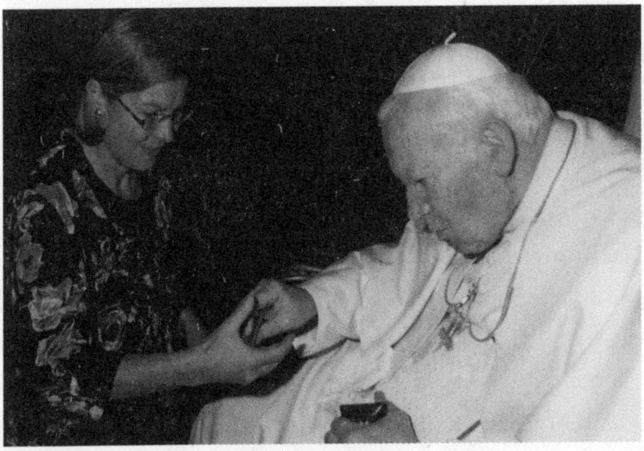

The Vatican was a generous donor. Kathi meeting Pope John Paul II.

Although the Flood Damage Rehabilitation Committee had been Caritas's main North Korean partner from the beginning, there was always interest in trying to find a way to collaborate with the Catholic Church in North Korea, given that Caritas was a Catholic organization. Although I am not Catholic, I had been raised with Christian values, and whenever I happened to be in Pyongyang on a Sunday, I made a point of attending services. This was also because I wanted to be completely transparent with the North Koreans about the Catholic foundation of Caritas. Moreover, I was curious to see whether the Church, which, before Kim Il Sung took power, had already entered the country and put down deep roots, was still playing any meaningful role.

On my travels, every so often I would stumble on traces of its once-large presence. On one occasion, traveling with a Canadian delegation, we were taken to a building, and as we sat down, it was immediately evident that we were sitting on what had been church benches. While visiting Sepo County, in Kangwon Province, I spoke with older people who recalled foreigners living there decades ago. It turned out that Sepo had once hosted Benedictine monks. The Benedictines, who arrived in Korea in 1909, built monasteries, seminaries, and small centers to provide social services in the province. Indeed, the campus of the Wonsan Agricultural University, also in Kangwon, originally had been a Benedictine abbey. The religious origins were evident in the large, impressive structures with arched windows—a classic example of traditional Catholic architecture.

Yet these were faint echoes of a presence that, apart from the one Catholic and two Protestant churches in Pyongyang, had largely disappeared. In fact, most of the Benedictine monks and sisters had been either imprisoned or executed after Kim Il Sung took power in the North. Several dozen German missionaries who had been jailed then were eventually repatriated. The congregations at the three churches were small and made up mostly of older people. There were no children. When I asked why, the North Koreans said that most kids had organized activities on Sunday, but it was clearly an excuse to cover the fact that the government, which had long viewed organized religion with suspicion, simply did not allow children to attend church.

Thus, it was more than a little remarkable that in November 1999, the North Koreans agreed to my request to allow a visit from two senior Vatican officials: Monsignor Celestino Migliore, the Vatican's undersecretary for relations with states, who had visited Vietnam and China, and Monsignor Paul Gallagher, at that time a Southeast Asia specialist at the Vatican Secretariat of State. During their five-day stay, we visited a hospital in Kujang County, in North Pyongan Province. We then traveled to Wonsan, in Kangwon Province, where we visited an orphanage, a boarding school for nine hundred children, and a baby home. Bouncing along the potholed roads in a four-wheel-drive automobile, the two priests were impressed by the beauty of the country but saddened by the realities of how people lived and how hard it was to survive. They were touched by what they saw in the residential childcare institutions, especially the stunting of the children at the boarding school, who had not received enough to eat and were small for their age—a sign of long-term food deprivation.

Pope John Paul II was a strong supporter of Caritas's work and had arranged for a contribution of nearly $300,000 to support our efforts in North Korea. Indeed, in 2002, while attending a Caritas meeting in Rome, I was invited to join a private Mass with the Holy Father at the Vatican. When he spoke to me, he made clear his interest in and concern for the humanitarian situation in the DPRK. Most of the $300,000 went toward the purchase of one thousand metric tons of peas, which, with their high protein content, provided valuable nutritional benefits. In Wonsan, a handover ceremony was held to mark the delivery of the peas. We were pleased that the North Koreans apparently had not objected to the marking of each bag with the Vatican coat of arms along with the Caritas logo. Because I had been involved in communicating the complicated bag design to the supplier in Bangkok, the two priests had nicknamed me "the bag lady," who had successfully arranged the shipment of what we jokingly dubbed "the holy peas."

The two priests also met Vice Minister of Foreign Affairs Ri In Gyu and other foreign ministry staff, as well as officials from the state-established Korean Catholic Association, including Thomas Han In Chol, the association's director of external affairs. While he was clearly part of the government's apparatus for controlling religion, Han struck us as having quite a good knowledge of the church's history, activities, and beliefs. He told us that of the three thousand Catholics in North Korea, eight hundred were in Pyongyang. When Migliore asked about Catholics in the rural areas, Han said there was no Catholic community life or churches, but some people were, in his words, "leading a Catholic life in their homes." Interestingly, in a later conversation, a church official told me that young people were taught the *juche* idea at school, and that the meaning of *juche* was "love for human beings," and thus similar to Christianity. It was as close as any North Korean ever came to openly admitting that the Kim cult and the worship of the national ideology were indeed a kind of religion.

The big question on the agenda of the two Vatican officials was whether the government would allow the stationing of a foreign priest in Pyongyang and the possible training of local priests. Han acknowledged that not having an ordained resident priest created problems. But he said any foreign priest would need to be able to speak Korean and "be aware of the Korean situation." To me, this was an oblique but clear signal that this idea, if it were ever to materialize, was still a long way off, and complicated negotiations would be required to make progress. Indeed, on a visit to the church in 1998, when I had casually asked the same question, I was told that "people would feel strange" in the presence of a foreign priest. Interestingly, after the historic North-South summit in June 2000, members of the Catholic Priests' Association for Justice in Seoul—who, incidentally, had been the organization to deliver to me the hundreds of thousands of dollars in cash in a McDonald's bag during the early stages of the famine—were allowed to conduct a service. But as of this writing, there is still no resident priest in Pyongyang.

Because the two priests were not going to be in Pyongyang on a Sunday, it was not possible for them to read Mass at the Catholic church, even if the North Korean authorities were prepared to allow it. They did, however, conduct a Mass at the Polish embassy on a Friday evening before a dinner hosted by the Polish ambassador for the delegation and a group of foreigners. It was a special occasion.

A year later, I arranged for Migliore to return to Pyongyang, this time accompanied by another priest working in the diplomatic service of the Vatican, Bueno Aires native Monsignor Luis Mariano Montemayor, as well as Duncan MacLaren, the secretary general of Caritas Internationalis. Together, we traveled to Wonsan to learn more about how the peas purchased with the Vatican's contribution and delivered on Migliore's visit the previous year were being used at various children's institutions. As we set out from Pyongyang, Migliore stressed to me that he and his colleagues wanted to learn how humanitarian aid worked and were eager to meet a wide variety of people to better understand the situation on the ground. In our meetings, during which he and his colleague were full of questions, he said that I should do most of the talking whenever it concerned aid distribution issues. We visited a nursery, a kindergarten, a family, a hospital, a distribution center, and a boarding school. It was gratifying to see that the peas, with their high protein input, had reached the intended beneficiaries.

Although the Caritas assistance in Wonsan was making a difference, it was clear that more help was needed. The suffering of the people, often behind closed doors, was not over. Winter was approaching, with temperatures set to plummet to minus twenty to thirty degrees Celsius. Despite some improvements, many people were facing hardship. In the hospitals, each of which had a pungent smell—a mixture of disinfectant, soap, and body odor—we saw broken windows covered with plastic and cardboard, not enough heating materials, no fuel, perhaps a little electricity, not enough warm blankets, and hardly any food. The medicine cabinets were empty. The medical services remained on the brink of collapse. Few people would go to the hospital, and with the limited food supply, it was scary to think of the implications of another cold winter. I wondered how long people would have to endure such a terrible situation.

The visits of the two Vatican priests had created a protocol problem for the North Koreans. Because they weren't aid workers, and because of the diplomatic sensitivity of any dealings between the Vatican and Pyongyang, our group was assigned two interpreters—one from the FDRC as usual, for the Caritas secretary general and me, and another, from the foreign ministry, for the church officials. After a day of meetings and visits, we spent the night at the Wonsan Tongmyong Hotel. The next morning, on the way back to Pyongyang, we stopped at an outlook on a hill. Monsignor Migliore told me to come to what he called "confession corner." What had I done? I wondered. But Migliore had a smile on his face, so it could not be that bad. He said that Mr. Kim, the foreign ministry interpreter, who had no experience with aid visits, had complained about me. Migliore said Kim had told him, "Ms. Kathi speaks too much. In our country, women are to speak only after men, and only if asked to do so!" It was a revealing insight into how strong traditional attitudes remained in North Korea, at least among officials. Migliore and I had a good laugh, got back in the car, and returned to Pyongyang.

In a sign of North Korea's gradually expanding openness to foreigners, Monsignor Migliore was invited to return in 2002 and was again allowed to celebrate Mass at Pyongyang's only Catholic church. The members of the small congregation at Changchung Cathedral who attended for Migliore's sermon were largely elderly. I had no way of knowing what proportion of those who were at the service were genuine Catholics, or who had just been told to attend to fill out the numbers because foreigners were going to be there. But as I watched the faces and body language of the people there, I had no doubt that for some, their faith was real. Elderly women, wearing lace mantillas that traditional Catholic women use to cover their heads, eagerly came forward to receive Communion. And when Migliore, speaking through a translator, said that he was bringing greetings from Pope John

Paul II, I could sense the response among some worshippers, similar to when the priests from the Vatican had celebrated Mass on their 2000 visit.

In conversations during the previous three years, I had tried to explore whether the Catholic Church could become a meaningful partner in the Caritas aid effort. As early as 1997, it was evident that Church officials had been given permission to encourage aid contributions from overseas, but the FDRC had made clear that it was responsible for overseeing the international relief effort. By 1998, though, officials of the Korean Catholic Association (KCA) appeared to expect me to bring on each of my visits some kind of aid for them to distribute. When I did not do so, my relations with them became somewhat cooler.

From the beginning, I had been skeptical about the Church's ability to act as a recipient and distributor of aid, and it clearly lacked the authority to conduct any monitoring activities. Still, in 1999, we launched a trial project in which we delivered 260 bicycles to the KCA. When I followed up on subsequent visits, however, I was told that the bikes had not been given to the Catholic community in Pyongyang as initially agreed upon. Instead, officials said, they had been distributed to Catholics in the countryside. It remained unclear to me whether the bicycles had been given away, sold, bartered, or simply taken by the government. I was disappointed but hardly surprised, and the episode confirmed my judgment that while it was worthwhile to continue to develop a relationship with the Church, the real aid would have to keep flowing through the FDRC.

That same autumn of 2000, in between regularly planned visits, I was sitting in my Hong Kong office when a fax arrived from Pyongyang marked "urgent." Another shipment of peas—this one not purchased with Vatican funds—had just arrived at the port of Nampo, only for the North Koreans to discover much of it was rotten. It was the first time we had encountered such a problem, and I was alarmed. For the North Koreans, with their always ambivalent attitude—wanting but deeply suspicious of external help—it raised questions about our entire aid effort. I worried that if they felt we could no longer be trusted to provide aid goods in an acceptable condition, our broader operation might face problems.

I rushed to Pyongyang, accompanied by Bangkok-based trader Hugo Hörndli and the Chinese supplier, Gary Zhang, as we had sourced the peas in China. We were taken almost immediately to Nampo, where we were met by officials from the FDRC, the Foreign Commodity Inspection Bureau, the Food Aid Liaison Unit, and the World Food Program. The shipment consisted of 1,218.6 metric tons of peas and 754.5 metric tons of lentils. From the moment we arrived, the appalling stench made clear that a large proportion of the peas was rotten. I felt terrible and was determined to get to the bottom of the problem and find an acceptable solution.

It turned out, the Chinese supplier admitted with considerable embarrassment, that more than ninety metric tons of peas were from the previous year's crop. They were over a year old, likely the reason they had gone bad. Moreover, whoever had assembled the shipment had added stones to the rotting peas. Although it remained unspoken, the suspicion was that this was a deliberate attempt to cut corners by adding weight to the shipment without having to provide as many peas. It was a huge embarrassment. Along with Hugo and Gary, I formally apologized and pledged that extra care would be taken with future shipments. To my relief, the North Koreans did not display overt anger or seek to score political points with the situation. Rather, they seemed eager to find a pragmatic solution. We agreed that the lentils were in good condition and could be sent for immediate distribution. As for the peas, after extensive discussion, Caritas agreed to provide 120 additional metric tons in the next shipment, and to pay the FDRC $10,000 in cash to cover storage, labor, disposal costs, and the inconvenience the shipment of rotting peas had caused.

By the end of the day, I was exhausted but very pleased to have found common ground and a way forward. It was a lesson to me that despite the North Koreans' reputation as being difficult customers, it was possible, with goodwill and flexibility, to work through problems and find practical solutions with them.

This display of pragmatism coincided with a growing flexibility and openness as the broader international environment changed and more countries began to establish or expand contact.

After years during which Russian had been the main foreign language in the country, I noticed an upsurge of interest in learning English. In hospitals, for example, I began to see that the signs for different departments, which had usually been in Korean and Russian, were now in Korean and English. Even in remote rural areas, teachers were beginning to offer basic English lessons. I saw schools where signs in English were affixed to various objects—desks, chairs, books, doors, windows, even trees—to help students learn. At a meeting with Ministry of Education officials, they expressed interest in cooperating more with Caritas, including asking for help in acquiring English-language books. They also told me they were considering trying to bring a couple of native English teachers to Pyongyang. At the Ministry of Foreign Trade, Caritas financed and provided more than one hundred books on economics, in English as well as in Chinese and Korean. Interestingly, the Korean-language books came from the South, but the North Koreans did not object.

Another sign of the changed mood was evident when Caritas decided in November 2001 to conduct in Beijing a five-year review of its North Korean program. The FDRC not only did not object but was very supportive, and offered to send two officials to participate in the Beijing meeting. To me, this was a very positive sign—a reflection of the FDRC's growing interest in professional exchanges, overseas training, and exposure visits. Also taking part were two Caritas members from South Korea, as well as representatives from the Canadian Foodgrains Bank, the Catholic Agency for Overseas Development (CAFOD), the United Nations' Office for Coordination of Humanitarian Affairs (OCHA), and Caritas Secretary General Duncan MacLaren. It was encouraging to see the cordial interactions between the two sets of Koreans, underscoring the goodwill that the June 2000 North-South summit had generated.

But long-standing sensitivities remained. When one international participant raised the issue of random-access monitoring, unaware of what a sore point it was, the infuriated North Koreans stormed out. I had to spend an entire morning listening to their complaints, nodding sympathetically, assisted by three-quarters of a bottle of whiskey that we consumed together, before they grudgingly agreed to return. Nonetheless, the meeting was extremely productive, reaffirming the Caritas commitment to North Korea and my own leading role in the effort, as well as laying out a future strategy focusing not only on food aid but on agriculture and health.

I had long had a special interest in helping the disabled, going back to my early work in China with Deng Xiaoping's paraplegic son Deng Pufang. On my first visit to North Korea, in 1995, I was allowed, to my surprise, to visit a school for the disabled. Although some government services did exist for children with a vision or hearing impairment, there were no major national organizations to assist the disabled, who were generally pushed to the margins of society. Indeed, in traditional Korean thinking, disability was viewed as kind of payback for past wrongdoing.

On subsequent trips, I repeatedly requested permission for Caritas to be allowed to provide help for the disabled. In the process, I learned that the government did look after the blind and deaf, as well as disabled war veterans, but that care was minimal. Moreover, at a time of famine, the issue clearly was a low priority. Indeed, on a trip in late 1997, some English-language books I had brought with me about disability were confiscated and held at the airport, and only released after a considerable delay. Although I was regularly told it would not be possible to collaborate with schools or centers for the disabled, I continued to raise the issue, stressing that in the current crisis, the disabled were among those most in need.

Then I learned that the North Korean government in July 1998 had established what it described as a "civil society organization" to represent the rights and interests of people with disabilities. Initially this body was known as the Korean Association for Supporting the Disabled (KASD), but subsequently it was renamed the Korean Federation for the Protection of the Disabled (KFPD). Its creation marked a sea change in official attitudes toward disability and opened the door to cooperation with international NGOs, including Caritas. In March of the following year, I held my first meeting at the KFPD office, where I received a warm welcome. Officials expressed appreciation for the books and other materials I had brought on previous trips. We discussed several ideas for collaboration, and I asked them to submit one or two proposals for us to consider. They also expressed interested in learning more about the China Disabled Persons' Federation and, given my past connections, asked if I could arrange a proper introduction. I was happy to do so, as I believed that there were enough similarities with the Chinese experience of creating services for the disabled that it would be a valuable first step for the North Koreans. Indeed, this became the beginning on an ongoing collaboration between the two organizations that would continue for many years.

In the coming years, helping the disabled in North Korea would become one of my primary interests. But in 2001, the focus remained on the overall situation, which was still precarious. In April, at the end of my thirty-third visit, I drafted some notes for a series of press interviews. By now, I had become a regular source for a number of influential journalists, and sought to use my unusual access and insights to help shape a more nuanced picture of North Korea. It was a delicate balancing act to acknowledge the grim realities on the ground—essential to keep the donations flowing—without angering the always prickly North Koreans.

My single page of bullet points provides a thumbnail description of how I saw the situation then. I emphasized the continuing crisis in the medical sector, the disastrous state of the country's infrastructure, including water and sanitation systems, and the continuing prevalence of hunger and disease. But I stressed that international food aid was making an enormous difference, providing an opportunity to shift the focus from emergency relief to rehabilitation and development. I noted that for the overall situation to improve, though, the cautious opening of the previous year needed to continue—with the international community reciprocating. Finally, I stressed that the money our latest drive would raise (the goal was around $3 million) would go not only for food but for agricultural inputs such as fertilizer, plastic sheets, fuel, small tractors, and other machinery in the hope of reviving the still-devastated agricultural sector. At the bottom of my notes, I had scribbled a short reality check that our donation target would be "very likely difficult to achieve."

But for me, there was no choice but to carry on. And I was heartened by the fact that, as one UN official in Pyongyang told me, I had helped save hundreds of thousands of lives. Indeed, a North Korean official turned to me one day and declared, "Miss Kathi, you are the Mother Teresa of North Korea!" I was mortified. But deep down, I used that knowledge to help keep me going amidst all the obstacles, setbacks, and frustrations.

CHAPTER EIGHT

Trees, Potatoes, and Fish

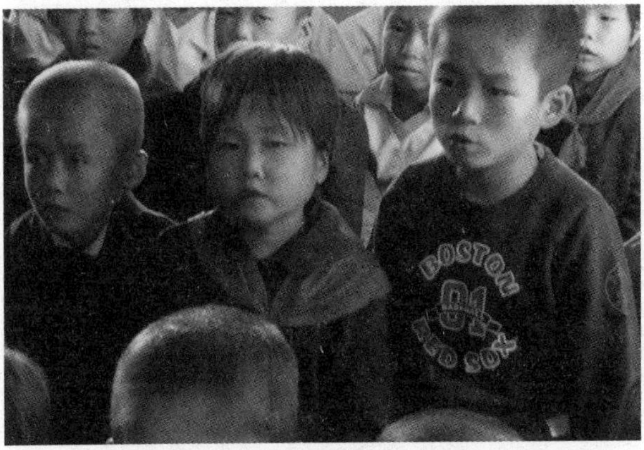

A young North Korean boy wears a Boston Red Sox baseball team shirt. How did he got it?

In July 2002, the North Korean government introduced the most significant changes in economic policy since the creation of the DPRK in 1948. Overnight, the government declared that prices would henceforth be determined largely by supply and demand, and signaled that it was considering abolishing the food rationing coupon system. Wages were dramatically increased to cushion the impact of the rise in the cost of living. Small private plots were declared legal, and farmers were officially allowed to grow crops on these small pieces of land and sell or barter them for profit at farmers markets. At the same time, the government showed a growing tolerance for the large numbers of people who already had been selling goods and services on their own as a coping mechanism during the famine.

Moreover, economic decision-making was in part decentralized, giving local industrial and agricultural managers more authority. The government devalued the North Korean currency and announced plans to develop special economic zones to attract foreign investors. Following the thaw with South Korea in the wake of the North-South summit of June 2000, a fledgling zone already had been established in Kaesong near the DMZ, and plans were underway for a second one at Sinuiju on the border with China.

Officially, the word "reform" was never used. Given the way so much of life in North Korea was framed in ideological terms, the measures were described as a creative adaptation of the *juche* ideology. And it remained unclear whether the moves were simply an attempt by the state to both regularize and assert control over the unofficial markets that had proliferated throughout the country, or whether they presaged deeper, more meaningful change.

There had certainly been indications that Kim Jong Il was serious about seeking new ways to fix his broken economy. In 2001, in a sign of his interest in hybrid market-communist systems like that in China, he spent a week in Shanghai, where he visited the city's gleaming new stock exchange and several joint ventures between Chinese and foreign companies. He also gave a speech that year in which he declared that "no one should follow the way people used to do things in the past. We should make consistent efforts to meet the requirements of a new era."[2]

Given the rigidity of the North Korean system, and despite many question marks as well as likely opposition from skeptics within the DPRK leadership, I felt that the policy change marked a positive step forward. I was not alone in hoping this would be followed by reforms in other areas—finance, taxes, the labor market. I was acutely aware of the need for deeper systemic change, but also of how destabilizing such a process could be in a system as rigid as that of North Korea.

In August 2002, shortly after the new measures were announced, I spent a month with a foreign colleague from the FALU and a local guide and interpreter, traveling 4,600 kilometers by jeep, mostly on dirt roads scarred with potholes. Starting in Pyongyang, we first went north to South Pyongyan Province, then across the peninsula to Kangwon Province, before heading up the east coast to South Hamgyong, Ryanggang, and North Hamgyong near the Russian border. The areas we visited, especially on the eastern side of the country—mountainous, with little arable land—had been among those worst hit by the famine, and they remained the focus of most of Caritas's humanitarian work. Because I had by now spent so much time in these provinces, I had gotten to know variety of provincial and local officials, which made the process of assessing needs and providing and monitoring aid considerably less difficult. I was encouraged by at least some of what I saw. Although the roads, dotted with broken-down vehicles, were in dreadful condition (heightening my greatest fear in all the years I visited North Korea: that I would be in a road accident), I did observe more trucks and many more bicycles. I was amused when our guide, reflecting North Korea's deeply ingrained male chauvinism, was shocked to see a woman driving a car. Along the roadside, there were many more stalls with people bartering and selling. Some were run by individuals. Others, I was told, were actually run by work units seeking to take advantage of the changed atmosphere.

I also was surprised to see people wearing more colorful clothes, including T-shirts with images, logos, or writing. One little boy wore a dark blue T-shirt with "Red Sox"—the name of the American baseball team from Boston—written in red framed in white on it. I presumed the T-shirts had come from China. In many villages, farmers had more livestock—oxen, geese, dogs, goats, rabbits, pigs, and chickens—and I saw small private plots where maize, string beans, potatoes, peppers, and a variety of other vegetables were being grown. In cities and towns, I noticed that supplies in shops seemed more plentiful than before, and customers were busy comparing the variety and prices of items. When I asked, most people expressed enthusiasm for the new policies. Suddenly, terms such as "cost-effectiveness," "management," and even the once-scorned "profit" entered the vocabulary of ordinary citizens.

Indeed, in some ways, the most striking change was the erosion of decades of propaganda about how the state would always provide everything, accompanied by the slow emergence of a market-oriented mindset. This was coupled with a growing interest among my North Korean interlocutors in life outside the country, to the point that I now began to bring with me VHS cassettes of Western movies that I purchased in Hong Kong. I would discreetly hand them over in a brown envelope. On several occasions, foreign diplomats subsequently mentioned to me how surprised they were that North Korean officials were so familiar with the latest hit films. I had to suppress a smile.

Nonetheless, the changing environment could not disguise the fact that North Korea remained very much a country on the brink. Despite the somewhat encouraging signs, the catastrophic impact of the famine years remained visible. Infrastructure was crumbling. Apart from the appalling roads, water supplies in many places were erratic, leading to an increase in diarrhea and other intestinal diseases. The health system remained in terrible shape, with acute shortages of drugs, medical supplies, and basic equipment. For every well-stocked shop packed with consumers, I saw many more with broken windows covered by plastic or cardboard. Most families I visited said they were lucky to eat meat once or twice a year.

While those in the countryside had the possibility of growing their own food, it was clear that residents of urban areas remained extremely dependent on food aid for survival, a fact underscored with every visit to a nursery, kindergarten, childcare facility, or family. In one of the areas most devastated by the famine, Chongjin, a dreary industrial city in the far northeast dotted with shabby Stalinist-style buildings, officials from the Flood Damage Rehabilitation Committee said they had been forced briefly to reduce rations again to 150 grams a day—barely enough for survival. The shortage of protein remained particularly acute, they told me, with one egg a month allocated per person. Many people were still relying on an alternative food mixture of seaweed, dried vegetable stalks, mushrooms, potato leaves, and herbs. Few could remember the last time they had had meat. Fish also was a rarity despite the sea nearby.

Not surprisingly, in schools, nurseries, and orphanages, stunted children were the norm. At one boarding school outside Hamhung, a staff member told me, "I have children. A child here is much smaller than mine were at the same age." Of the children at this school, 40 percent were orphans and 30 percent had one parent. The remaining 30 percent came from families with parents so ill or otherwise unable to cope that they had been forced to send their kids here. Mr. Rim, the principal, told me that aid from Caritas and other international agencies—oil, beans, maize, flour, rice, sugar, and canned fish—had been crucial in keeping the children alive, and that some had begun to show noticeable improvement. Still, to see nine-year-old children who barely looked six haunted me and made my heart ache. I wondered what kind of future they would have.

Moreover, it was evident to me that the new measures, although a step in the right direction, had the potential to create a host of problems. While individuals were being given more personal responsibility and thus felt more in charge of their own destiny, the cradle-to-grave security system, which had, in theory at least, been a central underpinning of the North Korean system, no longer existed. Families now had the challenge of managing household budgets and paying for their own rent, gas, water, and electricity as well for clothing and, above all, food. Yet prices of most staples were now rising sharply. For those with the means to purchase items, the upshot was a greater variety of goods available and a better standard of living, but there was a real danger that many people would slip through the fraying social safety net. What would happen to those in obsolete factories or without a backyard garden to grow vegetables for sale or other means to benefit from a more entrepreneurial environment? Some families I visited told me they were now spending up to 80 percent of their income on food.

In addition, the new measures were reinforcing a shift away from the uniformity I had observed on my earlier trips, creating greater disparities among geographic regions and types of citizens: between Pyongyang and the rest of the country, between urban and rural people, between farmers and workers. To me, though, the changed situation only made our work more critical. As I wrote to Caritas in a report at the end of my 4,600-kilometer journey, "What remains very clear is that the need for humanitarian assistance has NOT changed. The support for the weak and vulnerable will have to continue. In fact, needs are very likely to grow with more people having coping difficulties due to the changes."

Despite the easing of the famine, malnutrition was still a major problem. Even though the North Korean authorities had vowed not to allow the United Nations to conduct a second nationwide nutrition survey, due to their anger at how the results of the first one, done in 1998, had been presented, by 2002 they had changed their minds. Once again, teams of international humanitarian workers and their North Korean colleagues fanned out across the country. What they found was a situation noticeably better than during the depths of the famine, but one in which levels of acute and chronic malnutrition were still high, with one-third of all young mothers surveyed either malnourished or anemic. It made clear the continuing importance of the work of Caritas delivering food aid, especially to children and pregnant and nursing mothers. This included delivering to virtually all the country's forty provincial residential institutions for children. In one room at the Chongjin Orphanage and Baby Home, for example, four out of eighteen infants I saw were badly malnourished. I was used to such scenes, but on this visit, I kept thinking, *Will they survive? Will I ever see them again?* The staff there said international food aid had been an absolute lifeline, but apart from food, they also needed clothing, especially shoes for winter, and toys. The orphanage didn't even have enough cups and bowls, so the children were forced to eat their meager meals in shifts.

On the same visit to Chongjin, I met Mrs. Lee, a thirty-three-year-old textile worker married to a steelworker. She was eight months pregnant and proudly told me that she had gained five kilos during her pregnancy. She credited food aid for her improved diet and thanked us profoundly for the assistance provided. I also visited the home of thirty-year-old Mrs. Kim, who had given birth to a baby boy in April. She too said the peas, wheat, rice, and oil from international aid agencies had made a big difference during her pregnancy, but that vegetables and meat remained in short supply. Occasionally, the family was able to buy a few eggs at the free market. She was giving her son rice porridge and whatever breast milk she had, but the child remained worryingly weak.

In another town, I met twenty-eight-year-old Mrs. Pak, the wife of a chemical plant worker, who was seven months pregnant. We were the first foreigners she had ever encountered, and in her drab apartment, she was visibly nervous. As she relaxed, she told us about her diet. Lunch on this day would be rice mixed with potatoes, and she had gained only three kilos during her pregnancy. As she expressed the hope she would have a boy, she turned to me and pleaded, "Please continue to give us rice and oil."

While the need for emergency food aid remained clear, I had become convinced that over the long term, North Korea's best hope for improving its situation—and avoiding a recurrence of famine—was to strengthen its own ability to feed and care for its people. I assumed that the government intended the July 2002 reforms to be a step in this direction. For Caritas, that meant a change in focus from merely supplying food to making rehabilitation a priority and beginning to emphasize development. As one official from our longtime partner the FDRC told me during a meeting, "We have to improve the capacity of the nation." He noted that supplying fertilizer was better than giving food aid, and renovating or replacing the fertilizer plant so the North Koreans could produce their own would be even better. One ton of fertilizer costs the same as one ton of rice, he said, but with a ton of fertilizer, eight tons of rice could be grown.

Initially, even though this shift in emphasis reflected what the North Korean government itself wanted to see, the FDRC, which jealously guarded its relationship with Caritas, was reluctant to help us connect with people at other ministries, such as agriculture, health, education, and forestry. Eventually, however, the FDRC staff realized they simply did not have the capability to address the many complex challenges and questions that arose as we sought to expand the nature of our engagement. Our access to ministries, professional associations, and educational institutions gradually became easier.

At the same time, building on their experience dealing with Swiss fish farmer Thomas Wettstein, the North Korean authorities asked me to help support the expansion of fish farming, since fish were an important source of protein. Partnering with the Swiss government, as well as with the United Nations Development Program (UNDP), we spent over $200,000 to upgrade three North Korean fish farms. On my visits to the farms, I was struck by how antiquated everything was, and part of our effort involved providing more modern equipment. To reduce any chance that the assistance would be diverted, all the items were routed through the UNDP rather than going directly to the North Korean government. The farms produced trout and carp fingerlings that were then given to other farms for breeding. As part of our arrangement, the recipient fish farms agreed to provide 120 kilograms of fish per month to nearby children's centers and boarding schools.

With everything else on my plate, I did not have the time to conduct regular monitoring to determine whether the supplies of fish were actually being delivered. But some months later, while visiting a nursery, I noted a large container full of fish bones. When I asked, I was told the bones were kept, dried, powdered, and then sprinkled onto rice or maize as a good source of calcium. It was confirmation both that the fish were reaching the intended beneficiaries and that the North Koreans were still being resourceful, not letting anything go to waste.

On one visit to a fish farm, as I was observing a pond full of trout bred from eggs provided by the Swiss government, I played a joke on the North Koreans accompanying me. I suddenly exclaimed, "I am very disappointed!" My guides turned to me, horrified that I had found something wrong. I then said, "I had expected that there would be an image of the white cross of the Swiss flag on the back of each of the fish." There was a stunned moment of silence. Then, as they got the joke, they broke into laughter. One of them quickly replied, "Don't worry. We will ensure that each fish will have an image of the North Korean flag!"

In some quarters in Europe, however, our effort was no laughing matter. As I was sitting at my desk in Hong Kong one day between trips, the phone rang. A man identified himself as an official from the Bundeskriminalamt (BKA, or Federal Criminal Police Office) in Berlin. My immediate thought was, *Oh no. What have I done?* The official told me that the BKA had heard that Caritas was sending equipment to fish farms in North Korea, which sounded suspicious, and he demanded to know more. I explained the nature of the project, stressing that we were working through a UN agency and that we had in fact consigned the goods to UNDP. I mentioned Abu Salim, at that time the head of the UNDP Pyongyang office and the consignee of our donations.

"Abu Salim," the official sneered. "Does he even exist?" As the call continued, I made my displeasure known in the strongest possible terms. I never heard from the BKA again.

In 1999, as previously mentioned, a Peruvian agronomist named Roberto Christen had arrived in Pyongyang as a technical advisor to UNDP. As the focus shifted to recovery, the UNDP's role was becoming even more important, as was that of the Agricultural Recovery and Environmental Protection (AREP) program, which UNDP created to work exclusively on the agricultural sector in North Korea. Christen soon emerged as a leading figure in this effort, in which Caritas became deeply involved. Short, ebullient, with a wicked sense of humor, he had deep knowledge and vast experience all over the world. When we first met, I asked him where else he had worked. "Better to ask me where I have not worked," he shot back, as his answer would be shorter.

We soon became close friends, carrying on such intense conversations, usually about North Korea, that we often lost track of time. Indeed, one evening, with Roberto driving, we set off for dinner at a restaurant in Pyongyang, when we had to stop behind a truck. We were so engrossed in whatever we were discussing that it was only after ten minutes that we realized we weren't stuck in traffic. The truck had broken down, and we simply hadn't noticed it wasn't moving. On another memorable evening driving through the city with Roberto, as we jokingly compared notes about the many inconveniences of operating in the DPRK, he suddenly proclaimed in a loud voice, "Don't forget you are living in paradise here! In paradise!"

Despite his worldly cynicism, Roberto also established strong relationships with his North Korean colleagues, talking with them for hours about the ins and outs of farming. Having grown up on a farm in Switzerland, I also knew a lot about the subject, and was able to hold my own when dealing with agricultural issues—much to the surprise of the North Koreans, who could not imagine that a Western woman living in a big city like Hong Kong would know anything about agriculture. But my background proved increasingly useful as Caritas, in collaboration with the UNDP and AREP, lent its support to a number of projects aimed at promoting the recovery and development of the agricultural sector.

It was a sector that, in a mountainous country where 80 percent of the land was unsuitable for farming, had been struggling long before the famine. Moreover, years of intensive planting, coupled with the overuse of fertilizer, had left the soil seriously depleted. In a country that always had been susceptible to flooding from frequent heavy rains and typhoons, this vulnerability had been exacerbated by a lack of trees on hillsides, with many cut down so that crops could be planted. During the famine, this situation was made worse as desperate people foraged where they could for wood for cooking and roots, plants, herbs, and mushrooms for eating. Adding to the problem was an acute shortage of agricultural inputs—not just fertilizers but also pesticides and plastic sheeting as well as tractor tires, fuel, and spare parts for agricultural machinery. On visits to farms, I commonly saw rusting tractors sitting idle. When talking with farm managers, I soon learned not just to ask how many tractors the farm had. A follow-up question was crucial: How many were actually working? At one farm, I was told only six of fourteen were working, while at another one, only three of twenty-six were operational, sputtering along with parts cannibalized from other machines.

As with everything else in North Korea, I was aware that whatever Caritas did would be only a drop in the bucket, but we felt we could still make an impact. Replenishing the supply of trees was one area where we could help, again in collaboration with the UNDP and AREP. Caritas provided $189,000 for the rehabilitation of a tree nursery in Tongchon County, in Kangwon Province. The nursery had been devastated by the floods of 1995, with the land covered with debris and most of the saplings washed away. It remained a wasteland during the height of the famine, when the focus was on emergency food aid and neither the humanitarian community nor the North Korean government had the resources to devote to repair work. Now, however, with the aid of two ten-ton trucks, two tractors, a water pump, generators, three metric tons of imported seeds, fifty metric tons of fertilizer, shovels, picks, axes, and buckets acquired with Caritas funds, the land was restored and twelve tree species were being grown. Saplings were delivered to other farms eager to develop their own nurseries. Moreover, as North Korea became steadily more receptive to expanded international contact, we also paid for a trip the UNDP organized for officials from the nursery to visit Nepal to observe forestry techniques there.

We began supplying inputs to other farms as well. We donated fertilizer, plastic sheeting, water pumps, and a truck to the Suhung Cooperative Farm in Hamju County, in South Hamgyong Province. The farm managers told me that the inputs would mean the farm could produce an additional 1.5 metric tons of rice and maize per hectare. Officials there and elsewhere said that the plastic sheeting—which was needed to grow the seeds under prior to transplantation to the fields—was particularly important, as doing this seed propagation method increased the short growing season by about two weeks. But sheeting had been in desperately short supply for years, and it was used, washed, dried, stored, and reused in the following years. Indeed, several farm managers said that the last time they had received sheeting from the government had been in 1993. Even in the recently legalized free markets, finding sheeting was next to impossible, so the supplies from Caritas were crucial.

At the same time, with Roberto's guidance, Caritas provided a substantial amount of money to support a sweet potato starch extraction facility in Pangyo County, in Kangwon Province. As a crop that grew easily in higher altitudes and in cold and rugged terrain, the sweet potato, rich in carbohydrates, vitamins, and fiber, was particularly appropriate for North Korea. Moreover, potato starch can be made into flour for noodles, and preserving flour in the winter was much simpler than preserving fresh potatoes, which, if they freeze, are no longer edible. In the initial phase, $150,000 was used to procure sweet potato seeds from China, as well as the essential equipment to build the plant. The funds also paid for two DPRK technicians to be trained in China, and for two Chinese experts to come to North Korea and assist with the setup of the facility. In the second phase, funding was used to create a noodle production line, a starch-drying and virus-free sweet potato production facility, and a mini hydropower plant. The result, I was told by our North Korean partners, was the first fully operational starch and noodle plant in North Korea. By the end of 2001, it had produced its first one hundred metric tons of starch and soon was able to make an average of three hundred metric tons annually after the potato harvest.

From my earliest trips, Caritas had been providing clothing for needy children, and on visits to orphanages and other childcare facilities, I was repeatedly told this remained a pressing need. Instead of importing clothing, usually from China, it occurred to me that it might be possible to produce children's clothing inside North Korea. I raised the idea with the FDRC, noting that it could save on international shipping costs as well as support the local economy. The FDRC was supportive and connected me with the Pyongyang Women's Trade Center and Garment Factory. Initially, I had concerns that I was being sent to a North Korean version of the kind of garment sweatshops so common in places such as Cambodia or Bangladesh. But I was pleasantly surprised. The factory had large, airy, bright rooms, with 250 women sitting in front of antiquated sewing machines for eight hours a day. Many of them wore pieces of fabric over the sleeves of their sweaters to protect their own clothing. This reminded me of my childhood, when many people wore elbow sleeves to keep their daily clothing from wearing out. The facilities were not modern, but the working environment seemed decent.

Even more striking was that the factory was run entirely by women, including the energetic director, Mrs. Park, and her English-speaking colleague, Ms. Kim. Mrs. Park told me the factory had been established in 1994 with the help of the UNDP and the United Nations Development Fund for Women (UNIFEM). Starting with eighty workers, all of whom previously had been housewives, it had expanded to its current size despite the economic crisis caused by the famine and previously had received orders from China and Japan.

We reached an arrangement in which I would put in an order—say, two thousand sets of children's clothing. Once we agreed on a price, Caritas would make a down payment of 80 percent. With that money, the factory would send two or three women to China to purchase the material. I would often give them samples of colorful styles and lively patterns, but in keeping with North Korea's conservative culture, they wanted clothing in plain colors. In any case, off to China they would go, and a month later, the clothing would be ready to send to orphanages, boarding schools, and other residential childcare facilities. Word spread, and soon other NGOs also were placing orders. The government would take 30 percent, but the 70 percent left to the factory was more than the state allowed many other organizations to keep.

It was as close to a win-win situation as one could imagine for North Korea. Orders from Caritas and other NGOs were serving to strengthen industrial capacity and provide decent jobs. Working with the factory was helping to increase access to and understanding of international trade and markets—while producing affordable high-quality goods for distribution to those most in need.

To me, that a factory run by women even existed in Pyongyang was remarkable. The North Koreans did not play up this aspect, but Mrs. Park and her colleagues were confident, even feisty, in a way that I had not often seen, and the more they traveled abroad and dealt with foreigners, the more confident they became. Indeed, Mrs. Park told me she was hoping, with sponsorship from the United Nations, to attend a fashion fair in Hong Kong—something that would have been unimaginable at the time of my first visit to North Korea.

The changing atmosphere also led to some improvements in conditions for Pyongyang's small international community. For the first time, the government allowed UN and NGO offices to install computers with internet access, which made communicating with the outside world much easier. Moreover, the loosening of restrictions produced a sharp increase in the number and variety of restaurants in the capital. The range, especially for North Korea, was remarkable. Dozens of restaurants began to offer Western and Asian fare, from hamburgers to chicken Kiev to Korean staples such as cold noodles and kimchi. There were such abundant choices that Roberto Christen and a couple of international colleagues started compiling a guide, which they called *Eating Out in Pyongyang*. By the time Roberto ended his North Korea assignment in 2004, it would list over one hundred restaurants where foreigners and the North Korean elite could enjoy a good meal. The guide rated eateries with images of chopsticks, with one signifying poor and five excellent.

Among the best places was the Pirobong Restaurant in the Pyongyang Hotel, which served an extensive buffet with seaweed salad, miso soup, desserts, fruit, and cheese. "International hotel lobby ambience. Very clean and nice," the guide said. "Popular with the Pyongyang elite. Good service. So new it did not have a menu our first time there." Prices were high—a meal at the cheapest place was around six dollars, and the fancier ones charged much more—but the explosion of restaurants underscored the changes taking place, especially the emergence of an urban elite. It was not uncommon on weekends to see whole families, including children, enjoying themselves at a restaurant on Roberto's list. Ironically, after some time, Roberto came under pressure not to publicize the list. The pressure came not from the North Koreans but from some diplomats and UN officials. They worried that the list was giving the impression that North Korea was no longer a hardship post and their salaries and fringe benefits might be cut.

The contrast with conditions in so much of the rest of the country was profound. Indeed, on my forty-first trip, in February 2003, the FDRC acknowledged a continuing severe shortage of food supplies. At one meeting, I was told that the only international food shipment to arrive so far in 2003 was 2,200 metric tons of rice ordered by Caritas. WFP officials said that without major pledges, the food aid pipeline could dry up by midyear, risking a new food crisis just when it appeared the country was beginning to emerge from the previous one.

Adding to my concern was an abrupt change in what had been a promising international climate. The month of my visit, the Agreed Framework, the 1994 deal negotiated by the Clinton administration under which North Korea agreed to freeze activity at its Yongbyon nuclear reactor in return for promises of better ties, collapsed. The administration of George W. Bush, which had begun in January 2001, had from the start expressed skepticism about the deal. In early 2002, Bush had included North Korea, along with Iraq and Iran, in his so-called "axis of evil" and made a deliberate decision not to pursue the opening with Pyongyang that had emerged under Clinton. When the United States then found evidence suggesting that North Korea might be seeking to acquire components for a possible uranium nuclear program to complement the now-frozen plutonium one at Yongbyon, Bush spurned North Korean offers to negotiate about the matter and walked away from the Agreed Framework. North Korea then withdrew from the Nuclear Non-Proliferation Treaty and restarted its Yongbyon nuclear reactor. Tensions on the peninsula rose sharply.

CHAPTER NINE

The Red Dots

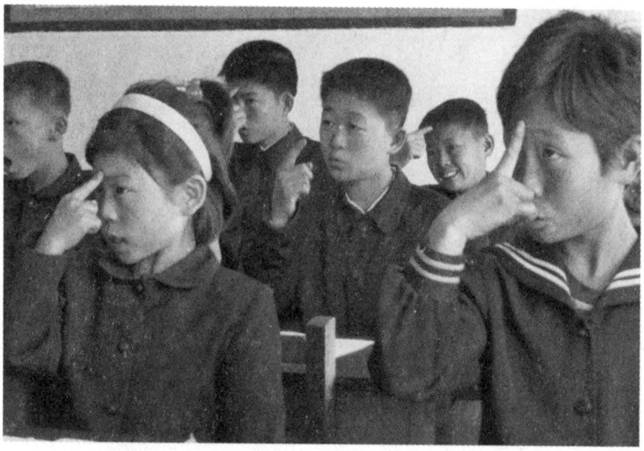

Deaf children learning sign language at a boarding school in South Pyongyan province.

Every year, Caritas would launch an international appeal for funds to support our work in North Korea. It was always an uphill struggle. By 2003, the worst of the famine was over, and the sense of urgency around the world had faded. With so many other crises across the globe, donor fatigue had set in. North Korea's dubious international reputation didn't help, and neither did the increasingly tense climate on the Korean peninsula. International media coverage often suggested that an outbreak of hostilities was looming. On my visits that year, I certainly noticed an uptick in anti-American rhetoric and more anti-American posters in the streets of Pyongyang. Moreover, air raid drills—long a regular occurrence—appeared to be more frequent and were being held not only in Pyongyang but in other parts of the country too. Yet I did not sense much difference on the ground and saw no evidence that North Korea was on any kind of a real war footing. Nonetheless, this combination of factors meant a sharp drop in donations. In 2002, we reached just half of our target. In 2003, it was the same story; by October of that year, we had raised only 50 percent of our $2.67 million goal to assist with food and medical aid, agriculture, and capacity building.

The acute humanitarian needs remained, however, and nowhere more so than in North Korea's barely functioning health-care system. On paper, the health-care infrastructure in North Korea was extensive—seventy-six thousand doctors; two hundred thousand health-care workers; hospitals at the provincial, county, and *dong* (district) levels; and clinics at the *ri* (village) level. Yet economic difficulties before the famine and the disaster of the past half dozen years had left the health-care system in dire condition. I usually visited at least one hospital or clinic on every visit, and often more. Even as the famine eased, the picture that I saw was grim. Health facilities routinely lacked drugs and medical supplies, functioning equipment, electricity, water, and, in the winter, heating. The absence of antibiotics and painkillers made even the treatment of routine ailments a challenge. Virtually every medical facility was sending staff into surrounding fields, forests, or mountains in search of leaves, roots, flowers, and berries to make traditional Korean medicine. It was a reasonable coping strategy under the circumstances, but hardly adequate.

At the two-story Kangwon Provincial Pediatric Hospital in Wonsan, for instance, Dr. Pak, the chief medical officer for a facility serving fifteen counties and two cities, greeted me in his humble office illuminated by one light bulb hanging from the ceiling. On one wall was a new UNICEF "Weight for Height" chart. He told me that although cases of malnutrition had decreased, the hospital was still caring for over a dozen children suffering from it. The most pressing needs, he said, were an X-ray machine as well as a water distiller and a backup generator, as power supplies were often cut.

As I was shown later that day around the Kosan County People's Hospital, where 10 percent of the patients were malnourished, I saw a single X-ray machine that dated back to World War Two. It had been years since the facility had the films required to use it. Other laboratory equipment was also old and hardly functioning. The hospital had no food for the patients, whose families had to bring their own. I often wondered how people who barely had enough to eat at home would be able to provide for hospitalized relatives. The Provincial Maternity Hospital in Chongjin, the capital of North Hamgyong Province, had no working incubators, making it extremely difficult to deal with premature births. The hospital also had only a makeshift operating theater, and running water was in such short supply that staff members were forced to bring in buckets of water from outside. Mr. Song, the director, gave me a list of three hundred items he needed. On my notes from a trip at that time, I wrote, "What a depressing place! I felt very miserable and helpless. I definitely would not want to be ill here!"

Indeed, I was struck by how many empty beds I saw at the various hospitals I visited. In contrast, there were often long lines at outpatient clinics. It was clear that people tried to avoid going to hospitals unless absolutely necessary, for obvious reasons, preferring instead to pick up medicine and return home. I was told there were no public markets or shops where medicines were sold, making the outpatient clinics the only source. Interestingly, an official rule required doctors to give patients only enough for just two to four days, making it necessary for them to return regularly for more. With supplies so limited, that was understandable to avoid waste, but it was also apparent that there was concern that medications might be sold on the black market.

However dispiriting, the grim scenes only reinforced my determination to help. Increasingly, the focus of our work shifted to hospitals and health care. This involved expanded cooperation not only with our regular partner, the Flood Damage Rehabilitation Committee, but also with the Ministry of Health and the World Health Organization. The other UN agencies on the ground in the DPRK, such as the World Food Program and UNICEF, were also interested both in what Caritas was doing and in what I was seeing, as my access was better than many others'. We regularly met when I returned to Pyongyang from field trips.

I relied especially on the WHO for guidance and advice, and we worked closely together to be sure our efforts were complementary, rather than overlapping. Of crucial importance, the UN agencies agreed that Caritas shipments to the DPRK could be consigned to them rather than directly to the North Korean authorities. As I was not always in the country, this enabled much more efficient tracking to ensure the supplies sent by Caritas were delivered to the intended beneficiaries.

With this kind of collaboration, we stepped up efforts to provide medical kits containing basic supplies and equipment, such as painkillers, antibiotics, and oral rehydration salts (diarrhea remained a chronic problem) as well as basic medical equipment, such as scalpels, blood pressure monitors, and stethoscopes. We gave village clinics a simple kit, and larger hospitals a more elaborate one. Maternity wards got a kit specifically designed for expectant mothers and newborns. We also provided both paper and cloth diapers, but were frequently told that the cloth ones, while in theory more valuable because they could be reused, were actually a problem because of an acute nationwide shortage of soap, which made washing them a major challenge. Vegetable oil or animal fat is a key ingredient in soap production, and both were in extremely short supply in North Korea. As a result, soap quickly became an important addition to our regular shipments to the DPRK.

Early on, the Ministry of Health had asked Caritas to provide ambulances. For reasons of cost, logistics, and practicality, I made clear that we did not believe importing ambulances made sense. Instead, I proposed bringing in bicycles for medical staff to get around the countryside. The disappointment on the faces of the officials in Pyongyang when I rejected the request for ambulances was evident. But on a visit to a clinic at a cooperative farm in South Hamgyong Province, I saw doctors using bikes we had donated to move around the community, visit sick patients, and administer vaccinations at schools and nurseries. They told me that the bicycles were the first the clinic had ever had, and it was clear that the staff were deeply relieved not to have to walk for miles to make house calls. I felt that my initial judgment had been vindicated.

One important aspect of our work with the ministry was a series of initiatives to renovate medical facilities—putting in new floors and windows, refurbishing operating rooms, and otherwise upgrading usually decrepit facilities. In the remote northeast, we worked with a half dozen hospitals but consistently had difficulty getting one in particular to implement any changes. I finally figured out the reason after noticing a painting of the hospital decorated with red dots in the office of the hospital director. I asked about the meaning of the dots and was told they identified every room that Kim Il Sung had set foot in when he visited many years before. Since then, the hospital had been seen not only as a medical facility but as almost a kind of sacred location. Local officials were terrified of making any changes to a place where the Great Leader himself had set foot. Eventually, I discovered they needed to request permission from the central authorities in Pyongyang before doing anything that would disturb the hallowed ground. To me, the episode was an "aha" moment—another reminder of the power of the veneration of the Kim family, and the way it could serve as a roadblock to otherwise sensible behavior.

It was not the only instance where I encountered challenges dealing with local officials. In many locations, repeated visits had enabled me to develop cordial relationships and build a degree of trust. But when I traveled to the northeastern provinces of North Hamgyong and Ryanggang, the most remote and inaccessible of all the country's provinces, especially outside the cities, I found that many officials were suspicious and unwelcoming. When the new head of the FALU, Umberto Greco, and I visited the maternity ward at the Hwasong County hospital, for example, the director, Dr. Chae, did not let me take photographs. Then he said he had not been informed that we wanted to see the rest of the facility and refused to let us look around further, even when I explained to him the importance of seeing more to be able to plan future aid shipments. But complaining about our presence did not stop him from requesting additional medical kits, diapers, bedding, and food.

Back at the dingy Kolmalsan Hotel in Chongjin, Umberto and I discussed our reception. North Hamgyong got very few foreign visitors, and we agreed that this explained Dr. Chae's less than friendly attitude. It would take time and more trips to forge the kind of positive working relationships we had with officials in other parts of the country, but we were both heartened by the fact that the Caritas aid had been received and that, even while grumbling, Dr. Chae had acknowledged it had been extremely helpful.

Overall, though, my access continued to expand. In 2004, I became, so I was told, the first foreigner ever allowed to visit a hospital for psychiatric patients: the Yongsan Psychiatric Hospital, also known as the Center for Mental Patients, located in South Pyongan Province. A spartan two-story concrete structure, dimly lit with a few light bulbs, it had an atmosphere so grim, I felt uneasy taking photographs. Like virtually all North Korean medical facilities, however, it was spotless. It had eighty patients, most of whom were young or middle-aged men wearing striped pajamas and lying in bed. To me, they looked lost and totally drugged.

The staff told me that the center had been established in 1987, much later than most North Korean hospitals, suggesting that an official decision to provide care for the mentally ill had been a relatively recent development. It had a carpentry workshop and a place where patients could paint and draw—a simple kind of occupational therapy. I was told that 80 percent of the patients stayed for two to three months and then went home, while the remaining 20 percent were sent to other facilities in nearby towns. It was not clear whether these other places were solely for psychiatric patients or simply regular medical facilities.

As in most North Korean hospitals, the supply of water and power was a problem, as was food. The staff complained that allocations from the government were not enough, and what was grown in the center's small garden could not make up the difference. They also told me of a severe shortage of appropriate drugs to treat psychiatric patients. But when they asked if Caritas could provide help, I was noncommittal. Privately, I was concerned that dealing with such a sensitive issue—people with mental disorders, requests for powerful drugs—was beyond the capability of Caritas to handle. When I returned to Pyongyang, I told my colleagues at the WHO about the visit. They had never been given access to such a facility, and it was far from clear that the North Koreans would agree to receive such help, even though they had expressed interest. Despite the obvious need, helping the mentally ill was an area in which the role of foreign assistance would remain problematic.

At ten minutes past noon on April 22, 2004, a massive explosion shattered the train station in the town of Ryongchon, fifteen kilometers from North Korea's border with China. The blast, estimated to be equal to eight hundred to one thousand tons of the chemical explosive TNT, was seen and heard as far away as in China. The station was obliterated, and hundreds of nearby buildings, including a primary school packed with children, were destroyed or damaged. Nearly two hundred people died, and over a thousand were injured. It was one of the worst disasters in the history of North Korea.

Just hours earlier, Kim Jong Il, having finished a trip to China, had passed through Ryongchon on his way back to Pyongyang. Had his official train been there at the time of the blast, he and his entourage likely would have been killed or injured. Not surprisingly, the timing fueled intense speculation that it might have been an assassination attempt. Later, an official North Korean report said it was in fact a tragic accident in which faulty electrical wiring had produced sparks that ignited several train carriages packed with ammonium nitrate.

As soon as I saw the news reports, I sent a note of condolence to the FDRC and offered to help. Within just a few hours—unprecedented speed for the North Koreans—a staffer replied, "Yes, please." Caritas immediately launched an appeal for $200,000 to help the city's devastated health-care facilities by providing furnishings, equipment, medical supplies, and drugs. I was pleasantly surprised that, despite the usual donor fatigue, donations soon exceeded that amount. In early June, less than two months after the explosion, I was allowed to visit the devastated city. The two-hundred-kilometer trip from Pyongyang took four hours over roads in appalling condition. I was struck by the numerous checkpoints and the guards deployed to protect the fields of rice and maize that we passed.

"Misery has taken up home in Ryongchon," I noted in my report for Caritas. Although located some distance from the blast, the Ryongchon County Hospital—to which I was immediately taken—had sustained major damage, with large cracks visible in the walls and many windows blown out. But it was still treating victims of the explosion, who were suffering from cuts, infected wounds, eye problems, headaches, and psychological issues. "At the peak, we had one thousand three hundred people for treatment," Dr. Kim, the Ryongchon County Hospital chief, told me. "It was the first time that I had to cope with such a disaster."

In addition to Caritas, the WHO, the Red Cross, and the Swiss Agency for Development and Cooperation (SDC), among others, joined the effort to provide help. So did the Swiss arm of the Adventist Development and Relief Agency (ADRA), operated by the Seventh Day Adventist Church, which had opened an office in Pyongyang in 1999. While Caritas decided not to get involved in supporting the actual construction work, ADRA offered to bring in foreign experts in hospital construction and provide other construction assistance, and the North Koreans quickly agreed.

By the time I arrived in Ryongchon, nearly ten thousand workers, including many soldiers, were involved in clearing away debris and beginning the task of rebuilding the city. In addition to two thousand family homes, a new primary school, a nursery, two kindergartens, and three secondary schools were under construction.

I would make three more trips to Ryongchon in the following two years. I was impressed by the hospital staff, whom I found to be friendly, engaging, and committed. It turned out, however, that the quality of the construction work was shoddy at best, and many of the new buildings soon began showing signs of dilapidation and decay. Moreover, progress in rebuilding the hospital was painfully slow. Because the plastering had been done in the winter, some walls had not dried properly, and many rooms and corridors had to be redone. Walking through the facility, I saw that the heating and electricity systems and other fittings had not been fully installed. Roof insulation was a problem, and the alarm and double locks on the storeroom for drugs suggested that security was a serious problem.

In my notes, I observed: "The Ryongchon officials, obviously incapable of supervising the construction of the new hospital, showed very little enthusiasm for moving the process forward speedily. For the local government, health services are low priority and people in need of hospitalization and treatment are the losers." Even months after the disaster, many items donated by Caritas, including furnishings, equipment, supplies, and drugs, were still in storage. At one meeting, I suggested that if the new hospital was not ready to reopen, perhaps the Caritas donation should be taken back and given to another hospital in North Korea. The officials present met the idea with indifference.

Although it was the international lead agency, the ADRA eventually left North Korea before the reconstruction work was completed. And it was clear to me that, even with the best will in the world, too many people and organizations had gotten involved to bring the effort to a successful conclusion. There was considerable confusion about the decision-making process and the lines of authority, further complicated by the many different sources of international financial support for Ryongchon flowing into Pyongyang. The result was that far too little was accomplished despite the urgent need. In my journal, I wrote, "The Caritas decision not to get involved in big construction projects had been the right one!"

For me, one important development emerged from my work at Ryongchon. With so many blast victims suffering eye injuries, Caritas had devoted considerable resources to helping people deal with eye disabilities, providing a fresh impetus to what was becoming an increasingly important priority for me—helping the disabled.

By the early 2000s, my initial encounter with the Korean Federation for the Protection of the Disabled—and especially my helping arrange for KFPD officials to visit China and meet their Chinese counterparts—had begun to lead to improved access, opening the door to expanded engagement. In addition, it also provided me with a deeper understanding of the inner workings of North Korean society in relation to an issue that was highly sensitive and about which there was scant knowledge.

For many years, the North Korean government had done little to acknowledge the existence of disabled people, and even less to help them, except in the cases of some visually or hearing-impaired children and victims of the Korean War decades earlier. Part of the reason was a desperate shortage of resources, but it also stemmed from a traditional belief, held in both North and South Korea, that disability was a kind of payback for something done wrong. As a result, many Koreans with disabilities and their families suffered from shame, hopelessness, denial, withdrawal, and depression. Moreover, human rights groups had reported that historically, disabled persons were housed in special facilities, often in harsh conditions, away from Pyongyang and other cities. There was no way to confirm such reports, but the lack of devices and equipment to assist those with disabilities, such as wheelchairs, crutches, and canes, not to mention the lack of accessibility on streets and in buildings, certainly hindered the integration of disabled people into mainstream society.

Yet attitudes were slowly beginning to change. In 1999, for the first time, a national survey on the situation of people with disabilities was conducted. By 2003, a new law was passed designed to protect the disabled, and the government pledged to expand the availability of wheelchairs, crutches, and hearing aids as well as the production of prostheses to help those with missing limbs.

The early KFPD China trip turned out to be an important turning point in this change of attitude. KFPD officials were able to learn from their Chinese counterparts at the China Disabled Persons' Federation, and told me they'd returned with a better appreciation of the importance and benefits of early intervention to assist children with disabilities. Yet facilities in North Korea remained minimal. Even in 2004, there were only three schools for the blind and nine for the deaf in the whole country. After repeatedly explaining that assisting the disabled was a key Caritas priority, I was finally allowed, for the first time since my initial trip in 1995, to visit institutions for the disabled, including one for the visually impaired and another for the hearing impaired in Hamhung. In the following months, I visited other schools.

The picture that emerged was depressing. The children I observed in classrooms and dormitories were all unnaturally small, and some appeared deprived or ill. I was told that the kids had a normal school curriculum, only conducted in sign language, with some limited speech training for the hearing impaired, while the visually impaired were learning Korean Hangul characters in Braille. In addition, they were also taught, if their condition allowed, haircutting, painting, sewing, carpentry, and photography. It was clear that the outdated and often dilapidated training equipment needed to be replaced. There were many other needs as well—for food, coal, blankets, kitchenware, and visual materials for teaching.

Slowly, I tried to expand my collaboration with the KFPD, and began to arrange support for the printing of dictionaries and reference books for the hearing impaired, and for the provision of blankets, winter clothing, and food to some schools. Yet questions soon arose about what kind of relationship the authorities would allow Caritas to develop with the KFPD and, indeed, whether we would be able to continue to work with the organization. A follow-up KFPD tour to China, for which most of the arrangements already had been made, was postponed.

It was hardly the first time that Caritas had been entangled in North Korea's complex bureaucratic politics. Since my earliest visits, the FDRC had been our main partner. I had previously encountered situations in which FDRC officials were uneasy with Caritas's developing separate relationships with other organizations. Now, it was balking at sanctioning an expansion of Caritas dealings with the KFPD. Further complicating the situation was the fact that the KFPD had been created, in the government's own words, as a "civil society organization." While it remained closely connected to the Ministry of Health and all of its funds came from the government or international donations, the KFPD did appear to have greater flexibility in terms of what it did and with whom it collaborated. I could understand why the FDRC was at first uneasy.

Luckily, I found a way to manage the situation by working through Handicap International (HI). Founded in 1982 and managing hundreds of programs in dozens of countries, that organization had begun dealing with the North Koreans in 1998, with activities coordinated by its Belgium branch. The focus was on improving physical rehabilitation services, facilitating vocational training, and supporting the KPFD in terms of capacity-building. Given HI's single-minded focus, it was logical that its main partner would be the KFPD. With my own interest in helping the disabled, I maintained close contact with the HI staff in Pyongyang, and I was grateful for their collaboration and assistance. On one occasion, when funding was needed to cover the KFPD's cost for printing a sign language dictionary and reference books for people with hearing problems, we sent the money to Handicap International. I also was able to use the HI email to have more direct communication with the KFPD. Eventually, the KFPD would assign a staffer to HI, making contact even easier. To my relief, my own dealings with the FDRC, forged over nearly a decade, not only remained unaffected but continued to improve.

CHAPTER TEN

"Anything Can Be Solved with Money"

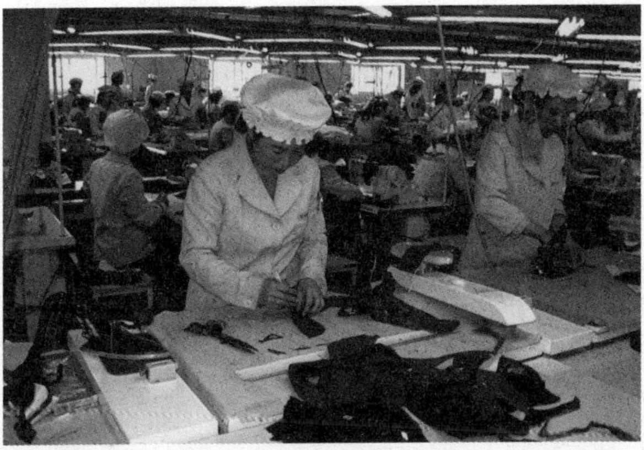

North Korean workers at the Kaesong Industrial Park, a project with South Korea, had an opportunity to earn more money.

In the summer of 2005, I made my forty-ninth trip to North Korea. When I had first visited a decade before, the country was reeling from unprecedented floods that, on top of its inefficient state-run economic system, engendered years of famine. Now, signs of change were everywhere. The most striking transformation, which had begun with the adoption of some economic reforms in 2002, was the emergence of officially sanctioned markets and an easing of state control over the economy. There were now some three hundred approved markets across the country, including several dozen in Pyongyang. The biggest was the Tongil (Unification) Market, a two-story structure near the center of the capital. Whereas previously, foreigners had been forbidden from visiting markets anywhere—indeed, when we would drive past a market in the countryside, my North Korean colleagues would simply pretend it wasn't there—by trip forty-nine, it was possible to wander through Tongil Market and take in the astonishing change it represented, although photography was not permitted.

The range of goods was, especially for North Korea, remarkable. Fresh vegetables, fruit, meat, fish, cigarettes, cosmetics, stockings, clothing, shoes, soap, TV sets, refrigerators, tools, spare parts, traditional Korean medicine, and many other items were available. Rice and maize technically were not allowed to be sold in the markets. They remained, at least in theory, available only through the government-controlled public distribution system. Yet with the right connections, I was told, such items could be acquired at markets or even from private homes. Moreover, I was struck by how many goods were imported from outside North Korea. The majority came from China, but on one visit, in just a few minutes, I counted items from over ten countries. Most of those countries were in Asia, but I even saw Migros chocolate from Switzerland. Almost all the vendors were women—indeed, the role women were playing in this emerging market economy was striking. I jokingly observed to a North Korean colleague that if North Korean women were to go on strike, the country would collapse in two weeks. He laughed and replied, "No, it would collapse in two days!" Almost all the saleswomen had small calculators, and intensive bargaining was common.

There was a noticeable spirit of entrepreneurship—suddenly people were exchanging name cards and asking about business connections. Making money had become a common topic of conversation, especially among the younger generation. I could feel a sense of liberation as people purchased in a market goods they actually wanted, instead of grudgingly accepting whatever meager supplies were on offer in state-run shops. The new atmosphere made people willing to articulate dreams and hopes in a way I could never have imagined previously. A cell phone or a trip abroad seemed to be among the most popular aspirations. As one of my North Korean colleagues said to me, "Anything can be solved with money."

Beyond the markets, I could feel a sense of fresh energy in Pyongyang. In a city where the most striking feature had long been the total absence of advertisements, the streets lined only with political slogans or images of Kim Il Sung, billboards suddenly appeared advertising a car called the Hwiparam

(Korean for "whistle"). The Hwiparam was the first car ever manufactured in North Korea, the result of a joint venture the government had signed with the Reverend Sun Myung Moon, head of the Unification Church, whose followers were known as "Moonies." Moon, whose family came from the northern half of Korea, had visited Pyongyang in 1991, meeting with Kim Il Sung and forged a warm relationship with the Great Leader. The upshot was the opening in 2002 of the Pyeonghwa (Korean for "peace") automobile factory. The plan was to produce the Hwiparam, an updated version of Fiat's Siena, initially primarily for export but with the hope that eventually the domestic market would grow. Pyongyang had few vehicles and little traffic, so it seemed hard to imagine that any North Koreans would be able to buy such a car. But the plant, the advertisements, and the opening of a car wash on the outskirts of the capital—something I had never seen before—were all signs of change.

So was the growing number of restaurants and bars, numbering over two hundred by 2005, including a few that stayed open twenty-four hours a day. As competition for business had become increasingly fierce, some were offering not only tasty food but also a variety of promotional gimmicks. One eatery was giving customers a complimentary "dish of the day" if they agreed to return, while another was promising discounts to repeat diners—practices that had previously been unheard of. At the same time, the rules under which most Pyongyang residents were barred from entering the city's main hotels, especially those where foreigners stayed, were relaxed, at least for some members of the population. With the entry of locals now permitted, one hotel began to rent out billiard and karaoke equipment as a moneymaking venture, and singing at the entertainment venues could be heard well into the night. To see people having fun and enjoying themselves was itself a striking change from the dour, grim atmosphere I had come to associate with North Korea.

The sense of change was noticeable in the countryside as well. As I visited farms and villages, I was told that decision-making had become increasingly decentralized, and managers at several cooperative farms said they now had more freedom to decide what crops to plant. "The mindset has changed," one told me. "We are becoming money-centered." The result was greater emphasis on cash crops that could be sold at local markets, such as tobacco, chili, vegetables, and fruits.

Moreover, private plots—the yield of which farmers could either keep for their own consumption or sell at markets—were expanding. I was struck as well by the spread of individual enterprise: people offering services such as shoe and bicycle repair, tailoring, wood delivery, and haircutting, and products such as ice cream. One manager noted that the people on his farm—who seemed to be dressed in more colorful clothes than on my previous visits—felt increasingly motivated, as they could see direct benefits to them from the new policies, including investments in new facilities and performance-related bonuses. Added one of his colleagues, "Economic management is easier. The changes were a surprise at first, but now we think differently. We are getting accustomed to a new reality."

There was a new atmosphere in the DPRK's international relationships as well. At Pyongyang airport, I noticed more flights operating, including for a new route to the Russian port city of Vladivostok. Moreover, the long-standing practice of security officers confiscating the cell phones of arriving foreigners and returning them only on departure had been discontinued. Foreign visitors could keep their mobiles, even though there was no roaming signal within the DPRK that could be used to make a call. It also was possible to rent a local mobile phone with a North Korean SIM card, enabling foreigners to call both internationally and domestically to other foreigners. Indeed, on one occasion, while visiting Hamhung in the far northeast, I used my rented North Korean mobile to call a colleague in Washington, who almost fell out of his chair in astonishment.

The emergence of surprisingly warm ties with South Korea was particularly striking. In the wake of the June 2000 North-South summit, aid from the South, especially supplies of fertilizer, had increased dramatically. In 2004, the Kaesong Industrial Complex (KIC) was launched. Located just across the Demilitarized Zone from South Korea, and financed largely by the South Korean company Hyundai, Kaesong was designed to draw South Korean firms eager to take advantage of cheap North Korean labor. A symbol of expanded North-South cooperation, it would become the most significant and successful special economic zone to operate in North Korea.

By 2005, more than a dozen South Korean companies were employing nearly five thousand North Koreans, and the waiting list of other South Korean firms eager to invest ran into the hundreds. The South supplied electricity, direct-dial phones connected the two countries, and every day, South Korean managers and engineers went back and forth across the border. In contrast to the typical North Korean factory, the facilities at Kaesong were modern, bright, and largely free of propaganda, and the North Korean workers—almost all women—enjoyed a ready supply of snacks, power, and clean, hot water. For these young North Koreans, exposure to a South Korean–style work environment must have been an eye-opener, and the fact that the zone appeared to please both governments was another sign of how tensions on the peninsula were easing.

But the Kaesong experiment with not without problems, including, improbably, tensions over a popular South Korean snack called the Choco Pie. The North Korean government had refused to allow South Korean businesses to pay workers for overtime in cash. As a result, South Korean companies began to use Choco Pies as compensation. Soon, the tasty treat was appearing at black markets across North Korea. For the authorities in a country still struggling to feed itself, the Choco Pies underscored the disparity between the impoverished North and the far wealthier South. It was not long before state media launched a campaign to warn citizens that the pies were harmful to health. Eventually, the pies were banned altogether.

But the Choco Pie spat did not disrupt the emerging thaw. The number of tourists from the South shot up sharply, with many visiting scenic Mount Kumgang, also located just on the Northern side of the DMZ, where Hyundai was also developing a lavish resort complex with hotels, restaurants, and a reunion center for divided families. In May 2005, the North even announced plans to open Mount Paekdu, the most sacred spot in North Korea's official mythology, to South Korean visitors.

Meanwhile, the diplomatic atmosphere also showed signs of improvement. After nearly three years of stalemate, in September 2005, six-party talks in Beijing involving the North, the South, the United States, China, Japan, and Russia produced a landmark declaration. It outlined a set of principles intended to resolve the long-running nuclear crisis, with the North committing to "abandoning all nuclear weapons and existing programs, and returning, at an early date, to the Treaty on the Non-Proliferation of Nuclear Weapons and to IAEA safeguards," while the United States and Pyongyang both agreed to "respect each other's sovereignty, exist peacefully together, and take steps to normalize their relations."

As the dynamic of internal change and external relaxation accelerated, I was grateful to see the signs of progress after so many grim years. Yet it was also increasingly clear that the winners in North Korean society were vastly outnumbered by those being left behind. In Pyongyang, a new elite was emerging, composed of high-ranking military, party, and state officials, and employees of work units involved in foreign trade or international organizations. They were augmented by a growing middle class—those vendors and entrepreneurs I had seen at Tongil and other markets who had benefited from the upsurge in economic activity not controlled directly by the state. As they flaunted their new wealth in high-end restaurants and cafés, showing off their mobile telephones and taste for expensive products, there was, I wrote in a report for Caritas, "a situation where, earlier, the deprivation was equally shared, but now there is a growing separation between the haves and have-nots. New vulnerability patterns are emerging, creating challenges for humanitarian aid agencies and the government. Caritas assistance remains crucial in such difficult times. Targeting of aid is becoming more important in order to reach those left out by the economic reform process. People can no longer depend on government rations or handouts and have to fend for themselves."

Indeed, for the average North Korean, life was still a grim struggle for survival. But the issue now was no longer just food availability but access to it. Those too poor to afford what was on sale at the markets remained dependent on a still barely functioning public distribution system, where the average food ration was a paltry 250 to 300 grams of cereals a day, providing just about one thousand calories. Although the 2004 harvest had been the best in a decade, over six million people were still in need of food assistance, by our calculations. Moreover, one result of the growing influence of market forces was rampant inflation, making many goods unaffordable for ordinary people. In some cases, families I met said they were spending 80 percent of their total income on food or relying on supplies from relatives in the countryside to have enough to eat.

On yet another visit to Hamhung in the far northeast, for example, I found that a kilo of rice in the market cost 950 North Korean won, while the average monthly salary for a nurse at the local hospital was between 1,100 and 1,500 won. No wonder people were struggling. How did they manage? Nonetheless, it did seem to me that the system must have had its own logic, and we foreigners were constantly frustrated trying to figure out how it actually worked.

The shortage of energy also remained acute. There continued to be periodic power outages in Pyongyang, often lasting hours at a time, while elsewhere, I found people still relying on candlelight or wood-burning stoves. I often saw trucks with engines that had been converted to run on wood or charcoal fuel, and few tractors were visible in the fields. Although the two textile factories from which Caritas had been ordering children's clothing were operating, the energy crisis meant that economic production in many places remained at a standstill, and the transport of goods and food was still a serious issue.

As I observed both the signs of progress and the overwhelming evidence of how far North Korea still had to go, I was struck by a noticeable change in the attitude about international relief efforts. With conditions slowly improving, the underlying tensions that had long existed between the authorities and the aid community appeared to be growing. North Korean officials increasingly spoke to me of the need to shift the focus from humanitarian assistance to development aid and capacity-building. On one level, I could understand their feelings. As I wrote in a report for Caritas, "The DPRK does not like to be viewed as an aid-dependent country any longer. Moreover, it was clear they resented the monitoring requests and foreigners that go along with the assistance." I was also aware that the effectiveness of development aid would require even greater dialogue, information, transparency, and accountability—all of which the North, based on past behavior, would likely be reluctant to welcome.

I frequently urged North Korean officials to find a way to move beyond emergency aid, as I had long believed in the importance of trying to provide the country with the kind of help that would underpin economic reconstruction and development and reduce the chances of another catastrophic famine. While we continued to provide food assistance, by 2005, Caritas had expanded its involvement in other projects, which already included farming, forestry, and fisheries. An additional program, in the town of Sukchon, in South Pyongan Province, trained farm mechanics and tractor drivers. We provided tractors, tires, and spare parts, and supported the training of over 150 people from several farms in the surrounding area. Some of those who had received training were now offering repair work services for other farming vehicles, raising hopes that the project could generate income and eventually become self-sustaining. This project was undertaken in collaboration with the Swiss government's Agency for Development and Cooperation (SDC), which had been operating in North Korea since the beginning of the famine and had opened an office in Pyongyang in 1997.

At the same time, we began supporting a women's garment cooperative in the eastern port city of Wonsan. Located on the ground floor of a decrepit building of residential flats, it had been a tailoring workshop until a lack of equipment led to its closure. Now, using sixty secondhand sewing machines and dozens of rolls of cloth provided by Caritas, women there were producing gloves for construction workers, overalls, and suits for both companies and individuals. The workforce was composed of two teams, each with forty women, all of them former housewives. As urban residents outside Pyongyang had long faced more difficulties than did farmers in the countryside, who could grow their own food and sell any excess at the market, I felt gratified that this project was helping ease the burden on a particularly hard-hit section of the population.

The DPRK government's receptivity to both projects was a sign of a broader interest in doing business, reflected in a request from the Ministry of Foreign Trade for Caritas to help stock a library. We provided books on economics, trade, and business in English, Chinese, and Korean. The Korean-language books all had been published in the South, but interestingly, the North Koreans had no objection as long as the books were sent via Hong Kong and not directly from Seoul. The library was on the fifth floor of the ministry. Apart from books, it had newspapers and magazines, although many were out of date, and officials said they could not afford to purchase new subscriptions. They said that around twenty people used the facility every day, and work was underway to create a computer link so people outside Pyongyang could access the collection—part of a countrywide intranet now under construction.

As I traveled across North Korea that summer of 2005, the government was reaching a decision with momentous consequences. In September, during the annual gathering of the UN General Assembly, North Korean Deputy Foreign Minister Choe Su Hon asked UN Secretary-General Kofi Annan to discontinue the World Food Program's emergency food aid program by the end of the year. More broadly, all organizations involved in humanitarian assistance were told that going forward, programs would be required to shift from emergency aid to development aid or else shut down altogether. And all foreign personnel from the dozen private aid groups operating in Pyongyang were ordered to leave or change their program to a development-oriented approach. In public, Choe said the decision was the result of a better harvest, and also a response to what he described as efforts by the United States and other Western countries to link humanitarian assistance to human rights.

As the shock waves from the decision reverberated throughout the aid community, there was widespread consternation and confusion. Jan Egeland, the United Nations' undersecretary-general for humanitarian affairs, told reporters that "abruptly halting humanitarian assistance programs at the end of the year would be potentially disastrous for the millions of people who benefit from the humanitarian assistance including food and medicines provided by the United Nations."

While disappointed and concerned, I was not altogether surprised, as my North Korean colleagues had been sending signals of their frustration at becoming overly dependent on external aid for some time. Moreover, in a sign of the government's changing attitude, in the preceding few months, many NGOs based in Pyongyang had faced problems getting permission to travel and visit projects outside the capital. Because Caritas had begun to shift from primarily delivering emergency aid to focusing on rehabilitation and development, North Korean officials made clear that we were welcome to continue our work, even as they asked other NGOs to leave. The fact that Caritas had not opened an office with staff based in Pyongyang—a step I had long opposed, convinced that as long we could regularly visit, the problems of being based there would outweigh the benefits—appeared to make it easier for the North Koreans to continue to welcome us.

As part of its new approach, however, the government said it would dissolve in December 2005 the Flood Damage Rehabilitation Committee, our primary interlocutor since the earliest days of the famine. This led in turn to the end of the Food Aid Liaison Unit that had been operating within the WFP, established and funded by a group of NGOs, including Caritas. The FALU had played a key role in monitoring the delivery of food aid, but the government made clear that from now on, it was no longer interested in such aid. Going forward, our new partner would be, at least for the time being, the country's National Commission for the DPRK for UNESCO, which had hosted me on my first visit in 1995. The unfortunate result was that the whole process of nurturing good working relationships and cultivating the trust so essential to being able to operate in the DPRK had to start again. I felt like things had come full circle.

One sign of the level of suspicion that still permeated so many of our dealings with the DPRK came when the FALU was wound up. Located in the WFP compound in Pyongyang's diplomatic quarter, the FALU office contained documents, correspondence, and other papers that had accumulated during the nine years of its existence. We were uncertain whether we would be allowed to take the papers out of the country—although the FALU was housed with a UN agency, no one there had diplomatic status—and did not want the papers to fall into the hands of the North Koreans. So we decided instead to burn the material. On a clear, chilly day in the courtyard of the WFP building, we consigned box after box to the flames. A photo shows me and a couple of colleagues with sheepish grins on our faces as we watch much of the written history of the organization go up in smoke.

Meanwhile, international organizations and NGOs were scrambling to figure out what to do. Some, whose mandates and funding were based solely on delivering emergency humanitarian aid, had no choice but to pack up and leave. These included, among others, the Adventist Development and Relief Agency (ADRA), the German Campus für Christus, the Canada-based Global Aid Network (GAIN), and the Italian NGO Cesvi. Those who wanted to continue suddenly faced the challenge of, in effect, repackaging themselves. They needed to meet North Korea's new requirements while simultaneously satisfying donors who had been willing to help provide food but who were much less comfortable with the idea of development aid that many saw as propping up the regime. In some cases, they presented the different focus as just a minor shift with a new name. Then the European Union got involved.

The EU had maintained an office of Humanitarian Aid Operations (ECHO) in Pyongyang since the earliest days of the famine in 1996. Now, in deference to the new North Korean regulations, the ECHO office was closed. However, an EU technical office remained open. To get around the new rules, this office offered to put NGOs eager to continue operating in the DPRK under its umbrella. With the arrangement, the organizations effectively gave up their old identities and were renamed Unit One, Unit Two, and so on. With these new public profiles, NGO staff no longer used their old name cards, and they removed logos with the names of their original organizations from their vehicles. It was in many ways just a facade, but the move enabled the North Korean officials tasked with dealing with humanitarian agencies to tell their bosses that the new rules were being implemented, while ensuring that at least some of those agencies, under the aegis of the EU, could carry on their work.

For me, the changes in North Korea coincided with a series of rather unsettling developments within Caritas. In the wake of Hong Kong's handover to China in 1997, and especially following the death in 2003 of the organization's longtime leader in the territory, Father Francesco Lerda, the feel at the office became increasingly different. The Hong Kong Chinese priest who succeeded Lerda repeatedly made clear his view that, regardless of Hong Kong's long-standing position as an international crossroads, locals should play an increasingly important role. I did not altogether disagree, but in fact there were fewer than a half dozen foreigners holding senior positions in Caritas–Hong Kong, an organization with thousands of full-time staff members. All the rest were locals, so I felt that in my case, the argument did not carry much weight. Nonetheless, I could definitely sense some resentment toward me over the fact that, as the organization's director of international cooperation and lead in dealing with North Korea, I had a higher international profile and a wider range of contacts around the world than anyone else in the office. This manifested itself in often unsubtle hints that a Chinese person should have my job. I began to feel that the writing was on the wall, and I might soon have to consider leaving.

At the same time, as South Korea's engagement with North Korea continued to accelerate, the Caritas branch in Seoul, known as Caritas Coreana, made a push to take charge of the organization's activities in the DPRK. In principle, the move made sense. I had long favored greater involvement by organizations from South Korea, with its potential to impact both the humanitarian effort and the burgeoning cooperation between North and South. At the same time, however, I was acutely conscious of how complex and volatile the politics of the Korean peninsula could be, and I knew that any North-South thaw could be reversed in an instant.

Moreover, the North Koreans had a long-standing prohibition on South Koreans' traveling outside Pyongyang. With projects dotted all over the country, I was concerned that the regular visits and monitoring activities that had taken up so much of my time would be severely limited—a development that could well undermine the confidence of the donors who were funding Caritas's efforts in the North. Weighing up the admirable idealism of my South Korean colleagues with the harsh challenges of getting anything done in the DPRK, I was concerned that giving Caritas Coreana the leading role might jeopardize much of what had been achieved.

Yet the cumulative impact of these developments was, in effect, to make me feel as if I was being pushed out—a feeling that intensified when the head of Caritas–Hong Kong offered me a new two-year contract, but with my role to be confined largely to fundraising. Although not bitter, I turned him down, noting in a letter that "I do not believe the new arrangement would work out. And the reason for this is that important components for a happy and productive working relationship are no longer in place. These include, for example, issues related to trust and transparency, as well as Caritas–Hong Kong's localization policy, and thus my job security." After twenty-eight years with Caritas, it was time for me to look elsewhere.

In mid-2005, I attended an international conference on humanitarian aid to North Korea held in Beijing. During one session, I happened by chance to sit next to the head of East Asian operations for the Swiss Agency for Development and Cooperation. As we chatted, he casually mentioned to me that the SDC was looking for a new director for its Pyongyang office, which had been set up in 1997. He asked me, "Why don't you apply?"

I was intrigued. Caritas and the SDC had cooperated on a number of projects. I had known all the previous SDC chiefs in Pyongyang, and we had even traveled together occasionally. This appeared to be an opportunity for deeper engagement with North Korea, with the resources of the Swiss government, at a critical turning point for the DPRK, as well an opportunity for a fresh start for me just when my circumstances at Caritas–Hong Kong had soured.

The job was officially posted in the autumn of 2005, and I submitted my application. While waiting for an answer, I made my fiftieth trip to the DPRK in March 2006. The international community had shrunk dramatically. Several NGOs had pulled out, and apart from the small number of diplomats, there were only fifty-eight resident foreigners—thirty-one from the United Nations, ten from a half dozen NGOs under the umbrella of the EU, and a few others. Those who remained spoke of the difficulty of getting permission to travel outside the capital, and of continuing uncertainty about their work. I held a series of meetings with our new official partner, the National Commission for the DPRK for UNESCO, and informed staffers that going forward, Caritas–Hong Kong would no longer be the liaison agency for the DPRK, and that this role would be taken over by Caritas Coreana in South Korea. The North Koreans did not object, but it was evident that they were not pleased. My trip notes say that "this statement was accepted without comment." Moreover, in our conversations, they were less than forthcoming about future working arrangements.

Nonetheless, as far as I was concerned, it was still business as usual, at least for now. In Pyongyang, I held meetings with the Ministries of Health, Labor, Agriculture, and Foreign Trade as well as the Fisheries Bureau. While other foreigners continued to have trouble getting permission for field trips, I was able to travel more than 1,300 kilometers by jeep, visiting the provinces of South Hamgyong, North Hamgyong, and South Pyongan, checking on a variety of projects and trying to determine what adjustments might be needed going forward.

One of the stops was Hamhung, the capital city of South Hamgyong. Devastated during the Korean War, it had been rebuilt under the guidance of East German architects and engineers in the 1950s, with the monotonous and ugly concrete slab structures typical of East German Plattenbau architecture. Hamhung had been particularly badly affected by the famine, and Caritas had been active there for a long time. I was put up at the Sinhungsan Hotel in the city center. My experience at the hotel was, I thought, a good reflection of the broader situation in North Korea. The hotel rooms had been renovated, and the hotel shop displayed an eclectic variety of goods—milk chocolate from Argentina, tins of sausage from Germany, jars of red cabbage and black olives. Yet the hotel had no running water, and just outside the front door, I saw children in rags begging. Meanwhile, I was being charged fifty-six euros a night. In a market I visited, the unofficial exchange rate for one euro was 3,000 won, meaning my room was costing, at the unofficial rate, 168,000 won per night. Yet the average monthly salary for a doctor was just 2,500 won plus occasional fringe benefits. It was a vivid example of the distortions in the country's still-struggling economy.

In Hamhung, I visited three hospitals, holding candid discussions with hospital officials about the government's decision to shift from emergency assistance to development aid and what it would mean. I remained uncertain whether the North Koreans themselves had any idea how in practice the transition was to be handled. For example, in Pyongyang, officials had told me that they were interested now in acquiring medical equipment, and rather than drugs, they wanted raw materials to develop a domestic pharmaceutical industry. But at the hospitals in Hamhung, the immediate need for drugs and medical supplies was obvious. It was not clear to me how a situation like this would be resolved.

The challenge of balancing immediate needs with long-term development also was evident when I visited a district hospital in the city. It had no tap water, limited supplies of electricity, and no generator. When I asked if the government was providing drugs, staff members began to laugh and said in Korean, "*Opsomida*," meaning "not available." At another hospital, doctors told me they also faced an acute shortage of drugs, apart from aspirin. The newest X-ray machine dated back to 1980. On their wish list were upgrading the operating room, acquiring diagnostic equipment such as an ultrasound machine or a gastroscope, and machinery to produce both intravenous fluids and traditional Korean medicine. It was clear to me that the government-mandated transition was not going to be easy and would likely cause considerable human suffering.

Despite the grim circumstances, back in Pyongyang, I was delighted and moved when both my Korean colleagues and members of the small international community staged parties at the Friendship Restaurant, a popular hangout located in the city's diplomatic compound, to mark my fiftieth visit. The Koreans had arranged for singing and dancing, with a female dance troupe wearing the traditional flowing *hanbok* dress. The Pyongyang office of the SDC arranged a cheese-themed evening featuring a Kathi Zellweger quiz. All the guests were given cards with good-humored questions about me. Among them: "What was the first song Kathi was challenged to sing on her first visit to the DPRK in 1995?" "How many years has Kathi lived outside Switzerland?" And, "What is the difference between Kathi's number of visits to the DPRK and her age (in months)?" To this last question, one guest sardonically answered, "Based on the number of visits—should be retired."

A month after returning to Hong Kong, I was offered the SDC job. But they wanted me to start almost immediately, and despite all the recent frustrations, I did not feel I could simply walk out on Caritas after so many years. I wanted to do what I could to smooth the way for my South Korean colleagues to take over, as well as to ensure that the projects on which I had invested so much time and energy were in the best possible shape to survive. To my relief, the SDC agreed that I could begin in October 2006.

In June, while attending a conference in Seoul, I informed Caritas of my impending departure. Many of my colleagues had surprised faces. "With some regret but also a sense of some accomplishments," I wrote in my resignation letter, "the time has come to move on." The SDC job, I continued, "will be a wonderful new challenge and a unique opportunity to undertake a greater commitment, having already been involved in Korean affairs for over ten years."

In mid-July, I made a final trip to North Korea on behalf of Caritas. Arriving in Pyongyang, I felt that the atmosphere was even more strained than on my previous visit. Even my normally hospitable North Korean interlocutors seemed withdrawn and reluctant to talk or share information. Adding to the tension, on July 4, 2006, two weeks before I flew into Pyongyang, the DPRK had launched seven missiles, including a long-range Taepodong with the potential to reach the continental United States; medium-range Rodongs, capable of hitting targets in Japan; and short-range Scuds, easily able to reach all parts of South Korea. The launches marked the end of a moratorium on missile tests that the North had observed since 1998, and it came as the diplomatic progress of the previous year had stalled.

Following the Bush administration's move to target North Korean assets in a bank in Macau just days after the signing of the September 19, 2005, agreement at the six-party talks, Pyongyang had walked away from the negotiations. When Washington rejected repeated requests for bilateral talks, the missile tests followed. While the launches—and the feverish press coverage they generated—fueled the perception of Kim Jong Il as reckless and bellicose, part of Pyongyang's motivation appeared to be to send a signal that absent diplomatic progress with the United States, the North had no incentive to continue observing its unilateral moratorium on missile and nuclear programs. The US response—to condemn Pyongyang at the United Nations and push for sanctions—only heightened the tension.

Despite the strains I felt, life in Pyongyang carried on. I was struck by what seemed to be more cars on the roads, while colleagues reported that the supply of energy was more consistent, and power cuts were fewer and for shorter periods of time. Renovation work was underway in several parts of the city, and large groups of workers were laboring away, encouraged by music blaring from loudspeakers, or sometimes from live bands. The sharp drop in the number of foreign residents had taken a toll on shops and restaurants, with the result that discounts, free dishes, or coupons for future visits were often on offer. And a wide range of goods was still available in the markets.

The dominant feature of that visit was the destruction caused by a new series of floods. Triggered by a typhoon, the floods left hundreds of people dead and thousands homeless, as well as ruined crops and damaged an already shaky infrastructure. The scene brought back memories of my first two trips in 2005, when the country had been hit by even more devastating floods that had proved to be the tipping point in the descent into famine. Driving again to Hamhung, I saw inundated fields, destroyed bridges, and vehicles that had gone off the road. The few remaining members of the humanitarian aid community in Pyongyang were more than willing to support the victims. The International Federation of the Red Cross and Red Crescent Societies began providing emergency kits through its North Korean counterpart, while the World Food Program offered food aid.

But the government indicated that, while grateful for any donations, it was not going to launch a formal appeal for international help. To me, it was a sign that, having just decreed an end to emergency assistance, the authorities did not want to signal any return to previous policy, even if it meant that people who needed assistance would not get it. I saw it as a worrying sign that the cautious movement toward greater openness had slowed and was in danger of being reversed. The diplomatic stalemate and the July 4 missile tests only heightened the tension.

It was in this uncertain climate in the summer of 2006 that I concluded my last trip for Caritas. Before leaving the organization, however, I was asked to fly to Rome for a meeting with colleagues at the head office and those from Caritas Coreana to discuss the handover of the North Korea portfolio. Despite my impending departure, the mood was cordial. Yet I was struck by the degree of skepticism among all but those from Seoul about the new arrangement. In our discussions, I and others emphasized the crucial importance of providing regular and reliable reports about Caritas projects in the North for donors, without whose help nothing would be possible. I also was concerned that the Caritas personnel from South Korea would not be as rigorous about the monitoring process as I had been. But they were determined to proceed, and motivated by the admirable—if, at least in my view, somewhat naive—view that as Koreans, even from the South, they needed to play a central role in promoting both economic development and North-South reconciliation. In any case, I wished them well and made clear that they should feel free to be in touch with me once I began my new job with the SDC.

As a Catholic organization, Caritas Internationalis has its headquarters within Vatican City. In the midst of one meeting, we were suddenly asked to go to the offices of the Vatican's secretary of state for a ceremony. Once we arrived, I was flabbergasted to be singled out and given the Order of St. Gregory the Great, established in 1831 and the highest award the Catholic Church can give a layperson—male or female, and sometimes to non-Catholics. It put me in quite exalted company, as previous recipients had included the writer G. K. Chesterton; Eunice Kennedy Shriver, sister of President John F. Kennedy and the founder of the Special Olympics; and the comedian Bob Hope.

Recovering from my astonishment, I told the gathering, "I am accepting this award with pride and humility. It is a great honor. But do I deserve such recognition? What I have achieved is all thanks to Caritas. So, I share this award with my Caritas colleagues and friends. North Korea is a special place, a strange country. The news from there is all negative and bad. It is so easy to forget that there are twenty-four million people in North Korea—struggling for survival, suffering, day by day. It is these people I care for. I hope that my new position with the Swiss government will give me even greater opportunities to contribute to the well-being of the North Korean people and to peace and reconciliation on the Korean peninsula."

After my twenty-eight years with Caritas, it was a bittersweet moment. As I looked back, I was amazed that in the previous ten years, Caritas and its donors, with me playing a central role, had managed to raise some $33 million in cash to provide food aid (66.6 percent); agricultural inputs (20.4 percent); assistance to the health sector (8.9 percent); other items such as blankets, shoes, clothing, maternity kits, and tools for UN/WFP food for work programs (4.2 percent); and assistance in capacity-building (0.9 percent). In all, over fifty organizations, a surprising number of them not religious, as well as many individuals had contributed. Even the Caritas office in impoverished Bangladesh had sent $500. One of the biggest supporters was the Irish Catholic organization Trócaire, which provided nearly 15 percent of the total amount raised. One hundred and fifty years earlier, from 1845 to 1852, Ireland had suffered a devastating famine. It was one reason why the crisis in the DPRK resonated so powerfully there.

I had worked especially closely with the Canadian Foodgrains Bank and the Mennonite Central Committee. Both organizations had contributed cash to Caritas appeals: the CFGB, $3.35 million and the MCC, $660,000. Beyond this, they had together contributed some 78,944 metric tons of food (mostly cereals, but also pulses, oil, vitamins and minerals for blended food, and spinach seeds). In addition, the MCC had donated canned meat, a dried soup mix, school and hygiene kits, comforters, kits for newborns, secondhand medical equipment, and sewing machines. Altogether, the in-kind donations from the two organizations were worth over $24 million.

Given the difficulties of operating in the DPRK, it was not an insignificant achievement. Thousands—perhaps tens of thousands—of lives had been saved. Walking out of the Vatican, I was deeply grateful to all those who had helped. I remain so today.

At the same time, I was eager to return to North Korea and take up my new position with the SDC. I knew it would be challenging but also, I hoped, full of exciting possibilities.

Then, just days before I arrived in Pyongyang, North Korea conducted a nuclear test for the first time. The shock waves reverberated around the world.

CHAPTER ELEVEN

Madame Grandmother

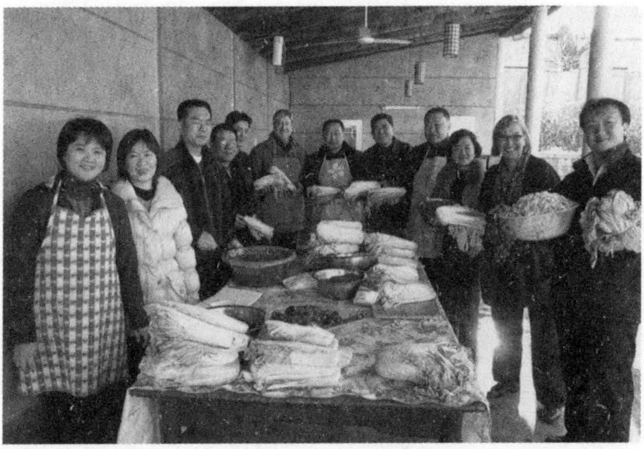

Tho whole SDC team in Pyongyang preparing Kimchi for the long winter.

When North Korea ended its self-imposed moratorium on missile tests with the launch of seven missiles on July 4, 2006, the political symbolism of doing so on America's national holiday was clearly intentional. The tests gave a strong boost to hard-liners in Washington who had long been advocating a tougher posture toward Pyongyang. The anger was shared, to varying degrees, in Seoul, Tokyo, and even Beijing. Within two weeks of the launches, the UN Security Council passed a resolution demanding that the DPRK halt all deployment and testing of missiles. For Kim Jong Il's regime, backing down in the face of such pressure was unthinkable. And so, on October 6, 2006, as I was in Switzerland following the Rome meeting preparing for my move to Pyongyang, the government of North Korea crossed the nuclear Rubicon and staged its first nuclear test, becoming just the eighth country to join the club of nuclear weapons states.

The test was widely seen as a game changer. It showed that the DPRK had basically mastered nuclear weapons technology and possessed enough weapons-grade plutonium to conduct a test while having some left over to make more bombs. Yet again, the UN Security Council met and passed a resolution denouncing the test and requiring all countries to block the transfer of materiel related to Pyongyang's nuclear and missile programs. Although not a member of the Security Council, and despite its official posture of neutrality, Switzerland joined in the condemnation, with the foreign ministry in Berne on October 9 denouncing the test as "counter to international efforts to prevent the proliferation of nuclear weapons and a threat to security in the region."[3] Across the globe, pressure grew to further cut off a country already subject to a host of international sanctions. Indeed, Switzerland became one of the first countries to publish a list of luxury goods to be banned from export to the DPRK, a step that particularly irritated the government in Pyongyang.

It was an unsettling backdrop against which to begin my new assignment, and I wrestled with a host of contradictory feelings. I was uneasy to see the increase in tension and concerned that nuclear weapons had become a reality on the peninsula—but equally worried about the plight of ordinary North Koreans. They had no say in their government's policies, and the vast majority simply were struggling to survive. I remained convinced that, even in the current crisis atmosphere, economic and humanitarian involvement not only would help people in need but might—however quixotic the sentiment may have seemed at the time—draw the DPRK into further international engagement and make some contribution, however modest, to lowering the political temperature.

So it was with a mixture of excitement, anticipation, and anxiety that, almost exactly a month after the nuclear test, I boarded an Air Koryo plane from Beijing to Pyongyang. I had taken this flight so often during my time at Caritas that it felt like traveling home. The creaky Soviet-built aircraft, the cabin staff with the Kim Il Sung and Kim Jong Il lapel pins, food barely good enough to fill your stomach, the propaganda magazines that were the only in-flight reading material—all made me feel oddly at home.

Among my fellow passengers was a group of left-wing South Koreans. Ignoring the international condemnation, they were journeying to the "enemy" capital, proudly displaying the Korean "reunification flag"—a white backdrop with the entire Korean peninsula in light blue—that originally had been designed to represent all of Korea when North and South were planning to field one team for the 1990 Asian Games. Although that plan fell victim to political disagreements, the unification flag had been used when the two Koreans marched together at the opening ceremony of the 2000 and 2004 Olympics. Under the current grim circumstances, I wondered if perhaps seeing this flag now was a positive sign.

For all the alarming headlines and heated international rhetoric, Pyongyang itself was curiously quiet. During the day, the weather was cool and crisp, the sky bright blue, and the trees dotted with colorful late-autumn leaves. On the city's streets, the female traffic wardens—whose robot-like movements had long been a source of amusement and astonishment to foreign visitors—were busy directing the few vehicles driving by. Despite the chilly weather, they were wearing their summer skirts. I learned that only on November 16 would they be allowed to change to the striking blue trousers, boots, and warm jackets with fur collars that constituted their winter uniform. Power cuts remained commonplace, and as evening fell, much of the city was dark.

With only a handful of foreigners now based in Pyongyang, a new arrival was a big deal. I was greeted warmly, and my Swiss colleagues from the SDC treated me to a welcome dinner with my favorite Korean dish, *dolsot bibimbap*—vegetables, minced meat, and a sunny-side-up egg artistically spread out on a bed of fluffy white rice and served with very hot red bean paste in a *dolsot*, or stone pot. It was good to be back, ready for a new adventure.

The Swiss Agency for Development and Cooperation was established in the 1960s. Operating under the Swiss Federal Department of Foreign Affairs, it has the mandate to implement the Swiss government's foreign policy on humanitarian and development cooperation, to "reduce poverty, foster economic self-reliance...and provide better access to education and health care services." It runs projects in many countries with wide-ranging cultural differences, such as Afghanistan, Burkina Faso, and since the mid-1990s, North Korea. In the latter, it was now supporting efforts to enhance food security by expanding the cultivation of hilly land, to promote greater crop yields through effective biological pest management, as well supporting a pilot agricultural credit scheme and a variety of capacity-building initiatives, including a plan to provide training for North Korean officials in the workings of international trade and a modern economy. From now on, together with my team of over twenty people, I would manage these and other programs.

The SDC office was split between two buildings that had originally housed the Hungarian embassy. After Hungary switched its diplomatic representation to Beijing, with an ambassador based there also accredited to the DPRK, the newly built facilities had been largely unused, so the Swiss government rented them for the SDC. We sublet half of the first building to the NGO German Agro Action. The other half was where the SDC's Korean staff members, international experts, and consultants worked. The ground floor of the second building housed the reception area, my office, my personal assistant's workplace, and storerooms. Upstairs was my apartment: an L-shaped living room with a TV in the corner, a dining room, a kitchen, a larder, and two bedrooms, each with its own bathroom.

Interestingly, our two buildings were not part of the larger Munsudong diplomatic compound, where most foreign embassies and international agencies were located. Instead, we were adjacent to just three other missions. The Romanians had a huge compound, a throwback to the heyday of fraternal socialist ties with North Korea. The Egyptian embassy was more modest, but the Iranian embassy was also large, augmented by a recently built mosque. Each of our compounds was self-contained and surrounded by walls, with North Korean guards at the gates to keep all but authorized locals out. While those who lived in the larger diplomatic area had only foreigners for neighbors, across the street from where I lived and worked was a large public housing estate, enabling me to at least get some sense of the rhythm of daily life for the average Pyongyang resident, and to feel slightly less isolated.

Monday, November 13, 2006, was my first day at work in Pyongyang for the SDC. After my twenty-eight years at Caritas, it was a strange sensation to be introduced to my new colleagues. In addition to me, there were four other foreign nationals—a deputy director, an expert who handled agricultural projects, an assistant who supported the agricultural expert, and an executive assistant who worked directly with me. More than a dozen North Koreans made up the rest of the team. Unlike during my early Caritas years in North Korea, when the Ministry of Foreign Affairs supplied most staff to international agencies, the authorities by now understood that an organization like the SDC, with its focus on development, required people with specific expertise, not just ministry bureaucrats. Indeed, whenever there was a change in personnel, we would be allowed to interview up to three candidates and make our own choice. By contrast, in China, even with its impressive economic achievements, staff members for foreign missions and companies were still assigned largely by the government, with the employers having little or no choice about who was sent to work for them.

Among my Korean colleagues were one who worked for the SDC's Agro-Processing and Marketing Support program, one in a pilot agricultural credit scheme, and two in the agricultural support programs. A dynamic young woman was focused on capacity development programs. In addition, we had an administrative-and-finance officer, a cashier, an interpreter, drivers, a mechanic, gardeners, cooks, and cleaning women. Most important was the liaison officer, the most senior staff member among the Korean team and my link to the Ministry of Foreign Affairs. I found my colleagues polite and always well-dressed, but a female SDC boss was something new, and I could sense their curiosity, tinged with more than a little anxiety. They appeared to be thinking, *Who is this woman? How will she manage? How will she treat us?* I knew it would take some time to gain their confidence.

Meanwhile, I began to settle in. My new position as an employee of the Swiss government meant that I had diplomatic status, including a new diplomatic passport. Soon after I arrived, an appointment was made for me at the foreign ministry, where, after filling out numerous forms, I was given my diplomatic card, making me an official member of Pyongyang's tiny diplomatic community. As a resident, I also was entitled to apply for a North Korean driver's license, and I would be able to use one of the office's eight vehicles.

Soon after my arrival, I set off for the traffic bureau with two local staff, where I went through a brief question-and-answer session described as the theoretical part of learning how to drive in the DPRK. Most of the questions were straightforward and practical, but one stood out. What was the correct behavior if, while driving, I saw one of the city's colorful traffic ladies hold her baton straight up? The answer was to immediately pull over and stop. The reason was that it meant the Great General—Kim Jong Il himself—was about to pass by. After the Q&A came ten minutes of routine driving to show that I knew how to operate a car. As I navigated the largely empty streets, the instructor engaged in animated conversation with the

SDC local staff. At the end, I was told that I had passed and that my license would be ready for collection in a matter of days.

On our way back to the SDC office, it became clear that the most important person in this whole process had been the one who helped with translation. A young, cheerful fellow whom I instinctively liked, he had told me soon after we met that as a child, he used to watch Russian and Chinese movies dubbed in Korean. He said that because the foreign actors appeared to be speaking in Korean, he was convinced his country's language was used everywhere in the world. It was quite a shock, he confessed, when he later learned this wasn't true.

I asked how I had done on the theoretical part of the driver's test. He smiled and said, "Well, Miss Kathi, I translated right!" Then I asked what he and the instructor had discussed as I drove around. Was it my skills as a driver? The answer was a resounding no. The whole conversation had been about the instructor's keen interest in Swiss watches!

In early December, the first snow fell in Pyongyang. The city looked like it had been coated in sugar, the white in striking contrast to the many old apartment blocks that appeared to have been recently repainted in light blue, pink, or lime green, making Pyongyang look less dismal than usual. The story making the rounds of the international community was that Kim Jong Il had ordered the buildings to be repainted after aides told him about the foreign media reports stating how drab the city looked.

The next day, the temperature dropped. It was an unfortunate time for the heating system in our building to break down, but that's what happened. Luckily, a mechanic from Switzerland had just arrived to service the SDC's fleet of cars—which he did in an outdoor garage where the temperature dipped to minus ten degrees Celsius. A jack of all trades, he also was able to get the heating on again, but we, like everyone in the city, faced regular power cuts. Although people said the situation was better this year than in previous ones, we, along with other foreign missions, had our own generator. Still, the cuts often required me to get up at night, put on a heavy winter coat over my pajamas, and walk across the compound to turn on the generator and the stabilizer, before huddling in bed waiting for the reassuring sound of power returning.

Even with the generator, the temperature in the office rarely exceeded fifteen or sixteen degrees Celsius, but I was struck that my North Korean colleagues seemed happy to come to work, as our premises were apparently still much warmer than their homes. The freezing conditions in most buildings in Pyongyang were brought home to me when I went to a meeting at the Grand People's Study House, the national library, located on Kim Il Sung Square next to the Taedong River. It was bitterly cold, and I shivered through the meeting with my winter coat on. I wanted to keep my gloves on as well, but writing notes with them was too difficult. At least the tea mugs served as hand warmers. Even in our office, we all had gloves, scarves, an extra sweater, and a torch ready on our desks, and, underneath the desk, winter boots, in the event that a fresh power outage made the temperature drop even further.

Barely a month after arriving in Pyongyang, I traveled to Beijing. This was to become a regular part of life for the SDC team, primarily because the Swiss government sent our mail and other important items to the Swiss embassy in Beijing. As a result, every five to six weeks, I or one of my colleagues had the chance to go to China to collect the diplomatic pouch and other supplies. It was a welcome, if brief, rest-and-relaxation break from the rigors of life in Pyongyang.

These trips to China involved a long and dreary twenty-four-hour train ride. Apart from a meager lunch, there was no service on the North Korean train, so I would manage with a bar of chocolate, three apples, a couple of bottles of water, and some packets of instant coffee. Hot water, at least, was made available from time to time. Passing through various train stations on one such visit, I noticed sacks of rice and maize piled high, presumably for use in the now-revived public distribution system. That evening, we reached Sinuiju, on the border with China. The city was pitch black, in striking contrast to the bright lights in the Chinese city of Dandong across the Yalu River. The next morning, we arrived in Beijing.

On that occasion, I held three meetings with Dante Martinelli, who was at that time accredited as Switzerland's ambassador to China, the DPRK, and Mongolia. As he visited Pyongyang only occasionally, I would in practice be the most senior Swiss official there. I would be reporting to him whatever insights I had gleaned on political and diplomatic issues, while dealing with SDC headquarters in the Swiss capital Berne on the substance of our development projects.

This arrangement had the potential to be complicated, but in fact worked surprisingly well. For me, the most important part of the trip was loading up on supplies that were not available in Pyongyang. I discovered that there was an Ikea shop in Beijing, where I spent hours buying a variety of household items and even some small pieces of furniture. When I checked in for my Air Koryo flight back to Pyongyang, I had seventy-six kilograms of excess baggage.

I returned to Pyongyang just before Christmas. Living so far from home for so many years, I always made a special effort to celebrate the holiday. We got a nice tree and put it outside the SDC building, decorated with 250 lights and forty red balls that had been in my shipment of personal goods from Switzerland. As I gazed at it proudly, I wondered if it was the only real Christmas tree in the city—as well as what my North Korean neighbors across the street must be thinking. We held an office Christmas party where we made raclette, the traditional Swiss dish with melted cheese and potatoes, using cheese I had brought from Switzerland. I also gave everyone a small gift, carefully wrapped in colorful paper. I had the impression that it was the first time my North Korean colleagues had ever received such a nicely wrapped gift. It helped to break the ice, as did my decision to make ten liters of *Glühwein*—mulled wine.

I found red wine at what was known as the Argentinian store. This outlet was near the Ryugyong Hotel, a 105-story structure started in the late 1980s and intended to be one of the tallest in the world, but its still-uncompleted status meant that the giant building towering over the city instead had become a symbol of so much that seemed wrong with the North Korean system. For some reason, the shop stocked imported products, including cheap Malbec wine from Argentina. With the mulled wine, the mood quickly became very lighthearted, and the cheeks of the North Koreans, whose fondness for alcohol is legendary, soon turned bright red. "Miss Kathi's *Glühwein*" after work at the SDC soon would become a tradition on cold Friday evenings in winter. Perhaps it contributed to the embarrassingly elaborate title that my North Korean colleagues started to use when they introduced me to other Koreans: Madame Grandmother Katherina Zellweger, country director of the Swiss Agency for Development.

On New Year's Eve that first year, I joined about fifty other expats at the still-vibrant Random Access Club, in the World Food Program building, for drinks, conversation, and a little dancing. Just before midnight, a few of us drove to Kim Il Sung Square. Despite the bitter cold, the vast space was dotted with people, some with families, others with their work units. As the clock struck midnight, we all exchanged good wishes for the New Year. Just fifteen minutes later, however, loudspeakers blared across the square telling the crowd it was now time to go home. As everyone dutifully departed, two grinning teenagers asked to have their photo taken with me, the blonde foreigner. A larger group of adults also gathered around our SDC jeep. They were curious but friendly. The experience reminded me of being in China in the early 1980s. I thought it was a good sign of a change in the political climate.

Early the next morning, the North Korean government invited ambassadors and heads of missions to mark the New Year by paying their respects before the embalmed corpse of Kim Il Sung. Following Kim's death in 1994, his preserved body had been put on display at the sprawling Kumsusan Palace, for many years his office and home. Now, Kumsusan had been transformed into a vast mausoleum—the physical and spiritual center of the Kim cult that was the glue holding the North Korean system together.

In formal dress, several dozen foreigners, some of whom seemed a little the worse for wear following the festivities of the previous evening, gathered in the bitter cold near the entrance to the palace at 8 a.m. We were then escorted through a series of vast marble corridors that led to a large room dominated by a white marble statue of the Great Leader, illuminated from behind by pink lights. Somber music played, while grim-faced members of the Korean People's Army stood next to the walls at rigid attention. After passing through a device that cleaned the soles of our shoes, and another machine that blew air at us to clean any specks of dirt from our clothing (while ruining our hairstyles), we were brought into the cavernous room where Kim's remains, dressed in a white shirt and a dark suit, were displayed in a large glass case. Each visitor was expected to bow three times, but not when they stood behind the Great Leader's head. I watched carefully to see who bowed and who did not. The ambassadors from EU countries kept their heads upright.

After this, we were shown a set of rooms where the North Koreans had installed Kim Il Sung's favorite train carriage as well as a bulletproof Mercedes-Benz that Kim Jong Il had gifted him. Then we walked through an exhibition containing his medals and some of the thousands of gifts that he had received over the decades. Eventually, we ended up in a room where we were asked to write something in a visitors' book. I don't remember my exact words, but it was something to the effect of how impressive the visit had been, and that I wished the people of North Korea well.

The official part of New Year's Day for the diplomatic corps concluded with our attendance at a concert held at the newly refurbished Moranbong Theatre, an imposing white building with four white columns towering over its front steps. The theater is located in the center of Pyongyang near the *Chollima*—a forty-six-meter-tall monument showing a flying horse famous in Korean mythology whose fighting spirit had long been invoked by the government. The acoustics in the theater were extremely good as we sat through a performance of songs and orchestral pieces with titles including "A Paradise of Socialism" and "A Bumper Harvest in the Chongan Plains." Incongruously, the concert also included part of the *Die Fledermaus* operetta by Johann Strauss and Rossini's overture to the opera *William Tell.*

Early on in my tenure, I made two trips outside Pyongyang. One was for three days to Pujon, a mountainous, thickly forested county in South Hamgyong Province, where the SDC was supporting some cooperative farms in an effort to boost agricultural production. Pujon had been an important area during the Japanese occupation of Korea as well as during the Korean War, and had long been closed to foreigners, but an exception had been made to allow the SDC to operate there. Although we stayed in what the locals had dubbed "the Swiss guesthouse," sleeping under portraits of the Great Leader and Dear Leader brought home that I definitely was not in Switzerland.

I also traveled to Ryongchon, where the Swiss government had contributed one hundred thousand Swiss francs to the Swiss arm of the Adventist Development and Relief Agency (ADRA), operated by the Seventh-day Adventist Church, for the reestablishment of the county hospital after the horrific April 2004 train crash and ensuing explosion. The hospital had been inaugurated in November 2006. At the entrance, I noted the usual pictures of Kim Il Sung and Kim Jong Il as well as their sayings on various banners. There were some real patients who appeared seriously ill, but a number of those presented as sick seemed quite OK.

Moreover, I did not notice any personal belongings or other signs of real patients I had seen in visits to other hospitals, and I wondered if these "patients" were just people who had been put under the bed covers for our visit. The donated equipment had arrived and was mostly working, although all Caritas logos had been removed, but to me the hospital seemed too big. With five buildings, upkeep would be expensive, draining scarce resources from caring for those in need. In addition, as in so many places in the DPRK, the heating was not working. The rooms were freezing cold. I felt bad that ADRA had left the country because of the new regulations requiring a shift to development aid, and thus could not help get the place in better shape.

Despite my years of involvement with North Korea, I had much to learn about the SDC, the nature of its work in the DPRK, and what was involved in my being, for all practical purposes, a member of the diplomatic corps. I spent hours reading documents and speaking with our expat staff and the local project officers to get up to speed. Every Friday, we had a staff meeting at 9 a.m. This was followed by a weekly interagency meeting, where the heads of all UN organizations, embassies, NGOs, and important foreign visitors involved in aid projects would share insights and trade information. From time to time, I also made a point of taking the local staff for dinner, which helped to break down barriers and create a foundation for positive working relationships. It was interesting to hear one of my North Korean colleagues express an interest in visiting Canada and the United States, while another wanted to see the countries of Scandinavia. It was clear that people assigned to work with foreign organizations had more knowledge and curiosity about the rest of the world, and were less influenced than other locals by the incessant propaganda that surrounded them.

It wasn't long before I had my first run-in with the Korean European Coordination Committee (KECCA), the SDC's counterpart at the foreign ministry. At a meeting, I was informed that if we invited North Koreans to travel abroad for study tours or training programs, in addition to all the other costs, the SDC was now expected also to pay the fee for the participants' North Korean passports, at thirty euros per passport. It was an unpleasant meeting. I insisted that as the SDC was covering everything else, this should be a local contribution. The committee members showed anger at my suggestion. I wondered if they were just testing how much more they could demand from me.

As the meeting continued, though, they admitted with some embarrassment that the reason for the request was that North Korean passports had to be printed outside of the country (presumably in China) and thus the North Koreans needed scarce hard currency to pay for them. Knowing that bigger issues would undoubtedly come up, not wanting to fight over what was, in the end, a relatively small amount, and aware that in the long run, building trust and cooperation would be crucial, I eventually agreed. But the conversation also made me wonder: if North Korea's passports were printed outside the DPRK because it lacked the special paper to print them on, was it possible that the fake US dollars the country had become notorious for spreading, the so-called super notes, also were being printed in another country? I had no way to know.

The idiosyncrasies of the North Korean system continued to manifest themselves. Early in the new year, two technicians from Switzerland arrived to connect the office to the server of the Swiss foreign ministry. This was a big development, as it meant we would be able to phone overseas free of charge instead of having to pay 3.70 euros per minute for using the local international phone connection. Also, our conversations would be much more secure. The wife of one expat staffer told me she had been phoning her elderly mother in France every Saturday afternoon. The two had always spoken in a mixture of English and French. While they were chatting one day, suddenly there was a click on the line and a little Korean voice pleaded, in English, "Please not to change languages." My colleague laughed the incident off. The person monitoring the call was, after all, only doing their job.

I was pleased with her reaction, because some among the foreign community had a difficult time dealing with the fact that, in all likelihood, everything was monitored. They would go out on their balcony for whispered conversations on what they considered sensitive issues. I felt I knew how to handle confidential information without having to act like that. Moreover, given the North Koreans' deep suspicion toward all foreigners, the less we behaved like secretive spies, feeding all their preconceptions, the better.

The installation of the server also allowed us much easier access to the internet and to international news. Until then, I had been relying on a short-wave radio I had purchased in Hong Kong. I would occasionally tune in to Radio Russia, Radio China International, and, especially around 2 a.m., the BBC or Radio Free Asia. It seemed clear that the North Koreans were trying to jam the signals of what they viewed as "hostile" outlets, and most of the time when I tried to tune in to these channels, the radio just produced static. But I did occasionally hear some news, including updates on the six-party talks aimed at resolving the nuclear issue. Despite the crisis caused by the nuclear test, the talks, involving the United States, the DPRK, China, South Korea, Japan, and Russia, were resuming in Beijing. I was not privy to any details, but it was clear in Pyongyang how important the nuclear test was to the regime's self-image. I saw new billboards with slogans in Korean and translated by my staff into English, saying, "Let us shine forever our becoming a nuclear power, a historic incident in the 5,000 years of our people's history."

Some diplomats and others speculated that the test might make North Korea feel secure enough to push ahead with more economic initiatives, while the North Korean media, in what seemed to me to be an opening bargaining position, stressed that it would not stop its nuclear activities unless the United States lifted financial sanctions. Still, I wondered whether, deep down, people in the North really felt the nuclear program was worth the sacrifice and, especially, the diversion of precious resources that otherwise could have been used to revive the economy.

Nonetheless, as I noted in my first monthly report to the SDC, "North Korea has changed and is more open in comparison to a decade ago. People now tend to speak about business and wanting to earn money. The social fabric of the DPRK society is changing with the appearance of more market and entrepreneurial activities. In today's DPRK, money matters because the government no longer can provide for all basic needs such as food, shelter, health care, education, and social welfare. People today have to fend for themselves: there are winners and losers." But I noted that many acute problems remained. "Inflation has become rampant and the black-market rate for Euros reached a level of around Won 4,000 while the official exchange rate is Won 200. Pay-offs are becoming almost 'normal' and sometime foreigners are also asked to 'contribute,' for example packets of cigarettes or cash," while the 2006 harvest was expected to be smaller than that of 2005.

It was a mixed picture, to be sure, but was nonetheless a dramatic contrast from the first time I had set foot in the DPRK in spring 1995, more than a decade earlier. Perhaps, I thought, there might be cautious grounds for optimism, both about the broader situation and the prospects for our work.

Then came a bombshell by the Swiss parliamentarian Gerhard Pfister, a prominent member of the Christian Democratic People's Party in Switzerland who, in the wake of the October 2006 nuclear test, emerged as a vocal critic of North Korea. Supported by nearly a dozen other parliamentarians, Pfister submitted on December 20, 2006, a motion to the Swiss Federal Council demanding that the SDC end its development program in the DPRK. His motion denounced the North as a "totalitarian dictatorship" and accused the SDC of depicting North Korea's halting efforts at economic reform as a "success of Swiss development cooperation." In the wake of the nuclear test, Pfister declared, "North Korea does not show a 'tentative opening,' rather the opposite."

Having worked for Caritas, a Catholic agency, for almost thirty years, I was particularly disappointed that Gerhard Pfister and ten other parliamentarians who were members of the Christian Democratic People's Party—all Catholics—had made this motion. Moreover, it was precisely the kind of sweeping negative judgement that ignored a more complex reality. I, perhaps more than most, having made scores of trips and now residing in Pyongyang, was well aware of the nature of the North Korean system. But beyond the slogans and the saber-rattling was a society of twenty-four million human beings, most living in conditions of acute distress, and I remained convinced that engagement could help ordinary people while continuing to gradually increase the country's connections with the rest of the world in a way that perhaps could contribute to an easing of tensions.

Both houses of the Swiss Parliament would need to approve the motion for it to become government policy, so in the short term nothing changed. But Pfister's campaign set in motion a protracted political battle over the fate of the SDC in the DPRK that would cast a long shadow over my entire time in Pyongyang.

CHAPTER TWELVE

Barking Rabbits

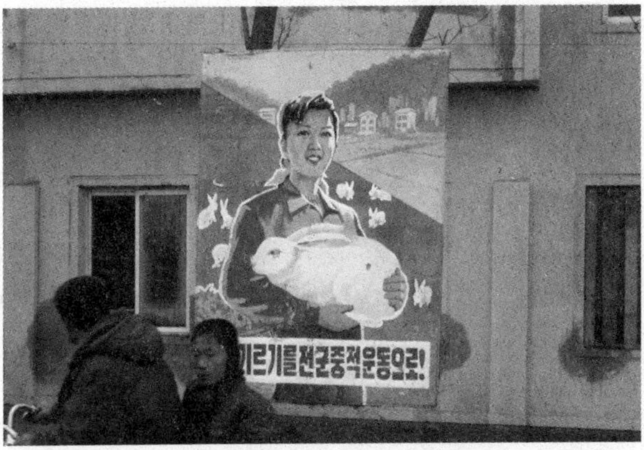

To improve the diet of the population, the government promoted raising grass eating animals.

One thing that became clear early in my tenure in Pyongyang was that I did not need an alarm clock. Every morning at 6 a.m., loudspeakers would begin to blare, pumping out rousing music and government propaganda. Sleep was no longer possible, so I would get up and start my day. In my journal, I noted "how lucky I was to have been born in Switzerland and not into this."

The loudspeakers were but one aspect of the state's seemingly non-stop efforts to mobilize and indoctrinate the population. Driving across Pyongyang for various meetings during the late winter and early spring of 2007, I regularly saw thousands of children rehearsing for the Arirang Mass Games, an extraordinary spectacle held periodically at the city's Mayday stadium. On previous visits, I had attended a number of these events, where up to one hundred thousand people would participate in highly synchronized displays of gymnastics and singing. This was punctuated by the creation of a kind of giant human mosaic composed of performers flipping colored cards in unison to form giant images of whatever happened to be the regime's current propaganda priorities. Sometimes the theme was agricultural or industrial production, but increasingly, the focus was on national defense, with images of soldiers, rockets, and missiles.

Dwarfing mass events in other communist countries, the Arirang Mass Games were an extraordinary form of social control, mobilizing huge numbers of people, mostly students, inculcating loyalty to the leader and demonstrating the clout of the regime. As I was from a country where getting students to stand in a straight line for gym class was often a challenge, it always took my breath away to observe the discipline—indeed regimentation—that was a central characteristic of the mass games.

Each performance required months of rehearsal, and many children had to give up not only their spare time but school time as well. Large groups of youngsters marching, chanting, and engaging in drills became a regular feature of the Pyongyang landscape. I often wondered what these kids and their families really thought. On the few occasions when foreigners were able to speak with either the children or their parents, the standard family response was to express pride at the honor of being selected. There appeared to be little resentment at the demands that participating in the Arirang games required. Indeed, for youngsters brought into Pyongyang from the countryside, I wondered whether the rehearsals meant better food and more pleasant circumstances than they were used to. Whatever the behind-the-scenes arrangements, the Arirang games became one of the DPRK's biggest tourist attractions, and visitors were always asking whether it was possible to go. I never met a foreigner who attended who did not come away impressed and astonished.

In one respect, the games reflected the pride many North Koreans felt now that the country had joined the nuclear club. They also helped to shore up loyalty to the leader and system as the DPRK confronted a sweeping range of new sanctions following the October 2006 nuclear test. These included a UN Security Council resolution prohibiting the export of military supplies from and the import of luxury goods to North Korea. The EU added its own measures, while Japan banned all trade and barred North

Korean vessels from its ports, shutting down a long-standing ferry connection. The tiny foreign community in Pyongyang also felt the impact, as it was increasingly difficult to import goods. Sometimes, the ban on items that conceivably might have had dual civilian and military use seemed excessive. Pig-breeding equipment we ordered from Germany was held up, as well as a steam boiler purchased in China. At the SDC, we were even unable to bring in an air compressor for car repair purposes.

On the diplomatic front, however, the news appeared less bleak. Despite the nuclear test, the six-party talks involving the United States, North Korea, South Korea, China, Russia, and Japan resumed in Beijing and led to an interim agreement under which the North agreed to verifiably disable its Yongbyon plutonium nuclear reactor. At the same time, the North Koreans sent other signals indicating a desire for better relations with the United States, including an invitation for the New York Philharmonic to visit Pyongyang in 2008.

On the domestic front, though, North Korean society remained, as I wrote in an early report to SDC, in dire straits. In early 2007, we heard reports of epidemics of scarlet fever, measles, and rubella, particularly on the east coast—outbreaks made worse by the collapse of childhood immunization programs during the famine years. Overall, the country's infrastructure continued to crumble, power cuts were routine, and I started noticing that ground-level and first-floor apartments or businesses in Pyongyang were often barred and heavily locked, a sign that crime was becoming a concern.

The food situation also was worrisome. It took the North Koreans until March 2007 to provide the international community with figures for 2006 grain production. Unlike in previous years, the government did not permit the United Nations' World Food Program and Food and Agriculture organization to participate in assessing crops, with the result that many of us were skeptical of the figures. A separate assessment by the WFP concluded that in 2007, the country faced a grain shortfall of a million metric tons. Not to mention, the food distribution system still was barely functioning, and the markets, where those with money could get almost anything and those without were deprived, further accentuated the inequality.

In the face of these grim circumstances, I continued to be struck by the resilience and surprising good humor of so many of the North Koreans I encountered. It reinforced my belief that it was wrong not to try to help ordinary people who were not responsible for the failings of a state over which they had no control. But it wasn't an easy task.

As head of the SDC office, working closely with my international and North Korean colleagues, I was in charge of four major initiatives. The first was a program to support North Korean agriculture through a variety of innovative measures, including using new techniques to combat pests and boost output, devising ways to expand the area available for cultivation, and employing technology to help with the planning and monitoring of farmland.

The second was a capacity development program that included the Pyongyang Business School, where foreign experts came to run workshops on international business practices for young North Korean businesspeople and officials, and which sent a variety of groups for courses, conferences, and training programs outside the country. The goal was to improve professional expertise in the fields of international cooperation, economics, business, and agriculture. We also ran projects to improve the food supply by supporting agro-processing and -marketing, as well as a pilot agricultural credit scheme to improve economic performance by using market mechanisms to offset shortcomings in the planned economy.

Apart from the SDC, the only other international organization I knew of working on development projects was the United Nations Development Program (UNDP). The UNDP had been operating in North Korea since 1979. By the time I took up my SDC post, it was involved in a series of projects, from capacity-building to trade and agricultural development. The focus was on introducing North Koreans to modern technology in agriculture, such as using remote sensing to verify the extent of crops and using lasers to assess water levels during times of flooding. The goal was to help North Korea begin to transition from its old, inefficient Soviet-style agricultural system to a new, more modern, sustainable form of development. Like the SDC, the UNDP was providing the DPRK with a window into economic growth strategies used in other parts of the world, and I often met with my colleagues there to share ideas and insights.

In the spring of 2007, however, the UNDP became a victim of both its own internal flaws and the Bush administration's hostility to North Korea, resulting in a controversy that would leave the SDC as the only organization working on development cooperation in the DPRK. It began with a whistleblower, an Albanian named Artjon Shkurtaj, who was working as an operations manager at the UNDP's Pyongyang office. After he raised concerns of sloppy accounting with minimal safeguards within the UNDP, his contract was not renewed. Feeling aggrieved, he repeated his allegations to the US Mission to the United Nations. That led the Bush administration, already hostile to any efforts to assist North Korea's economic recovery, to support a US Senate investigation, which produced a report with a series of damning findings. The most serious was that North Korea had used a UNDP bank account to move $2.72 million to various diplomatic missions around the world, without informing the UNDP. There also was a set of broader allegations of mismanagement and lack of oversight. UNDP officials in New York made the situation worse by trying to downplay the problems rather than address them—which served only to further anger the Bush administration.

I was not altogether surprised to learn about the banking episode, as the DPRK had a long history of somewhat dubious international banking transactions. But I found the other allegations much less substantial. The US Senate investigators criticized the UNDP because North Korean nationals working in its Pyongyang office had been selected by the government, and their salaries were not paid directly to the individuals but to a government agency, which took a cut for itself. Moreover, the investigation claimed, the "UNDP was allowed to conduct on-site project visits only with prior notice and in the company of North Korean officials, [which is] contrary to UNDP best practices."[4] While acknowledging that the UNDP had successfully implemented development projects, the Senate investigation declared that "by operating under the compromised conditions set forth in this report, UNDP rendered itself vulnerable to manipulation by the North Korean government."[5]

To me, these other allegations seemed to be taking standard North Korean behavior and presenting it as some sort of shockingly nefarious scheme. Members of all international organizations had to obtain permission prior to traveling in North Korea and always were accompanied by government officials. However, the North Korean people also were not allowed to travel freely. Without travel permission, there was no travel outside of Pyongyang or the person's county of residence. All local staff were provided by the government as well, and for most international organizations, salaries were paid through the government and not directly to individuals. This had been the case as long as I had been dealing with the DPRK.

Despite these less than optimal arrangements, my own experience had shown that the North Korean authorities occasionally were capable of considerable flexibility. At the SDC, for example, we paid our staff their monthly salary directly to them in cash (euros). They would sign for the payment, and what they did with the money after that was beyond our control. The SDC also would provide field trip allowances to staff members traveling out of Pyongyang. I was always puzzled that my North Korean colleagues did not ask for the funds at the time of the trip, but rather for the money to be paid at the end of the month.

Interestingly, I would later learn that staff members who were entitled to the travel allowance would pool the extra funds and share it with those who worked solely in the Pyongyang office and did not travel. It was a touching example of "socialist sharing"—something I suspected would not happen in most Western societies. Moreover, although our local staff were, like those at the UNDP, assigned by the government, they had genuine professional expertise, not least because it would have been a severe loss of face if the authorities sent someone who was not professionally competent.

In addition, the government began to give us three choices to fill each open position, allowing us to review résumés and conduct interviews before making a hiring decision. New staff would be on an initial three-month probation period. Although it happened only once during my time, that gave the SDC the option of letting go someone who did not work out. The SDC's headquarters in Berne also required me to do annual staff evaluations—something that was unheard of in North Korea. To reduce the awkwardness and manage concerns about losing face, I told my North Korean colleagues they also could evaluate me. Most of them viewed working at the SDC as a privilege. I usually found them committed and conscientious and had few complaints. In their evaluations of me, they generally described me as "tough and fair"—which I found gratifying.

Yet with the UNDP facing sweeping condemnation as part of the Bush administration's broader hostility to engaging with North Korea, which clearly included a strong disapproval of the whole idea of providing development aid, the organization suspended its operations in the DPRK in March 2007 and withdrew seven of its nine foreign staff members. The two who remained were tasked with carrying out a detailed audit, which hopefully would clear the UNDP of the allegations that its funds had been diverted to the North Korean regime.

The departure of the UNDP in what I saw as a largely politically motivated exercise significantly reduced the size of Pyongyang's international community. Even with the large number of personnel at the Russian and Chinese embassies, the total number of expats in the country was now barely three hundred. The atmosphere was gloomy at the weekly interagency meetings, where we gathered to exchange experiences and ideas. For their part, the North Koreans were furious, with the official Korea Central News Agency denouncing the UNDP for "succumbing to outside pressure" from the United States.[6]

For the SDC, it meant losing a key partner, and it left me leading the only organization still working on development cooperation. Just months into the job, I and other SDC staff had lost like-minded colleagues with whom we could share ideas, questions, and concerns. I also was worried that the UNDP episode would provide additional ammunition to those in Switzerland who were campaigning for an end to the SDC's own work in the DPRK. I felt like an ever-darkening cloud was hovering over what my colleagues and I were trying to accomplish.

Despite the difficult circumstances, I threw myself into the job. My mood was lifted by the approach of spring. Winter in the DPRK is particularly dark, cold, and grim. When the first flowers began to appear, everything seemed brighter and more hopeful. I also enjoyed the beautiful flute music of a man who, as the weather got warmer, would stand on a balcony in the apartment building across the street every evening and play.

A key early priority was to further consolidate a positive relationship with my North Korean colleagues, with the goal of making everyone feel that they were part of a single team, not foreigners on one side and Koreans on the other. One opportunity arose on March 8, International Women's Day. After attending a long and boring formal ceremony in the morning, I invited all the female members of our staff, from office workers to cooks and cleaners, to have lunch at my apartment. It was the first time that many of them had been in the residence of a foreigner.

I welcomed them by making several Swiss dishes, including *rösti* (potatoes), as well as baking a cake. Aware that they might find the food strange, I made sure that kimchi was on the menu as well. And I told them they should feel free to look around—which they did, examining my shoes, handbags, the contents of my closets. The genuine goodwill, symbolized by the flowers my whole team had delivered to me earlier that morning, was one small step toward forging real human contact, despite the restrictive environment. And my frequent conversations helped not only to bridge barriers but to foster an understanding of what the red lines were—what one could say or do without getting oneself or one's local colleagues into trouble.

Navigating cultural differences was a constant challenge. I knew from my earlier visits that blue jeans were considered the worst example of capitalist American decadence—to the point that a foreigner wearing jeans would make any meeting with the North Koreans more awkward. Therefore, I had to advise those at SDC headquarters, as well as consultants and other visitors, to leave their jeans at home. Culinary habits also proved tricky. On one occasion, we were taken for lunch and our hosts asked, "Do you like rabbit?" to which I replied, "Yes, I haven't had rabbit in a long time." But when the meal was served, the meat tasted nothing like any rabbit I had ever eaten. I had a sinking feeling in my stomach. Turning to the guide, I said, "Are we by any chance eating *barking* rabbit?" It took him a moment to realize what I had said, at which point his face turned bright red, and he raced into the kitchen. The dog meat was removed, and we were instead served kimchi rice.

This was hardly the only time I was served dog meat. It still is considered a delicacy in North Korea and in South Korea and China, and I was invited to several dog meat dinners. Indeed, some restaurants in Pyongyang specialized in dog meat dishes. Often treated as the guest of honor at many gatherings, I found it hard to refuse. To cope, I would imagine I was eating something else, a dish that I liked—and I would wash down the meal with copious amounts of beer. This North Korean culinary taste also was evident when my colleagues and I visited various children's institutions. When we asked whether they had animals, they would list rabbits, goats, sometimes chickens or an ox, and occasionally a few dogs. I never told my foreign colleagues what the fate of the dogs would likely be.

I knew that during the famine, people ate not only dogs but cats and any other animals they could get their hands on. I thought of this when a skinny tiger cat with long legs and watchful eyes began appearing at the SDC compound, meowing loudly and insistently. She was friendly to us foreigners, but the minute my Korean colleagues arrived, she scampered away, reappearing only when they had gone home. I wondered if she had had bad experiences with local people, been chased or beaten, or even if she had figured out that she might end up as someone's dinner.

I called her Dusty, as her coat was always coated with dust. I began to feed her, mostly with canned pork produced in North Korea, which she ate very, very reluctantly. In my journal, I wrote, "It must have been a very old pig." I became quite fond of her and looked forward to her regular evening visits to my apartment. Then, a few weeks later, she was gone and never returned. To my journal, I confided, "Where, I wondered and feared." I had to admit that I missed her.

CHAPTER THIRTEEN

Pests

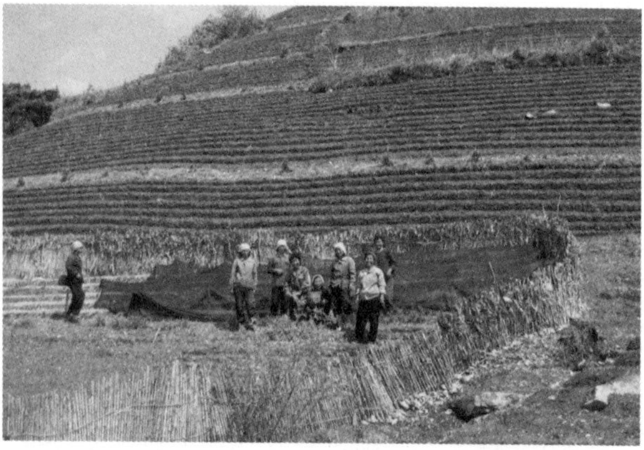

A user group working hard at SDC's Sloping Land Management Program.

In April 2007, Adrian Schlaepfer, the assistant director of the SDC, arrived for a weeklong stay. Thin, mustachioed, and good-humored, he was the highest-ranking SDC official to visit since I had started the job. He came to Pyongyang amidst continuing political pressure in the Swiss Parliament for the SDC to terminate its development program. In a reflection of the widespread skepticism about the DPRK not only in Switzerland but more broadly, Schlaepfer told me that the foreign passenger sitting next to him on the Air Koryo flight from the Chinese capital had joked that the local time in Pyongyang was "an hour ahead of Beijing but fifty years behind."

In our conversations, we brainstormed ways to counter the pressure. We both agreed that North Korea was a special case, but I hoped that by showing him around Pyongyang and outside the capital, he would share my assessment of the value of what we were doing. Schlaepfer had visited once before, in 2003. He told me now that he was struck by the sense of change, observing that the dour looks and instant suspicion directed to him as a foreigner four years earlier seemed to have dissipated. Rather than turning away, people seemed much friendlier. Indeed, when we took a ride on the Pyongyang subway, a gleaming transport system that was frequently shown off to foreign visitors, he recalled that in 2003, while on a train, a mother had slapped a child who had expressed curious friendliness toward him. This time, a child came forward, smiled, and said hello.

One evening, I took him to a soiree—a mass dancing event held in Kim Il Sung Square to mark the Great Leader's birthday. We were pulled into the square by the eager participants and made to dance with them. However tightly controlled, it represented a brief moment of human contact—but so great were the suspicions of the SDC program that Schlaepfer worried about being photographed dancing with a North Korean, an image that would only provide more ammunition for the critics back in Switzerland.

In our meetings with government officials, the North Koreans expressed the desire to continue our cooperation, and said they were especially interested in learning new methods and techniques both for agriculture and for broader economic development. Still, we faced many problems—not least their reluctance to share what we felt was essential data on how our projects were going. Nonetheless, the overall tone was upbeat, and Schlaepfer issued a strong public defense of our program to counter the barrage of negativity from those pressing for the SDC to pull out.

In a strongly worded statement posted on the SDC website, he confronted the critics head-on. "Probably no other SDC partner is so enigmatic and so little known as North Korea," he began. "And doubts are repeatedly expressed about Switzerland's engagement there, with questions like: are there any meaningful approaches for long-term development partnership in this country with its planned economy, backwardness, and secretiveness? Given the context, is it at all possible to initiate change?" But then he answered his own question, noting that "a recent on-the-spot appraisal confirms…there are many promising signs of changes in progress behind the façade—changes the SDC is actively supporting with its special programs… reason enough to maintain the development partnership between North Korea and Switzerland."

One of the most intriguing changes—in which the SDC was deeply involved—was taking place in North Hwanghae Province. Located south of Pyongyang, the province had long been considered part of the breadbasket of North Korea. Yet, reflecting the broader topography of a country with limited arable land, much of the province was made up of hilly, and often sharp and jagged, terrain. During the famine, food and energy shortages led desperate people to cut trees for fuel, and to try to grow whatever crops they could on the steep slopes. The result was a dramatic decrease in forest cover in the whole country, reduced, by the estimate of one Swedish aid group, from 8.2 million hectares in 1990 to less than 6 million by the early 2000s.[7]

This, coupled with the intense, haphazard cultivation of the hillsides, often without adequate fertilizer or appropriate seeds, caused widespread soil erosion and environmental degradation, leading to declining soil fertility, landslides, and flooding. The upshot was a project with the unglamorous name Sloping Land Management, which had the potential to boost food supply and, in the process, gradually help to modify the state's strict management of land, giving local citizens more individual opportunities.

Most farmland was controlled by the Ministry of Agriculture, known for its cautious approach to new ideas. But the Sloping Land Management project was conducted in collaboration with the North Korean Ministry of Land and Environmental Protection (MoLEP), which I found to be much more open and flexible. The idea was to reverse soil erosion and degradation and boost crop yields in the many hilly areas dotting North Hwanghae Province. The method was based on creating user groups, usually housewives or homemakers, sometimes elderly men or even people with disabilities, all with no stable employment. These were people mostly from the nearby villages and towns who had no background in farming, and for whom this was an entirely new experience. That's where the SDC program came in, providing advice, guidance, and practical help as these non-farmers struggled to understand the land. Each group was given ten to twelve hectares of sloping land and the right to decide what to do with it. The work was backbreaking, but whatever the group grew went not to the central government but to local families, who could use it themselves or barter or sell it.

Securing official approval for such relatively independent community-based groups had not been easy. It required protracted negotiations, in which the SDC had made the case that the benefits—increased food production and addressing environmental problems such as land degradation, floods, and soil nutrient depletion—were worth trying to modify previous government policy. The project had started in 2004 with three user groups in Suan County, in North Hwanghae Province, and by the time I began at the SDC, it had expanded to several dozen groups, with hundreds of members in five counties. The user groups could decide for themselves what to plant, and started to grow potatoes, sweet potatoes, upland rice, winter wheat, spices, and many kinds of vegetables. They soon also began to plant trees and shrubs that produced apples, peaches, pears, nuts, berries, and medicinal ingredients.

During my years at Caritas, the vast majority of my work involved hands-on management of projects around the country, requiring regular travel outside Pyongyang. Now, with my team, I was running an organization responsible for multiple initiatives in many areas. I spent much time in the capital, keeping abreast of everything and dealing with senior North Korean officials, the SDC head office, and numerous foreign visitors. Nonetheless, I made regular visits in the company of SDC agricultural and forestry experts to follow the various sloping land projects and other initiatives. I looked forward to them, because the hilly terrain reminded me of Switzerland, as the sloping landscapes looked like a mosaic, with small patches of diverse crops and a variety of plants, more or less spaced according to the gradient of the slope and the soil quality. It brought back childhood memories of my parents' farm in the hills of the canton of Appenzell Ausserrhoden.

It was clear that having a voice in what to grow and how to manage the land, being able to produce their own trees and plants, stabilizing the slopes, diversifying crops, and improving the food supply were having a visible impact on the North Koreans. As one group leader told me, "We now have enough to eat and plenty left over to sell." The program didn't just provide food; it helped them to earn money for daily necessities, including clothing or school items for children, as they could sell or barter their harvest at the farmers' markets. On one visit, my colleagues met Mrs. Kim, the leader of Sloping Land Users Group Number Seven in Suan County. She had recently joined this newly created user group to help feed her six-person family. "In the past," she said, "we were very much dependent on cultivating maize only, in a traditional way. We also cultivated crops without any clear land use plan, and the productivity was low. Now, we are cultivating a diversity of profitable crops while planting many trees and establishing ecological contour strips and grass belts to ward off erosion. We have developed a land use plan together with the support of the project management team, the land use plan designers, and the relevant county institutions. Our profit is much bigger now."

There also was a noticeable psychological effect: The local people began to express opinions on what they felt was necessary and beneficial, rather than just following orders. It was fascinating to watch the reaction of higher-level officials. In a society where everything was done in a top-down fashion, they appeared to find it an eye-opening change. The positive results strengthened the case that this was a valid supplemental approach. However, officials indicated that while the experiment would be tolerated—and many agreed with me that it had a lot of value, especially since the food situation remained precarious—they made clear that it could never become a mainstay of agriculture. That would remain the task of the centrally run collective farms.

To enhance the effectiveness of the Sloping Land Management program—and spur further interest within the North Korean system—the SDC also organized a series of workshops in Pyongyang. Here, we brought together local and foreign experts and people from relevant ministries, with the focus usually on highly technical matters. We also produced reference material, handbooks, and leaflets in both Korean and English to further popularize the initiative.

At the same time, to strengthen technical capacity, we pioneered two collaborative programs with China. One involved the China office of the International Center for Research in Agroforestry (ICRAF). The ICRAF had experience and expertise. When staff sent specialists to the DPRK, the Chinese, given the many similarities between the two countries, fit in well and interacted easily with their North Korean counterparts.

In addition, we were able to send people from the MoLEP, our local project partner, for long-term training to the Kunming Institute of Botany in southwestern China. The institute, affiliated with the Chinese Academy of Sciences, is a leading center of research on agroforestry. One of its top professors, Xu Jianchu, an internationally recognized expert in developing solutions for mountainous landscapes and degraded lands, was the main point of contact. Initially, three North Korean experts spent a full academic year there, with a midcourse break back in Pyongyang, and others would follow. The goal was to build a solid base of knowledge for the MoLEP to develop the sloping land initiative. While we at the SDC did not emphasize this point to our counterparts in Pyongyang, exposing North Koreans to the outside world was another—and not insignificant—benefit. To me, it was clear that the authorities were aware of this but understood the need and the value, despite the risks, of sending people abroad.

As the program expanded, Xu played an increasingly important role. He was both a specialist and an advocate, and made, in my view, major contributions both to expanding knowledge and to making the sloping land initiative more politically palatable. Thoughtful, good-humored, and enthusiastic, he was skilled at interacting with the still somewhat suspicious North Koreans. One of his strengths was that he could deal effectively with people of all backgrounds. Making two-week visits to the DPRK at regular intervals, he would spend time both in Pyongyang and in the countryside. He would explain to the user groups, most of whom had no experience working the land, both conceptual and practical ideas for how to manage the hillsides—what trees, shrubs, and fruits to plant to produce the maximum result, conservation measures, and so on. He worked as well with local scientists and experts, making a special effort to equip them with presentation skills so they could explain the idea of sloping land management to more senior officials in North Hwanghae Province or in other provinces who had heard about the initiative, or those in Pyongyang, as well as foreign visitors.

I remember being struck by the higher level of sophistication of the thirteen people who had spent time at the botany institute in Kunming. Before they attended the program, they would simply write on a blackboard. Upon returning from it, they would offer well-designed PowerPoint presentations that provided much more engrossing explanations, especially to foreign visitors. Indeed, the North Koreans were so grateful for Xu's efforts, they awarded him an honorary doctorate.

In comments to the World Agroforestry Center, Xu noted that "with similar experiences and history, our Chinese staff were well-placed to work in DPR Korea. It was important to have people with an understanding of the technical, institutional and socio-political context. What we have managed to achieve so far has had a dramatic impact on people's lives and the local environment. Previously malnourished communities are now producing their own trees and growing chestnut, walnut, peaches, pears, and other fruits and berries as well as medicinal bushes. They have more food and vitamins and are earning income through trading."[8]

As more areas in North Korea adopted sloping land management techniques, the results became increasingly visible. This was brought home to me during periodic trips I would make from Pyongyang to the eastern port city of Wonsan. Making the drive across the peninsula from west to east, almost always we would take a break at a small rest stop. It had a lovely old pagoda-like building and a beautiful view. In the famine years, the surrounding hillsides had been bare, the trees having all been cut down for firewood. Now, however, I could see not only trees but sloping fields with maize and other crops. The value of this innovative approach for North Korea was literally and figuratively taking root.

While significant, the sloping terrain comprised only a small proportion of North Korea's total arable land. In the larger, less hilly fields, collective farms grew staple crops such as rice and maize. But, on top of all the other problems, agriculture in North Korea involved serious dangers from pests. The maize crop was particularly susceptible, with insect pest damage in some areas leading to a halving of output or more. The chief culprit was *Ostrinia furnacalis*, a species of moth known more commonly as the Asian corn borer. Found throughout Asia, it could cause devastating losses, as the moth's larvae fed on all parts of the maize plant. In a country still facing chronic food shortages, the corn borer posed a serious threat.

To combat this danger, the SDC partnered with the Swiss office of the Center for Agriculture and Bioscience International (CABI) in Delémont, an international nonprofit devoted to providing scientific and technological expertise to promote food security, on a project called Integrated Pest Management (IPM). Traditionally, to the extent that it had acted, North Korea had targeted the Asia corn borer with chemical pesticides. However, between a shortage of pesticide ingredients and the environmental damage—to the land and to humans—that was a less than ideal solution. In contrast, IPM involved, in effect, beating nature at her own game by using other insects that were the natural predators of the corn borer to attack corn borer infestations.

Rather than trying to eradicate everything through the use of pesticides, in this case the project involved employing the *Trichogramma*, an extremely small parasitic wasp (four or five of them could sit on the head of a pin) that lays its eggs inside the eggs of larger insects, especially the corn borer moth. After hatching, the *Trichogramma* kills the pest moth and then searches for other pest eggs into which it can lay its eggs. The technique offered a way to reduce or avoid economic losses due to pest damage, and also an opportunity to reduce pesticide use and the resulting negative impact.

As was often the case, not all North Korean officials or farmers embraced a program that was so new and different from what they were used to. One particular stumbling block was a long-standing preference for using chemical pesticides. This was coupled with a cavalier attitude about the risks. Many North Koreans did not believe in wearing protective clothing when using pesticides. Indeed, one farm manager told me that one of his staff who was in charge of pesticides used to sleep in the room where the chemicals were kept, because it was warmer than other rooms in winter. This person, I was told, passed away from inhaling poisoned air. To win them over, the CABI held a workshop to demonstrate how a person not wearing a protective outfit could be exposed to the poison of chemical pesticides. The instructor asked the North Korean participants to put on white paper jumpsuits. The tanks normally used for spraying pesticides were instead filled with red water. When the hoses were turned on, the North Koreans saw the red dye on the outfits and on their skin. They were shocked and gradually began to change their minds. Before long, the objections started to fade.

Once the North Korean embraced IPM, its use expanded significantly. *Trichogramma* mass production technology from China was introduced, and a series of training courses established. These included workshops in Pyongyang and the countryside, consultations with Chinese experts, and a study tour to Switzerland for one small group. The hands-on training sessions for farmers involved over a thousand people. At the same time, instruction manuals were prepared and the authorities agreed to introduce IPM into the curriculum at the Pyongyang Agricultural University and other educational institutions with agriculture programs.

In the countryside, a dozen small facilities were set up to produce *Trichogramma*. The process was complex. A collection of *Trichogramma* eggs was glued to a paper card. The cards were then attached to maize plants in the field. The timing was crucial, as the *Trichogramma* had to emerge when pest eggs were present. But with the correct timing, the emerging *Trichogramma* would kill the corn borer before it was able to damage the maize. The results were dramatic. On pilot farms, the average yield of maize in IPM plots was 28 percent higher than in the traditional cultivation system, and the number of Asian corn borer larvae decreased by almost 65 percent. So enthusiastic was the government that, with support from the SDC, plans were made to establish an additional twenty *Trichogramma* production facilities, with the goal of enabling around one hundred maize-producing collective farms to implement IPM. The target was a potential 20 percent increase in maize yield over nearly twenty thousand hectares of land.

Maize wasn't the only crop that benefited from SDC-supported pest management programs. Another was the staple of the North Korean diet: cabbage. Especially during winter, when it is made into kimchi, the national dish of salted and fermented vegetables, it is a crucial source of vitamins, minerals such as potassium, and beneficial bacteria that helped to boost the immune system. Working with the Korean Plant Protection Institute (PPI) of the national Academy of Agricultural Sciences, the SDC was deeply involved in introducing the concept of integrated pest management for cabbage production. The main staples in North Korea are rice and maize, with cabbage also playing an important role. Every citizen consumes annually between 120 and 150 kilos of cabbage, usually processed into kimchi. Courses on IPM were started at the national agricultural university, and the PPI identified five farms for pilot projects. Ten scientists and twenty-five trainers fanned out to spread IPM knowledge to hundreds of team leaders and farmers.

The focus of the initiative was on the use of BT, the abbreviation of a common bacteria found in the soil known as *Bacillus thuringiensis*. Occurring naturally, the bacteria is relatively inexpensive to process and safe for humans, birds, fish, and most beneficial insects. But it is lethal for pests that infect cabbage. By replacing chemical pesticides with natural ones, not only could higher yields be achieved but people would be protected from the harmful effects of chemicals. The SDC helped to support facilities for the mass production of the BT pesticide, the use of which was combined with that of a parasitic wasp called the *Diadegma semiclausum*. This kills the pest species by laying eggs in the moth caterpillar and then destroying the parasitic larvae.

At first, several thousand wasps were reared in Switzerland and brought to North Korea to be released on five pilot cooperative farms over a period of two years. In the meantime, we worked with the Korean Plant Protection Institute to develop domestic capacity. The effect of the overall cabbage initiative was dramatic. Plans were made to use IPM techniques in all thirty thousand hectares of cabbage planted in the country, which had the potential to increase the harvest by an additional 225,000 tons of healthy cabbage.

One farm that enthusiastically embraced the IPM technique was Ryuli. Located in the Miru Hills area of North Hwanghae Province, just one hundred miles southeast of Pyongyang, it consisted of 450 hectares of arable land tilled by just over seven hundred farmers. Ryuli was one of several locations the government had proposed to the SDC as potential program sites. We chose it—and six others in the Miru Hills—also because of its closeness to the capital. It could be easily visited on a day trip, making engagement and monitoring significantly easier. Some previously started projects farther away often required staff to stay for up to a week, which was much harder in terms of time, travel, expense, and keeping an eye on what was going on.

Ryuli was a cooperative farm. Unlike on state farms, where workers were given a monthly salary, on cooperative farms, the farmers received an annual allotment of food but just a small additional yearly salary. This made them much more open to ideas about how to boost food production, especially since, as they were located in the breadbasket of North Korea, they were under pressure to produce more to help feed the cities. In most cases, up to 90 percent of output was delivered to the public distribution system.

My frequent trips to Ryuli provided valuable insights about conditions outside the capital. The road was a jumbled collection of concrete slabs, always in bad condition, ensuring a bumpy ride. There was hardly any traffic. Trucks, some powered by wood, would move slowly, transporting both goods and passengers while pumping out giant clouds of smoke. However uncomfortable riding in those trucks looked, it was evidently better than walking, although I also saw a lot of people carrying heavy loads trudging by the side of the road, passing large numbers of broken-down vehicles.

Ryuli also was a pilot site for other SDC-backed initiatives, including one to promote crop rotation. The practice, which involves not planting the same crops in the same place in back-to-back years, is a valuable way to replenish depleted soil and also helps to ward off pests. Most North Koreans, however, were unfamiliar with the concept. They were used to growing the same staple crops in the same place every year. The farm manager explained to me that he remained anxious about leaving a field fallow, for fear of losing a harvest that was still needed in a time of continuing food uncertainty, and also was anxious about fulfilling the government-set production target.

The project had started before my arrival, in 2005, with a ten-hectare pilot plot of land to be used in a four-year rotation cycle of main food crops such as maize, wheat, barley, and potatoes. By 2009, the farm had expanded the crop rotation area to a quarter of its fields. After a few years, the result of alternating crops was a 30 percent increase in maize yield, and less soil degradation. Other farms began to follow suit, including several others in the Miru Hills area. As my colleagues collected data on these trial plots, the assessment was that the rotation program was proving successful, significantly boosting yields. With the success at the local level, the hope was that senior officials in Pyongyang would embrace the initiative and agree to popularize it throughout the country.

As with the sloping land project, I could see that taking responsibility for doing something new was having an important psychological impact on the North Koreans. The farm manager I saw turned out to have quite an entrepreneurial spirit. On one visit, he gave me a sweet jelly candy to taste. It was a dark brown square made with dried acorns. It did not taste as bad as it looked. Indeed, it reminded me a bit of the gummy bear sweets I ate in Switzerland as a child. The manager told me that he made the sweets to earn some extra income. He would sell these to families, as the sweets were popular with children, who had hardly any candy to enjoy. Sugar was very precious, often not available, or prohibitively expensive.

Promoting sustainable agriculture—using sloping land, pest management, and crop rotation—was a key element of the SDC's programs. Overall, despite the many pitfalls, cultural challenges, and the overall difficulty of operating in the DPRK, I felt the results were generally encouraging. But in other important aspects of our work, we encountered significant problems. In the wake of the government's 2002 moves to slightly ease central control over the economy and institute measures that, while never officially called reforms, did indicate some desire to modify the system, the SDC had looked for ways it could help accelerate this process. The result was two initiatives. One was a pilot project called Agro-Processing and Marketing Support (APMS). The idea was that over three years, the SDC would lend its support to efforts to identify potential business opportunities and transfer know-how in technical and managerial terms to support agro-processing enterprises and link them to financial institutions. The goal was to create added value for the producers and improve farmers' livelihoods by allowing for the more effective marketing of products.

We identified a number of what we thought were promising opportunities that the SDC could support—including a small factory producing chopsticks, horseradish cultivation in the Miru Hills, a cheese and yogurt processing facility, and blueberry production in Samjiyon, near Mount Paektu in the far north. In a region where blueberries grew in abundance, the hope was that they could become a source for flavoring yogurt.

In 2007, we arranged for a Swiss specialist to visit and provided some Swiss blueberry plants. On one trip back to Switzerland for an ambassadors' meeting, I was asked to bring a container of the Samjiyon berries to be analyzed in a Swiss lab. I flew straight to Berne for the meeting, but when I opened my suitcase, I was horrified to see that the blueberries had not only spilled out but begun to ferment. Everything in my bag was stained a deep blue—clothing, shoes, presents for family and friends, even the suitcase. I raced to the dry cleaner to beg for help. She shrugged her shoulders and said that only my black clothes could be cleaned. The rest were a total loss. I was lucky no one at the meeting commented on what must have appeared to be my funereal garb. Another container of berries was later shipped to Switzerland for analysis, but it turned out they did not have enough sugar content to work for flavoring yogurt. As for me, since then, I have never been able to bring myself to eat blueberry yogurt.

The blueberries' low sugar content turned out to be the least of the problems with the Agro-Processing and Marketing Support initiative. The projects we backed were plagued by a lack of reliable energy sources, logistical bottlenecks, and no access to foreign currency, which was needed to import even the most basic spare parts and equipment. In one case, a potato processing operation, each factory needed just one hundred to two hundred euros a year for imported parts, but the authorities did not make available even this modest amount.

More broadly, it became evident that there was a vast conceptual gap between the way the SDC saw these projects and the attitude of the government. While the North Koreans were eager for practical inputs, they had no conception of what "market mechanisms" meant. Indeed, one senior North Korean official said to me, "If it were 'agro-processing' without the 'marketing,' it would be easier." It turned out that there wasn't even a clear Korean word for "marketing," and while my SDC Korean colleagues did include the word in our documents, it was missing from some official North Korean paperwork. In crucial ways, despite the goodwill, we were not speaking the same language. What we in the West took for granted was utterly alien in North Korea's state-run system. The initiative soon ran out of energy.

It was the same case with another project, a pilot agricultural credit scheme in cooperation with the loan department of the Central Bank. The underlying thinking was to improve economic performance by using market mechanisms to offset the shortcomings of the planned economy. The goal was to improve food security and increase the wealth of sub-workteams, the lowest work unit on cooperative farms, by giving them loans for viable small-scale agricultural and nonagricultural activities such as services and businesses. The hope was that the sub-workteams could sell their surplus product on local markets.

With the SDC's financial support, a fund was created for imported inputs and equipment, while the Central Bank created a separate fund to provide sub-workteams with the cash to purchase domestically available inputs, equipment, and services. The interest rate for the credits was fixed at 5 percent. But from the beginning, the nature of the North Korean system hobbled the initiative. For one thing, there were no market-oriented banking institutions in the countryside, where bartering remained prevalent. In one case, during Adrian Schlaepfer's visit, we were taken to a local branch office of a bank, where we were surprised to see crowds of people filling in forms. But I suspected that the whole scene may well have been staged for our benefit. In addition, the credits were managed largely by the cooperative farms, not the sub-workteams, hampering the teams' ability to experiment with new ideas.

Meanwhile, the Ministry of Agriculture retained its de facto monopoly on the supply of agricultural inputs and the setting of production targets, making all decisions on distribution and prices. The sub-workteams were forced to sell what little surplus they had to state-run shops at a fixed price well below market prices. Moreover, contrary to the agreement, in the first phase of the project, over 90 percent of all loans were used to increase grain production for the collective farms or the public distribution system, further marginalizing the small-scale units that were intended to be the primary beneficiaries.

The problem underlying these many frustrations and misunderstandings was the idea that two such sharply different approaches—that of the SDC and that of the North Koreans—could somehow harmoniously work together. As I noted in a report to the SDC, "all partners were well aware that consolidating the planned economy and socialist principles with best practices in microfinance would be difficult. Expectations were often not realistic, from both sides." The North Koreans thought the SDC was there just to support the existing system, which basically meant providing needed inputs. "From our side," our report continued, "too many believed that once the efficiency and success of our approach was demonstrated, common sense would prevail and gradual systemic change would start. This proved not to be the case; systemic change is still not possible, and every technical change is gradual and takes very long."

With the benefit of hindsight, it was clear that the SDC had read too much into the 2002 economic measures, which by 2007–2008 had come almost to a halt. It was not easy to determine precisely why that was the case. In all likelihood, there were elements in the regime opposed not only to any loosening of central control but to shifting resources from the military to the civilian economy. The external situation, with the Bush administration blocking moves toward better relations, may have been a factor as well. But in any case, the reformist momentum that started in 2002 had stalled.

Looking back, I realize that we should have been more modest and careful in our approach. For the North Koreans, even what we thought were incremental measures had been too radical a step away from their state-run system. More broadly, the experience underscored for me just how long and slow the journey to promoting meaningful change in the DPRK would be. The SDC was really the pioneer in development cooperation there, but we clearly underestimated how steep the learning curve for both sides would be. Given the dominance of the planned economy, identifying areas where individuals could be motived by incentives without arousing the suspicion of the system was a challenge. The North Koreans did not appreciate that, unlike with humanitarian aid, the process was not simply the foreign partner delivering handouts—imported inputs and cash for local production and other expenditures. Engagement needed to be a two-way street, which was problematic for many in the DPRK. Indeed, even in the terminology used, one lesson was the need to avoid references to what could be seen as politically questionable. In retrospect, talking about "market mechanisms" made the program harder to implement. Just as the word "reform" was not used in 2002, we perhaps should have found different language to alleviate North Korean suspicions.

Still, with three out of five agricultural initiatives showing signs of success, I was not discouraged. And other aspects of the SDC effort, focusing on promoting greater international engagement, continued to move ahead.

But hovering like a black cloud over all our endeavors was the political threat to the entire program. Setbacks such as those encountered in the credit program and the agro-processing project provided further ammunition to critics in Switzerland. We carried on well aware that even as we advanced multiple programs that helped expose North Koreans to the outside world, politics in Switzerland increasingly were threatening to put development cooperation with North Korea in jeopardy.[9]

CHAPTER FOURTEEN

Hunger for Learning

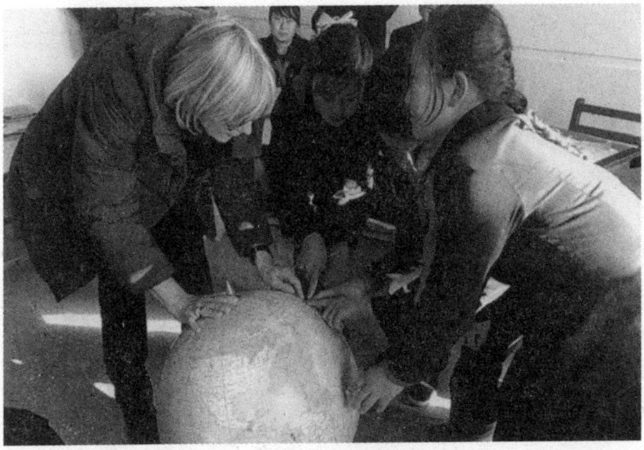

At a school for children with impaired hearing, Kathi helps students find Switzerland on the globe.

One morning, I was driving from the SDC office for a meeting at the People's Palace of Culture, a ponderously large building often used for meetings and workshops—Kim Jong Il had hosted visiting South Korean President Kim Dae-jung there during the first inter-Korean summit in 2000—when suddenly a jeep with UN license plates urgently signaled that I should pull over. Baffled and more than a little concerned that I might be in some kind of trouble, I did so. A young Korean man jumped out and started to gesture and talk rapidly. It turned out he was a local employee at a Pyongyang UN office, but I couldn't figure out what he was saying until my interpreter explained. Not only was I *not* in trouble, but the young man had recognized me, presumably from the diplomatic plates on my car—number seventy-three for Switzerland, and zero one for head of mission—and he wanted to thank me on behalf of his wife, who had attended a training program organized by the SDC and was now successfully running a local restaurant. He wanted to convey how grateful they both were. Offering me her name card, he encouraged me to come for a meal at her restaurant.

The episode was just one example of the impact of the Pyongyang Business School, a program that I felt was among the most positive during my entire tenure at the SDC. The idea of the business school was to train mid-level North Koreans officials engaged in commerce and a few officials and academics about how the world of business—especially outside the DPRK—actually worked. The school had been cofounded with the SDC in 2002 by Felix Abt, a Swiss national who was among the tiny number of Western businessmen (there were no women) who had chosen to be based in Pyongyang, where he ran the office of the Swiss-Swedish automation and power technology giant ABB. Bursting with energy, blunt, and direct, he had managed to win the confidence of the North Koreans. After prolonged discussions, which had to go up to the Ministry of Foreign Affairs and the cabinet, he had been able to get official approval for a series of courses that would explain how the world of international business really worked.

At a time when there was cautious optimism that North Korea, emerging from the famine, might be considering some modifications to its economic policy, Abt was able to secure financial and other support from a number of European companies, including his own. He brought in executives from ABB, the German chemical giant BASF, and other organizations to give presentations. The head of human resources in Asia for BASF, for example, ran a session on human resource issues.

From the beginning, my predecessors at the SDC in Pyongyang had supported the program. But in the wake of North Korea's October 2006 nuclear test, the Western firms that Abt had enlisted got cold feet and, in view of the widespread international condemnation, withdrew their support. By the time I arrived, only the SDC was keeping the program afloat. Yet I was a strong supporter. The project made me think of the efforts I had been involved in during the late 1990s at George Soros's Central European University in Budapest. Almost a decade later, it was still evident to me that the vast majority of North Koreans had little idea of even the most basic business concepts, such as marketing, international accounting, and logistics, let alone subjects such as e-commerce and trade outside the country's tightly sealed borders. Even with the controversy caused by the nuclear test, and despite the obvious political sensitivities involved in any effort to explain the capitalist world, my own conversations with North Korean officials suggested a continuing appetite for learning from abroad and engaging internationally. Abandoning the business school would serve no purpose, I felt, so I did what I could to keep it going.

I was aware that the learning curve remained steep. Indeed, even after the change in economic policy in 2002, the word "reform" was still too sensitive to be used, so people talked about economic "adjustments." And the word "profit" seemed absent from the North Korean vocabulary altogether. But the level of interest in the business school remained high, to the point that some applicants for the three-days-a-month, yearlong course had to be rejected for a lack of places.

With most of the Western firms pulling out, the SDC enlisted the Hong Kong Management Association (HKMA), a body that describes itself as "the leading professional organization advancing management excellence in Hong Kong and the Region," to take over teaching the various modules. Offering business training, including MBA and doctoral programs and individual courses in conjunction with leading universities around the world, the HKMA seemed like a promising partner. This was particularly true because the HKMA members we enlisted were ethnic Chinese, had received international training, and had done business in China, most notably in joint ventures. Their experiences in China gave the lecturers we invited the understanding and sensitivity to handle the delicate task of engaging with the DPRK. Moreover, their Chinese connection offered a degree of political reassurance to always anxious North Korean officials.

Most sessions of the business school had around thirty participants, coming from government offices, ministries, companies, and even universities. To ensure a wide variety of students, we limited each interested organization to two participants per cycle. All of them had to pass a basic English proficiency test. In almost all cases, the school exposed the students to ideas that were utterly alien to them. These included, as one course syllabus noted, "strategic management, marketing concepts and strategy, major export markets for DRPK companies, advertising and promotions management, buyer behavior, cross-cultural management, operations and logistics strategy, manufacturing systems management, managing e-commerce, accounting and financial management, new enterprise development, and organizational behavior and human resources." The material was largely indistinguishable from what a standard MBA covered.

In the early days, Felix Abt, who had a strong feel for North Korean sensitivities and whom the authorities trusted, helped play a role as gatekeeper. As was the case with other visiting foreign experts, we had to look over the curriculum vitae of prospective outside lecturers to ensure that they would be acceptable and that the course content would not create problems. Much of that content was highly technical, but sometimes intervention was required. One issue was the tendency of some lecturers to reference Samsung or other major South Korean companies. Out of deference to North Korean sensitivities, we had to ask that the lecturers replace such references with mentions of big Chinese or international companies. Even an American firm like Apple was OK, but to highlight those from South Korea was too much. North Korean officials also strongly hinted that references to the economic reform programs in China and Vietnam be omitted.

At the end of each program, the students took a final exam consisting of fifty multiple-choice questions. They also were assigned a group project. For many, coming from the notoriously siloed North Korean system, this was their first experience in being part of a team composed of people from different work units and organizations, let alone one in which the students had to come up with the initiative themselves rather than simply hearing the professor dictate a received truth. Learning how to network among themselves and engage with the visiting lecturers became very important parts of their experience. One participant told me he had been pleasantly surprised to discover that colleagues from other institutions, with whom he had previously never had contact, faced similar problems. As a professor from Kim Il Sung University acknowledged, the experience was an eye-opener, especially the new interpersonal connections. "The course was very people-oriented," he said. "I am impressed by the teaching methodology, the attitude to work, and the energy of the lecturers. I still have a lot to learn. I will change the way I teach."

The business school curriculum was later packaged as a 728-page book, in both Korean and English, called *International Business and Management—a Handbook*. With information in North Korea so tightly controlled, and the internet and email services not available to most of the participants, the thousand copies of the book we printed became a valuable and sought-after resource. We made a point to display copies prominently at the SDC library in our office, to which SDC staff, as well as both local and foreign visitors, had access. The book joined several other SDC publications in both languages, including one called *Agroforestry Technology Management* and another called *Rabbit Rearing Manual.* Moreover, in addition to the regular classes, we organized a host of one-off workshops on topics such as strategic management and sustainability.

Whatever the expectations—and, given North Korea's less than stellar international reputation, I am sure they were hardly all positive—most of the HKMA lecturers were pleasantly surprised by the eagerness and enthusiasm of their students. As I noted in a report to the SDC, "The Hong Kong lecturers are pleased with an eager student body, claiming that it is a joy to teach these young North Korean professionals."

Considering the potential sensitivities, classroom discussions proved surprisingly robust. In part this was because the participants were not of university age—college students in many Asian countries were known for not talking in class but simply writing down everything the professor said—but mature adults with significant professional experience. While the topics often were quite technical, the conversations were often intense—to the point that meal breaks were occasionally ignored so that the classroom debate could continue.

The participants were almost uniformly thrilled with their experience. In my notebook at the time, I recorded a host of positive reactions. "I understand the world trends in business now much better," one participant said. "Consumer orientation is of special interest to me. My boss appreciated what I have learned." Said another, "I work at a bank. We give a lot of loans. Now I have learned to evaluate a company, look at the leadership and the quality of management, and so on. The lecturers gave us academic theory and practical examples. It was easy for us to learn." A third declared that "I want to open a new business immediately and apply customer orientation and all the tools I have learned." One young woman summed up the value of the experience this way: "The professors of the Hong Kong Management Association are great. I am dreaming of becoming a businesswoman. I received a lot of new tools from this course. Patriotism is not enough. We need to think in business concepts."

For me, such reactions were proof that the business school experience, despite the limitations, was a positive one that would be internalized, stay with the participants, and not easily be erased, whatever their circumstances going forward.

As we proceeded through what would become four cycles of the business school during my years at the SDC in Pyongyang, we explored the idea of embedding the program in a local academic institution. Despite some exploratory discussions, however, we could not find a suitable partner. My foreign colleagues and I wondered whether this was due to the unreadiness of the authorities to include a course touching on so many sensitive topics in one of their institutions of higher learning, concerned that it could open the door to unwanted foreign influence or capitalist thinking. Although somewhat disappointed, I was actually relieved. With its quasi-independent status, I felt the business school enjoyed a degree of freedom—to hire the visiting HKMA lecturers and shape the curriculum, for example—that might not have existed if it had been part of a local university.

While it is difficult to quantify, the program's impact was real. Shops and restaurants, including the one run by the wife of the man who had stopped me on the road, were increasingly competing for customers. One North Korean bank, headed by a man who had attended the course, introduced debit cards—a radical innovation. Another set up North Korea's first advertising company. The hope was that other attendees also would become agents of change.

The business school was only one of several initiatives aimed at facilitating North Korea's engagement with the rest of the world under the general heading of "capacity development programs." Another was established in coordination with the Centre for Applied Studies in International Negotiations (CASIN). Founded in 1979 and based in Switzerland, CASIN focused on training government and business officials around the world in the mechanics of negotiation, diplomacy, and conflict management to help them devise better policy options. As the DPRK expanded the number of countries with which it had diplomatic relations and became deeply involved in the complex process of the six-party denuclearization talks in Beijing, it was not altogether surprising that the government was interested in a program that would improve the skill set of its increasingly overworked diplomats.

The CASIN initiative predated my arrival in Pyongyang, but it was still going strong. More than a hundred young diplomats over several years had been sent for a few weeks of intensive training in Geneva. In 2009, courses tailor-made for the North Koreans began in Switzerland at the University of Basel's Institute for European Global Studies and the Institute of Federalism in Fribourg. Not surprisingly, there was more than a little cultural confusion as the North Koreans experienced life in Switzerland, and I often heard of episodes when I debriefed delegations that had returned to Pyongyang. In one case, a delegation leader emphasized how stressful it was going from one appointment to the next. She would always ask the Swiss train conductor how many stops before her group needed to get off. The conductor invariably would say he didn't know but would give her an exact time when she could be confident the train had arrived. The woman did not believe what she was being told, only to discover that being on time precisely to the minute was a characteristic of Swiss train travel!

At the same time, the SDC provided support for two foreign ministry officials to attend a course in Switzerland on international peace mediation. It was the first time the DPRK had participated in such a course. For a country where belligerence was the default position in many of its international dealings, the very idea of the course was a novelty, but the North Koreans were open to participating. The course involved lectures, discussions, and even role-playing. I would have liked to see the North Korean diplomats having to act out being diplomats of other countries.

Another project involved bringing eleven young diplomats to the University of Basel for a four-week training course to better understand European integration. Given the challenge the Korean peninsula faced in terms of forging any degree of cooperation, let alone the often floated but never even remotely realized idea of an inter-Korean federation, the North Koreans were interested in the subject. They had an opportunity to visit Brussels, Belgium; the Council of Europe in Strasbourg, France; and the United Nations Office at Geneva, Switzerland. The trip clearly had an impact. As one participant who was involved in developing policy related to Korean reunification noted, "Federalism is needed to protect cultural diversity; important elements of federalism are equality, harmony, and legitimacy. A federal constitution is pivotal for this purpose; constant inter-Korean contacts and negotiations are inevitable processes and will be a long-term task." After returning, another participant told me, "I have so much I could talk about. I believed I knew something about the European Union, but I discovered I knew almost nothing. What I have learned will help me in my work, help me with the cooperation with the EU countries."

Separately, we arranged to send four experts in the energy sector for a three-month course in Switzerland covering topics such as project management theory, hydropower plant design, and renewable energy development. Given the persistent energy shortages in the DPRK, this was a particularly valuable program. The energy experts also requested access to special geotechnical software. This was to be used to assess and analyze land and soil resources to improve forecasting and modeling for agricultural production. But in the prevailing international climate, we at the SDC were concerned that providing the technology might violate the numerous sanctions in place against the DPRK. Nevertheless, after we checked with the Swiss government's State Secretariat for Economic Affairs to make sure no sanctions would be violated, we provided the software. One long-term result was that a law on the development of hydropower passed in 2008, which those who participated in the training program played a major role in drafting.

The authorities in Pyongyang also expressed interest in training programs for lawyers and personnel in the banking sector. I had no illusions that any of these sessions in Switzerland would lead to rapid changes in the DPRK's foreign or domestic policies, but I felt they represented an important step in building trust and relationships, a necessary development to further engagement. Moreover, Switzerland was probably the only country the DPRK felt comfortable enough with to allow its officials to travel and participate in such activities. Apart from occasional Swedish projects, I knew of no other nation that had been given as extensive opportunities.

This was part of a broader trend in which, through their presence in the DPRK, international organizations such as the United Nations, foreign embassies, NGOs, businesses, and the SDC provided the North Koreans with what amounted to on-the-job training. Whatever the organization, the North Koreans assigned to it often stayed for two or three years. During that time, they absorbed ways of operating and thinking to which they previously had not been exposed. Moreover, many had little familiarity with technology but soon were able to operate computers and other tools. The dynamic was hard to measure, but being there and observing it, I was convinced it was having an impact in ways that might continue to play a role after these people resumed their work inside the North Korean system or abroad, if the government were to post them there.

Despite the government's willingness to allow officials to participate in courses in Switzerland, I always detected an undercurrent of anxiety in

Pyongyang about the consequences of exposure to the West. This unease, however, was much less the case when we dealt with fraternal socialist allies such as China, Vietnam, and Cuba, so the SDC made a point of arranging programs in those countries as a way to expose the North Koreans to the outside world, but in less politically sensitive environments. Our main partner in China was the University of International Business and Economics (UIBE) in Beijing. We sent several dozen North Korean experts, from the Ministry of Finance and a variety of other financial institutions, there. The training modules included an introduction to the Chinese business environment, law and business, and sustainable development. It was most participants' first trip outside the DPRK, and seeing Beijing at a time when the Chinese economic boom was fully underway was as much of an eye-opener as the content of the actual courses. As one astonished North Korean participant observed upon arriving in the Chinese capital, "Things here are indeed the way you have been telling me!"

The Beijing courses were based largely on case studies. Chinese MBA students had researched some, described in a textbook compiled by one of the professors. The cases dealt with what, for the North Koreans, were sensitive topics. One focused on a mining disaster, another on a company that had been cheated, yet another on a corruption case. Interestingly, unlike at the business classes held in Pyongyang, the professors in Beijing were not asked to avoid mentioning South Korean firms, and were easily able to mention them in some of the case studies. The only explicit restriction from the authorities in Pyongyang was that under no circumstances were the teachers to mention that Kim Jong Il's son and prospective heir, Kim Jong Un, had been educated in Switzerland.

I met with each group before they left for Beijing and stressed that this was a serious course where they were expected to put in the work and not simply enjoy themselves in the Chinese capital. In general, they performed well. I was pleased that our colleagues at the UIBE reported that the participants, while somewhat cautious in some of their classes, were surprisingly open in other settings, such as over meals or beers or in the evening, talking freely and asking good questions. Moreover, most of them spent considerable time doing research on the internet (to which they would not have had access at home) or in the university library.

In collaboration with the SDC office in Hanoi, Vietnam, we also arranged for five officials from the Korean European Coordination Agency

(KECCA) of the North Korean foreign ministry to visit that country. The focus was on dealing with foreign aid donors and on technical, business, and vocational training. The North Koreans expressed keen interest in the Vietnamese model of development, but given that country's openness to foreign investment, trade, and tourism, and adoption of market-oriented economic reforms, it was hard to see how much would be relevant to the DPRK. Moreover, there was a not insignificant culture clash. Some of the North Korean visitors later privately expressed shock and distaste at what they saw as the dirt, chaos, and disorder on the crowded streets of Hanoi, bursting with motorcycles, cars, and seething masses of humanity. It was a far cry from what they were used to on the sterile streets of Pyongyang, where the traffic wardens had hardly any cars to direct. Still, the Vietnamese were the warmest of hosts, and repeatedly expressed their willingness to collaborate if the North Koreans were interested.

When the SDC arranged for a North Korean delegation to visit Cuba, there were no such ideological concerns. The two countries had been allies ever since Fidel Castro recognized the DPRK shortly after seizing power in 1959. Although separated by 12,500 kilometers, they remained united in their anti-Americanism—given the Korean War and the US effort to overthrow the Castro regime during the Bay of Pigs invasion in 1961, both saw themselves as being on the receiving end of American attacks—as well as in their enduring commitment to a socialist order that had collapsed or been reformed almost beyond recognition elsewhere. Still, we felt that with its somewhat less rigid social system, more international connections, and more vibrant economy, Cuba might offer North Korea something useful. So in mid-2008, five North Koreans, accompanied by Mayling Chan, an old friend of mine from Oxfam Hong Kong whose husband was Cuban, set out for Havana.

The goal was to understand the Cuban approach to farming and markets. Over two weeks, the group visited cooperative and private farms, state enterprises, and a variety of markets, and met with officials and experts. They spoke with farmers who were allowed to cultivate private plots, vendors selling goods from mobile carts on the street, ministers, and policymakers. They were especially struck by the people who they saw simply setting up streetside stalls evidently without any official permission and selling bananas, oranges, and tomatoes.

Many of the discussions were highly technical, especially when it came to the subject of biological pest control, which was one of the areas where the SDC had been most active in the DPRK and was quite advanced in Cuba. The North Koreans were eager to learn more about the Cuban experience, and studiously wrote almost everything down during their meetings. And when given a chance to shop, they stocked up on Cuban rum and cigars. When Mayling asked why they didn't focus more on the Chinese approach, as China was much closer geographically, one of the North Koreans responded that "the Chinese are more self-centered" and reluctant to share details of their experiences. It was a rare glimpse into what I and many other observers had long suspected—that despite the two countries' fraternal ties, multiple tensions plagued North Korea's dealings with China beneath the surface.

More generally, there also were some spirited ideological exchanges with the Cubans. The North Koreans, despite acknowledging that their cooperative farm system was not working well, still expressed concerns that Cuba's market structure allowed those with more money to get better food and more consumer goods, while those with less did without. On another subject, when discussing environmental protection, the North Koreans explained that people in the DPRK were "told" and "educated." The Cubans responded that this seemed to be all about control, and they had not heard the North Koreans talking about "working with" the community. It was another revealing moment, in which the Cubans came across as more open and liberal than the North Koreans. But the discussions were good-humored. It was clear the North Koreans felt comfortable in Cuba, and there were frequent references to the two countries' long-standing friendship.

It was not always easy to track the career paths of the many North Koreans who had the opportunity to participate in these kinds of programs. Upon returning, many often disappeared back into the North Korean system, with little opportunity to engage with foreigners. Anecdotally, however, it became clear that at least some of these once junior officials were promoted, presumably in part because of their international experiences, to more senior positions. In some cases, they were assigned to North Korean diplomatic offices or trade missions abroad.

We did seek to maintain some connection with those who had participated, inviting them to receptions, film screenings, and other diplomatic events—sometimes with unexpected consequences. The British embassy at one point organized a screening of the American TV show *Desperate Housewives* and invited both their local staff and some other officials to attend. Afterward, one North Korean official was absolutely convinced that all Western women led lives of luxury, full of mystery, passion, and illicit romance. It took some effort to explain that this was not the reality they would encounter should they have an opportunity to travel overseas.

CHAPTER FIFTEEN

Boogie-Woogie and Kim's Salon

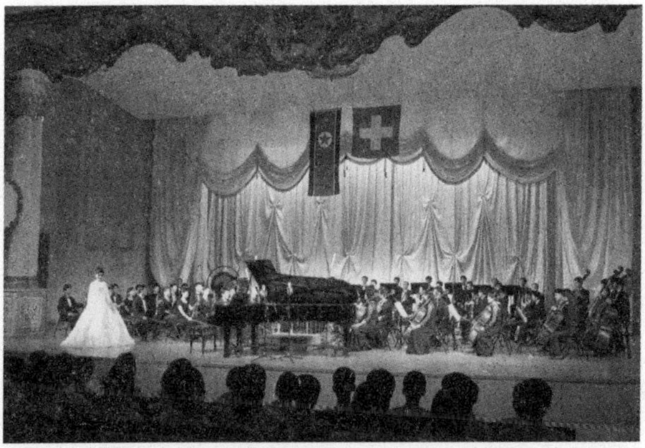

Swiss National Day 2011, featuring a concert with a visiting Swiss artist and the Pyongyang Philharmonic.

A large Swiss flag—a square with a white cross on a vivid red backdrop—hung from the wall. Next to it was the flag of the DPRK. From the ceiling dangled bright red balloons, each with a white cross. In front of the flags, a microphone was mounted on a rickety stand. Tables loaded with food—mostly Korean, plus plates of cheese from Switzerland, each cut into small pieces and adorned with a Swiss flag on top of a toothpick—were dotted around the room. The setting was the RAC, the Random Access Club, which, during the worst days of the famine, had been the favored—indeed the only—gathering place for Pyongyang's small and sorely beset international community. The premises were located inside the building housing the World Food Program. Until the collapse of communism in Eastern Europe, it had been the site of the Bulgarian embassy.

It was August 1, 2007, a hot, steamy day. With more than a little anxiety, I was about to host my first Swiss National Day reception since moving to Pyongyang. For diplomatic missions, especially in a country like the DPRK, national day events were not only a chance for some socializing with other members of the foreign community, but a rare opportunity for relatively relaxed interactions with North Korean officials. As the head of the SDC in the country, I was the most senior member of North Korea's eight-member Swiss community. On this day, only two of those eight besides me were in attendance. With the rest likely away on summer leave, the three of us joined about a hundred other people from embassies and humanitarian organizations, as well as local SDC staff and a handful of officials from the European Department of the North Korean foreign ministry and other local partner organizations.

The proceedings began with the playing of the national anthems of both countries on a tape recorder piped through the RAC's sound system. Then I played a CD containing a recorded message to all Swiss overseas (roughly 10 percent of the country's 7.5 million people at this time lived abroad) from Switzerland's president, Micheline Calmy-Rey—an annual ritual. The sound of ringing church bells preceded the president's message. For us, it evoked home. The North Korean guests, unused to religious music of any kind, simply seemed startled.

Then, wearing a red jacket and white trousers—the Swiss national colors—I nervously stepped up to the microphone.

"Excellencies, ladies, and gentlemen," I began, "it is my most pleasant task today, for the first time, to greet you on the occasion of the Swiss National Day."

Most of my remarks were about the origins of Swiss independence and some of my own childhood memories of the holiday. But I then shifted to mentioning Switzerland's role in the world—its pursuit of peace, its work to alleviate need and poverty, and—pointedly—its respect for human rights and democracy. In terms of Korea, I stressed as well the SDC's continuing presence in North Korea since 1997. And, I emphasized, Switzerland was "committed to involve itself more—if the Koreans wish us to do so." It was a deliberate signal to the DPRK that we would be open to enhancing cooperation if the opportunity were to arise. I concluded my remarks by proposing a toast to the friendship between Korea and Switzerland.

Kim Chun Guk, head of the foreign ministry's European Department and the most senior North Korean official in attendance, then rose to speak. His tone was friendly, reflecting the relatively good state of bilateral relations, and he expressed the desire for a further improvement of ties. He too concluded with a toast but added to the standard language of friendship a wish for good health for North Korean leader Kim Jong Il.

The formalities concluded, I sat down at the VIP table next to Kim Chun Guk and other high-ranking guests. While mostly an exchange of pleasantries, our conversation did involve a certain amount of business—discussing the state of various SDC projects, with my gently pushing for greater access. But it was mostly a convivial occasion. The atmosphere was further lightened because an accomplished Swiss jazz musician was providing live music. Louis de Saint-Gall, a curly-haired, twinkle-eyed artist, sculptor, guitarist, and piano player, was one of my oldest friends. We had met in St. Gallen even before I moved to Hong Kong for Caritas in the late 1970s and had stayed in touch over the years. I was eager to see him again and arranged a visit that would coincide with National Day so he could entertain the guests.

For this trip, Louis had actually built a guitar. It had an Asian motif—the sound hole was in the shape of a gingko leaf—and the neck was detachable, enabling him to easily carry it on the plane. I had tasked him with bringing cheese and chocolates from Switzerland, and at my request, he had stopped in a shop in Hong Kong run by a Swiss butcher and collected a large number of Swiss sausages usually made for Hong Kong's Swiss community. I did not offer these on Swiss National Day but saved them for a series of other social gatherings that I had arranged during his weeklong stay.

While I was busy with my diplomatic duties, Louis had been watching the North Korean guests closely, noticing, among other things, that some were stuffing bananas and other food into their pockets to take home to their families. And that the bottles of Swiss Appenzeller schnapps were soon empty. Then he began to play. Though an excellent singer, he recognized the political sensitivity of words in North Korea, and decided that music would, under these circumstances, serve as a more universal language if the lyrics of the songs he was performing were omitted. I certainly understood why, as his selection was, especially in a setting like this, more than a little radical.

He ran through a litany of jazz classics: "All of Me," "Sweet Georgia Brown," "Autumn Leaves," and boogie-woogie blues, among others. He and I were both struck by how much the North Koreans seemed to enjoy the beat and rhythm, since there were no politically sensitive lyrics to worry about. We could even see some of them discreetly tapping their feet under the table.

Louis played at a number of other social occasions during his weeklong stay, which included the obligatory trip to the DMZ, attending the Arirang Mass Games, and a visit to an art gallery. At the gallery, wowed by a particular painting, he exclaimed, "Crazy," which sparked a stern reaction from his North Korean guide, who thought he was being negative. Louis had to explain that in English, "crazy" can be a term of high praise. Overall, nevertheless, he and the North Koreans he met got on famously. Indeed, as he prepared to leave the country, the SDC foreign ministry liaison officer presented him with perhaps the greatest gift a foreign visitor could receive—a Kim Il Sung button of the kind all North Koreans wore on their lapels.

As a follow-up, a couple of years later, European Department head Kim Chun Guk was in Switzerland for regular bilateral meetings. I invited him and his small delegation to visit my home in Teufen, an hour outside Zurich, as we had some meetings nearby. Kim and his colleagues asked after Louis, and when I said he lived close by, they were very eager to see him. At that point, Louis was driving an MG convertible. When he arrived, the North Koreans, who had never seen a car like that, gasped in amazement. When Louis offered to drive Kim around the nearby mountain roads, the normally straitlaced diplomat beamed with pleasure. Although it was drizzling, Louis put the roof down, and off they went. When they hadn't returned after half an hour, I began to get worried. How could one explain an untoward incident to the North Korean (and Swiss) authorities? I was relieved when they finally drove up with big grins on their faces.

The annual bilateral "political dialogue" in which Kim and his colleagues were participating was a constructive one. The discussions covered, among many topics, possible collaboration with Swiss universities as well as climate change; the North Koreans asked if the SDC would consider assistance in the field of disaster preparedness regarding the latter. The group was taken to a technical school for the lumber industry, to a vocational college, and to a Swiss company that offered apprenticeships to fifty youngsters. I always had felt that vocational training would be of great benefit to the

DPRK, and was pleased to see the visitors exposed to how such programs worked in Switzerland.

The delegation included two members who had never been to Switzerland and one who had never left North Korea. They were overwhelmed by the beauty of the country, the general wealth, the well-functioning infrastructure (especially the always on-time Swiss trains), the access to so many international TV programs in the hotels, and the many free newspapers on offer at train stations. It was, for them, an entirely new world.

On their visit to my village, Teufen, with a little time before their departure, I suggested going to nearby St. Gallen, an old city and a UNESCO heritage site, with a famous library and cathedral. I was struck—and deeply moved—by Kim's response. "Miss Kathi," he said, "this is the only chance I will ever have in my lifetime to go there and do something like that." And off we went to St. Gallen.

When possible, I tried to continue my practice of making Swiss National Day as special as possible. In 2009, I invited Stefan Herzog, a Hong Kong–based Swiss chef, to cater the event. Before leaving Hong Kong, Stefan purchased twenty kilograms of sausages, beef, cheese, chocolate, and other ingredients. He also bought a box of twenty-five Swiss cigars. We requisitioned the kitchen of the Pyongyang International Club, and Stefan enlisted the help of a North Korean chef there who had worked in Eastern Europe years before and had some familiarity with Western food.

It took nearly two days for Stefan to prepare everything, and he encountered some predictable North Korean problems. He had made a chocolate mousse and, given the searing midsummer heat, put it in the refrigerator so it wouldn't go bad. Suddenly, there was a power outage—a not-infrequent event in Pyongyang. Stefan was paralyzed with fear. What if the North Korean officials attending the event got food poisoning—and blamed him? Luckily, all went smoothly. Stefan's food was a big hit, and the Swiss cigars he brought were gone in no time.

Watching the North Koreans grab the cigars, I was reminded of another occasion in Pyongyang when I had a cigar fiasco. The Cuban ambassador, with whom I was friendly, had given me a gift-wrapped box of Cuban cigars. One evening, I hosted a dinner, and some of the guests said that an after-meal cigar would be a nice treat. I piped up that I had a supply. I went upstairs to get the still-wrapped box and opened it in front of my guests. To my acute embarrassment, it was empty. I could only conclude that the ambassador had given the box to an aide to wrap—whether North Korean or Cuban, I had no way of knowing—and, assuming I would not go back to the ambassador and complain, the person simply had pocketed all the cigars.

That same year marked the thirty-fifth anniversary of the establishment of diplomatic relations between Switzerland and the DPRK. In late December, the Swiss ambassador to China, Blaise Godet, who was based in Beijing but accredited also to Pyongyang and Mongolia, arrived for a series of meetings and events. An experienced diplomat who had served as ambassador to Egypt, to the United Nations in Geneva, and in other important posts, he was round-faced, with a carefully trimmed beard and a good sense of humor. Thoughtful and articulate, he and I became good friends, and he made nearly a dozen trips during my time in the DPRK.

Switzerland had relatively good relations with North Korea. There were no outstanding bilateral disputes. The government in Berne did share the broader international concern about the North's nuclear and missile programs and human rights record—but we had also been, along with Sweden, Poland, and Czechoslovakia, a member of the United Nations' Neutral Nations Supervisory Commission created at the end of the Korean War to help maintain the armistice along the DMZ. Even though Pyongyang withdrew recognition of the commission in 1995, this still gave us a certain standing with the North Koreans. During this visit, Godet met with foreign ministry officials, and the vice foreign minister hosted him for dinner. In turn, the ambassador hosted a reception for nearly 150 people—resident expatriates and diplomats, the aid community, the SDC's international and local teams, and various other dignitaries. The highlight was the attendance of North Korean foreign minister Pak Ui Chun, a rare honor, as he normally attended events only at the Chinese and Russian embassies. It was a good opportunity to exchange views in a relatively relaxed setting.

"Political dialogue is a good thing," Pak told the ambassador. In an amiable mood, he noted that in 1995, Switzerland was the first country to offer help, and he expressed the hope that Swiss companies would invest in the DPRK. On the nuclear issue, he reiterated Pyongyang's long-standing contention that the program was the result of "US threats," and that Kim Il Sung had supported the denuclearization of the Korean peninsula. Godet noted that dialogue and confidence-building measures were crucial for the Korean peninsula, and offered the good services of Switzerland in any way that might be helpful to bring peace to the Korean peninsula. Pak said that North Korea was grateful that Switzerland had been willing to host meetings between the United States and the DPRK. While not directly challenging Pak, Godet also emphasized the importance of the Nuclear Non-Proliferation Treaty, from which North Korea had withdrawn in 2003. It was a fairly typical diplomatic exchange, but I always felt that each such discussion was a tiny building block toward more meaningful encounters.

The highlight of the anniversary events was the screening of the quintessentially Swiss film *Heidi.* For the occasion, we were able to rent a movie theater, and ordinary North Koreans were allowed to attend (although I had no way of knowing whether they had to get special permission or how they were chosen). Two versions of the film were shown, one made in the 1950s and the other a more modern one. Over 2,500 North Koreans watched the film, about a small girl who lives in the Swiss Alps with her goatherd grandfather. There was much laughter and tears as the audience enjoyed the timeless tale about love, family, and friendship. In the modern version, an ill-tempered aunt appears and takes Heidi with her to Berlin, where she has a daughter, Clara, who is the same age. The two teenagers initially don't get along, and Clara convinces Heidi that to be accepted, she must dye her hair blue. The North Korean audience was horrified by Heidi's blue hair, but it was fascinating to watch how mesmerized they were by the images of modern, sophisticated Berlin.

Overall, as I wrote in a report to SDC headquarters, "The message that tradition and modernity can go hand-in-hand was well understood. Local people enjoy and value such cultural exchanges, and moreover, such activities open small windows to the world to the isolated population here." Sometime later, my sister came to visit. She is named Heidi. The North Koreans she met, most of whom had seen the film, were thrilled. "Now we have a real Heidi," they exclaimed, and commented on how, just as in the film, she was a farmer's daughter! It added warmth to the already friendly reception my sister received.

One of my earliest, and most regular, visitors was Father Gerard Hammond. A native of Philadelphia and the son of immigrant Irish parents, he had been working as a Maryknoll missionary in South Korea since 1960—and as of this writing, is still there. I had gotten to know him during my time at Caritas, and he had participated in some of the meetings I attended in Rome and Seoul. A fluent Korean speaker, he often assisted my Korean colleagues with translations. Over the years, we became good friends.

Part of what spurred his commitment to Korea was a desire to emulate the Maryknoll missionaries who had served in Pyongyang until the early years of World War Two, some of whom died for their faith. Deeply committed to peace and reconciliation, he began working in the mid-1990s with the Eugene Bell Foundation, a United States–based foundation providing humanitarian assistance to the DPRK out of South Korea. Founded by a Korean-educated American named Stephen Linton and named in honor of a distant relative who had served in Korea as a missionary in the late 1800s, it focused on combating multidrug-resistant tuberculosis, which remained one of the biggest killers in the country. With his remarkable language skills, Hammond handled much of the foundation's administrative tasks and paperwork for the DPRK, keeping track of drug shipments, patient records, and so on.

It was a role that enabled him to travel to Pyongyang two or three times a year. A lively, jolly man with a twinkle in his eyes, he was always a welcome visitor. After so many years in the country, he seemed more Korean than American. When he happened to be in Pyongyang on a Sunday, he would conduct Mass for the foreign community. The service was held alternately at the SDC compound and the Polish embassy, as the Polish ambassador was a devout Catholic. I have vivid memories of Hammond sitting in the SDC library after Mass, surrounded by a crowd of children. Many foreign families brought their kids, and the priest, using a children's Bible that one of the mothers would bring along, would tell the age-old stories. The kids loved him, not only because of the warmth of his personality but because he could explain the stories in a simple, easily understandable way.

In 2011, he happened to be in Pyongyang again, this time over Easter, and read Easter Mass for foreigners at the Polish embassy. This was followed by a traditional Polish Easter breakfast for around fifty people. It was the first time since 1949 that Easter Mass had been celebrated in Pyongyang.

When he would stop by my office, as he did on most of his visits, he always made a point of greeting my local staff in Korean. They were absolutely astonished by his fluency in Korean, and engaged in polite chats, although, as was always the case, people remained very reserved in interpersonal interactions. I assumed they all had deduced he must have learned Korean in the South, but given the politics, none of them ever dared to ask.

But a foreign priest was only one of the wide range of visitors. In 2010, after four years of trying, I brought Kim's Salon to Pyongyang.

Australian Kim Robinson was known as a hairdresser to the stars. Since the late 1970s, he had run a salon in Hong Kong catering to celebrities, Cantopop stars, and other rich and famous people. His clients included supermodels such as Cindy Crawford and Kate Moss—even Princess Diana. Although no celebrity, I had been going to him since his modest start in the late 1970s at a shop in Hong Kong's long-since-demolished Furama Hotel, and he had remained my hairdresser even as his fame grew.

One day, shortly before I started my job with the SDC in 2006, I bumped into him on the street in Hong Kong and told him I was moving to Pyongyang. Kim's first reaction was, "Are you crazy?" But he followed this almost immediately with a request to visit. He had long been interested in visiting the DPRK and had made inquiries periodically during my years at Caritas, but my own work circumstances and the country's grim situation had made such a trip impossible then. But now, as a foreign resident of Pyongyang with diplomatic status, during a period of, by North Korean standards, relative openness to the outside world, I could invite people as my personal guests, although they still required official approval to get a visa. So I laughingly replied, "Of course—but only if you bring your scissors."

It took until 2010, but I finally secured permission from the authorities for Kim to accept my invitation to visit, which he paid for himself, as did all my visitors. He fulfilled his promise to bring his scissors—and a hairdryer too—and agreed to make his services available to expats as well as to local North Korean staff who worked for the small international community. Given his name, a common Korean surname, we thought it was highly appropriate to call his place Kim's Salon. We found a space in a building at the back of the main SDC compound and put up a sign, and with his modest equipment, Kim set up shop.

I spread the word at the regular interagency meetings the resident international organizations held every Friday, and soon, people began to sign up. In addition to members of the foreign community, a number of North Koreans, mostly staff members from the SDC and a few from other international organizations, asked Kim to do their hair. While the expats came simply expecting a high-class haircut, the North Koreans, especially the younger women, came with photos from fashion magazines or taken from the internet, to which they, as employees of international organizations, had some access.

In contrast, for ordinary North Koreans, access to any kind of information on Western hairstyles or almost anything else was just about impossible. Indeed, as Kim discovered when a North Korean guide took him around the city, hair salons in the DPRK had a selection of about a dozen officially approved styles, usually posted in grainy photographs on the wall, and all clients, men and women, had no choice but to pick one. Even if their knowledge of hairstyles was somewhat limited, however, most of the North Koreans were thrilled with the opportunity to have an expert with such a glittering international reputation do their hair, and they were happy to trust Kim's good taste. He had, after all, made a career specializing in Asian clients and knew a great deal about Asian hair.

One of the domestic staff members at the SDC, however, had a very specific idea in mind. Every Sunday evening, North Korean TV would broadcast about forty-five minutes of carefully edited international news. One Sunday, this staff member was very taken by a report from Germany. When I saw her arriving at Kim's Salon the following week, she announced with great pride that she wanted a haircut like the German president's. It took Kim and me a minute or two to realize that she was talking about German Chancellor Angela Merkel. Merkel was not exactly the most flattering role model for hair. A *New Yorker* magazine profile once described her as having "a helmet of no-color hair."[10] But I was tempted to send Merkel an email to tell her about her North Korean admirer. In any case, Kim, who rarely followed politics, had no idea what Merkel looked like, let alone her hairstyle, so additional research was required to keep my staff member happy.

Both North Korean men and women came to take advantage of Kim's presence. Given the language gap, there was usually little conversation or banter. One of the clients was a short, heavyset young man who preferred a bouffant hairdo like Kim Jong Un's. In 2010, Kim Jong Il's son Kim Jong Un was gradually being introduced to the North Korean people as the designated heir, with his photo beginning to appear in the domestic media before his broader international exposure. Later, Kim Robinson would say how much he had been struck by the resemblance of his client to the young leader, and he wondered if trying to look like the successor was a new fashion trend in Pyongyang.

Incidentally, other intriguing signs of the successor's emergence began appearing then. On January 8, 2010, all local SDC staff from the Ministry of Foreign Affairs were suddenly ordered to go to the ministry in the middle of the afternoon. No reason was given. When they returned, I casually asked, "Was it a good birthday party?" My North Korean colleagues were shocked. "How do you know, Miss Kathi?" they asked. I had heard rumors that January 8 was Kim Jong Un's birthday and had simply made an educated guess.

Another visitor was a Swiss animation artist whom I will call Jean. He was eager to develop a collaborative relationship with the Korean April 26 Animation Studio, the largest such studio in the DPRK. Although the fact was mostly unknown in the West, North Korea had for many years been an animation powerhouse. By the early 2000s, the studio employed over 1,600 staff and animated dozens of films—both domestic and foreign—every year, making it one of the largest animation studios in the world. One explanation for what otherwise seemed like a curiosity was that Kim Jong Il was well-known for his interest in all forms of cinema. Promoting cartoons was also a technique to inculcate the younger generation with the regime's ideology in an easy-to-swallow way.

In any case, after the Easter holiday in 2010, Jean arrived at my office in quite a distressed state. His tale of woe could have happened only in the DPRK. He told me that, since he traveled so much, he always sent his children in Switzerland postcards from wherever he was. This year was no exception. At his hotel in Pyongyang, he had purchased a postcard of the city's Juche Tower, a 170-meter-tall structure built to mark Kim Il Sung's seventieth birthday in 1982 and designed to honor the country's guiding ideology. Made up of 25,550 granite blocks, one for every day of Kim's life, and deliberately designed to be one meter taller than the Washington Monument, to which the North Koreans liked to compare it, it dominated the landscape of the capital.

To make the image into an Easter card, Jean, utterly ignorant of North Korean sensitivities, had sketched on the postcard little Easter bunnies climbing up the sides of the tower. When he gave it to the hotel reception with a request for stamps to mail it to Switzerland, he instead received a stern lecture about how he had insulted such an important national monument and was told in no uncertain terms that the card certainly would not be sent. Upset at the experience, he poured out his anxieties to me. I assured him that nothing more would happen to him—but his hope for collaboration with the animation studio evaporated. And even now, every Easter I think of this story and have a little laugh.

Hardly a visit with my foreign guests went by without some episode highlighting the idiosyncrasies of the North Korean system. In 2008, a half dozen friends from Hong Kong came after making arrangements with a North Korean tour agency. The tour guides showed them around Pyongyang and took them to all the usual tourist sights: the circus, with Americans portrayed as long-nosed villains; the giant monuments to the Kim family; restaurants where, despite chronic food shortages, they were served bulging plates of beef bulgogi and copious amounts of beer. When one of my friends asked a local guide the height of the giant bronze statue of Kim Il Sung where all visitors were taken to pay homage, the person responded, "The greatness of the leader cannot be measured in meters."

The group then traveled to see the North Korean side of the Demilitarized Zone. This trip usually involved a three-hour drive on an absolutely straight road from Pyongyang where virtually no other cars were visible, and a stop at the Panmunjom border, where South Korean and American soldiers were literally almost within touching distance. I had made the trip numerous times. On every visit, it brought home to me the starkness of the division of the Korean peninsula. Usually, the DMZ stop would be followed by an overnight stay at a hotel in the city of Kaesong, a few miles from the border.

During the evening after this group's DMZ visit, all of my friends got quite tipsy on a bottle of Bailey's liqueur which they had brought, and one of them, a Hong Kong businesswoman, composed new lyrics to the tune of the Beatles' famous song "Let It Be," to be sung at a farewell dinner for the group that I was planning to host at the SDC compound.

The new version went:

> When we arrived on Saturday our Mother Kathi came to us,
> Speaking words of welcome to Pyongyang:
> "You are here, you are here, in Pyongyang you are here,"
> Speaking words of welcome to Pyongyang.
> To the circus we did go to watch a most spectacular show
> Speaking words of awe, what a show
> What a show, oo-ah, what a show, ah-oo.
> We were so impressed with what they can do

The city is nice, the buildings humongous
The Great Leader is always among us
Speaking words of wisdom to you and me
Self-reliant, working hard, strong and brave, honest and smart
Follow the *juche* way with all your heart
Our guides are nice, their smiles are sunny, they bring us
food to fill our tummy
Speaking words of guidance, "Don't go far!"
The food is good, the beer is flowing, our heart for Korea
keeps on growing.
We'll be coming back to Pyongyang
To Pyongyang, to Pyongyang, we'll come back to Pyongyang
Thank you, Mother Kathi, we're your fans!

As my friends performed the song for me at the farewell dinner, our North Korean colleagues had a hard time understanding why we were laughing so hard.

A few days later, a member of another visiting group was doing exercises in front of a mirror in her room. Later, one of the hotel's cleaning ladies, seeking to be friendly, said to her, "You have a beautiful body." The cleaning lady obviously had been watching my friend on the hotel's internal monitoring system, and was blissfully unaware that, by her compliment, she was unwittingly revealing its existence. Doing morning exercises was quickly cut from my friend's daily routine.

A central part of my job was to act as a conduit between outside visitors and the North Koreans. Even with all the limitations on access and travel, and the frequent reluctance of our North Korean interlocutors to engage in candid discussions, I felt that the mere fact of expanded contact, however awkward, had its own value. Regular visitors included Swiss Ambassador Blaise Godet. Given the good relations between the two countries, Godet got, by Pyongyang standards, reasonably decent access. He was always able to see his counterparts at the foreign ministry. With my diplomatic status, he invited me to accompany him to these meetings, and we held lengthy discussions about them afterward. Godet said that while his interlocutors were cordial, they never went beyond their officially approved talking points, and he rarely came away with anything that he could not have learned from reading the official media.

The relatively warm ties did result in his being granted permission to travel, a privilege that officials routinely denied many foreign ambassadors who actually lived in the capital. The places he was taken to were the kinds I had been visiting regularly for years, such as farms, schools, and orphanages outside Pyongyang. As a relatively infrequent visitor unused to the DPRK, he usually returned deeply shocked by the level of poverty, and frustrated that everything seemed to be prearranged to ensure limited spontaneous interaction with the people he saw. But at least he was getting away from the capital, and the mere fact of travel contributed to his absorbing a better feel for the country.

Godet also tried to leverage the fact that Kim Jong Un had spent many years at schools in Switzerland. Even though the authorities never formally acknowledged this fact or mentioned it in any official documents, Godet frequently referred to the Kim family's special connection to Switzerland in his formal meetings, in the hope of using it in some way to advance the relationship. Here too, he ran into a brick wall. He never received any confirmation from his counterparts that Kim actually had studied there, let alone a follow-up to his queries. It was another example of the secrecy that dominated the North Korean system.

He and I had frequent long discussions trying to figure out what to make of the country. As a diplomat, he was more cynical, and occasionally told me he thought I wasn't critical enough of the regime and the system—possibly true, but it was much easier to be critical as a visitor than as someone living there and trying to manage a program effectively. I expected ambassadors to be critical. It was their job. But they also came and went, while I remained. He raised the same question that critics of the SDC program in Switzerland also were posing: Was providing development assistance simply freeing the North Korean government to devote greater resources to its military and nuclear and missile programs?

I acknowledged that it was a morally gray area, but my view was that, first, not providing the assistance hardly would compel Pyongyang to divert resources it felt were central to its own security. It would only make the lot of ordinary people, who had no choice about being born North Korean or about their present circumstances, even more miserable. There was, I believed, intrinsic value in trying to help those who were, after all, our fellow human beings, and who were suffering. Moreover, while I was as aware as anyone of the nature of the North Korean system, my goal was to try to get things done, to make programs actually work on the ground. In my position, denunciations, finger-pointing, and name-calling served no useful purpose. All it would do was reduce, if not sever, the access I had established during so many years of carefully building relationships. How would that help an ordinary North Korean? While Godet acknowledged that he would have been inclined to be tougher, he accepted that my efforts to forge empathy with the people were making a practical difference in the viability of the SDC's programs.

CHAPTER SIXTEEN

"A Difficult Place in Which to Do Business"

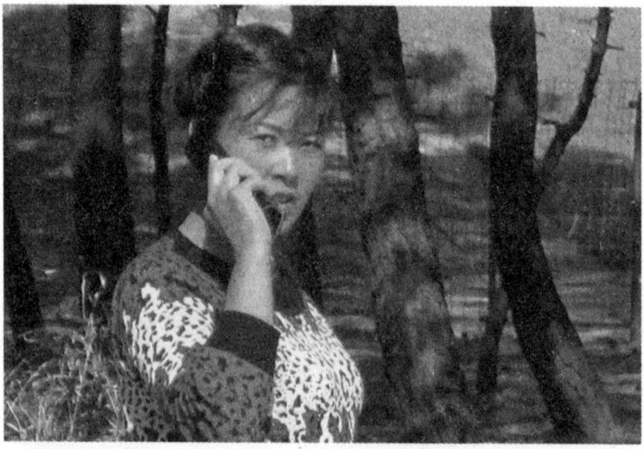

As the economy slowly improved, mobile phones became popular and an important tool for doing business.

In March 2008, the North Korean Ministry of Agriculture released harvest figures for 2007, which revealed that overall production was down by more than 1.4 million metric tons of grain from the 2006 harvest. It was a significant drop. Food was again becoming a serious concern. It had been a mild winter with little or no rain—bad news for spring crops. I picked up reports that even in Pyongyang, food distribution was becoming irregular. Traveling in the countryside, I found a visible increase in disheveled adults and scruffy street children. In the local markets, food prices were rising. The few foreign businesspeople traveling to Pyongyang were increasingly being asked to provide food as part of prospective deals.

The World Food Program estimated that more than 6.5 million North Koreans were suffering from food insecurity. As I noted in a report to the SDC, "The situation is fragile and could degenerate. Belt-tightening could become the motto of 2008 and 2009." Adding to the problem, South Korea—with whom relations had abruptly deteriorated after right-wing politician Lee Myung-bak became president in February 2008, a position he held until 2013—halted shipments of fertilizer, while China began to impose a 100 percent tax on its fertilizer exports. And the North Korean authorities initially turned down an offer of five hundred thousand tons of food from the United States, as no agreement on monitoring could be reached, although later in the year, this issue was resolved and at least some food supplies began arriving. Reflecting the dire situation, North Korean officials asked Switzerland for food aid, and the SDC approved a grant of one million Swiss francs for the World Food Program.

Still, the domestic picture was bleak. Although the international situation in mid-2008 was more mixed, it was also reaching a critical moment. In 2007, we had witnessed some real progress. In July, North Korea had shut down its Yongbyon nuclear reactor, and an agreement reached at the six-party talks in October committed North Korea to completely disable the reactor and provide a "complete and correct" declaration of its nuclear capabilities. Reflecting the more positive atmosphere, in early 2008, the New York Philharmonic had performed in Pyongyang—a breakthrough comparable to when the Philadelphia Orchestra in 1973 became the first American orchestra to perform in the People's Republic of China.

The New York Philharmonic's performance was probably the most talked-about cultural event in the capital in many years. Pyongyang put on its best face, illuminating many buildings and celebrating a generally festive mood that the authorities encouraged. The East Pyongyang Grand Theatre was filled to capacity, while hundreds of thousands more watched the performance on TV. The audience stood as the national anthems of both countries were played and both flags were displayed onstage. Emotions ran particularly high when the orchestra played "Arirang," a traditional folksong popular in both the North and the South. For Kim Jong Il, welcoming the orchestra was a signal of his desire for better relations with the United States.

I thought it was an interesting sign of the times that CD recordings of the performance, still technically illegal, were later on sale in local markets.

At the same time, though, the Bush administration remained divided between moderates who wanted to negotiate and hard-liners who wanted to confront the DPRK. One sign of this was Secretary of State Condoleezza Rice's decision to spurn the North Korean overture of attending the Philharmonic concert as a gesture of goodwill and reject Pyongyang's suggestion that its orchestra pay a return visit to the United States. North Korea's slowness in producing a declaration of its nuclear programs that would satisfy the hard-liners, as well as right-wing governments in Seoul and Tokyo, further complicated negotiations, although in late spring, the North did deliver nineteen thousand pages of documents, and then, in the presence of senior US State Department official Sung Kim, made the symbolic gesture of blowing up the Yongbyon reactor's cooling tower.

It was against this backdrop that I spent part of June 2008 in New York and Washington, DC. The Swiss embassy in Washington and the Swiss mission to the United Nations in New York arranged the trip. The goal was for me to meet as wide a range of people dealing with or interested in North Korea as possible and exchange insights and ideas. For me, as a supporter of engagement, it was a chance to make the case that there was more to be gained by talking with North Korea than confronting it.

My first stop was Washington, and it included meetings with Sung Kim, the head of the State Department's Korea desk, who had been invited to witness the destruction of the Yongbyon cooling tower. I also met with a senior official at the National Security Council who handled US government development assistance and humanitarian aid, and members of the Foreign Relations Committee in the Senate and the Committee on Foreign Affairs in the House of Representatives. The Swiss embassy even arranged for me and the embassy's military attaché to brief officials at the Pentagon, including the principal director for East Asia, who oversaw US defense policy for the region, and the US Army's country directors for Korea. For the Pentagon meetings, I passed through intensive security checks and was led down several levels deep into what seemed to me to be close to the basement of the huge complex. Never had I imagined I would be visiting the global nerve center of the American armed forces.

At all my encounters, I was received cordially, with not the slightest suggestion, even at the Pentagon, that my many years of involvement with

North Korea had in some way made me an apologist of or a sympathizer for the Pyongyang regime. Instead, at a time when, despite the internal policy debates in Washington, there was still at least some interest in exploring ways to expand contact with the DPRK, I found intense curiosity about my own experiences and observations. Indeed, the surprisingly high-level officials who met me were bursting with questions. What had changed in recent years? What was the food situation like? What kind of projects was the SDC involved in? My interlocutors were just as eager to learn about life on a more personal level, wondering about the size and nature of the expatriate community, how I got around, whether I could travel—even what I did in the evenings or on weekends. They also were curious about my own motivation for devoting so much time to North Korea. I explained that I always had liked challenges and been drawn to places where I could be something of a pioneer. Moreover, I felt my experiences working in China in the 1980s could act as something of a bridge. Above all, I believed that the people of North Korea deserved a better life and that if I could contribute to that, I should try to do so.

Not surprisingly, the discussion at the Pentagon focused on the North Korean military. I shared my impression that soldiers in the DPRK often were involved in civilian work, such as road construction, harvesting, or disaster relief. I also noted that the average foot soldier did not look particularly well-fed. I recounted an anecdote in which a North Korean defector I had met in Seoul told me that the final straw in her decision to flee came when both her sons returned from their military service badly malnourished. Despite the curiosity, as I noted in a report to the SDC, it was "still astounding how the DPRK [was] viewed—and most of the time in a negative way."

One reason, of course, was the country's abysmal human rights record. All of us living and working in Pyongyang were well aware of the nature of the North Korean regime and system. We were interacting with it every day and were familiar with the deeply troubling accounts from many North Korean defectors. But whether—and how—to address human rights concerns remained an exceptionally delicate issue for me and other colleagues engaged in humanitarian work. The North Koreans reacted to virtually any mention of the subject as an attack on their system and leader. For those of us on the ground seeking—in cautious, limited, but still at times successful—ways to improve the lives of at least some ordinary North Koreans, mentioning the subject of human rights almost invariably raised the possibility of jeopardizing everything we were doing.

Nonetheless, when the Swiss ambassador visited Pyongyang, or the two countries held their annual political dialogue, human rights always were on the agenda—and the North Koreans almost always reacted with anger. One particular sore point was the United Nations' Universal Periodic Review, a mechanism of the UN Human Rights Council created in 2006 to examine the human rights practices of all 193 member states. The North Koreans were exceptionally defensive about this process. I recall sitting in one meeting where North Korean officials blamed the United States for the entire exercise and then declared, "We will defend our socialist system based on the *juche* idea. We do not bow to pressure to give up our socialist system." One could really feel their anger. When challenged about why the North was devoting so many resources to its military while people went hungry, one official replied, "We may not have enough sweets to give to our children, but we need bullets to defend us."

When the United Nations asked permission for its special rapporteur on human rights to visit the DPRK, the response was equally furious. DPRK representative Pak Ton Hun declared the resolution was "a product of a political plot" and that the DPRK "categorically rejected" the mandate of the Special Rapporteur as a violation of its sovereignty.[11]

I explained to my American interlocutors that this was the atmosphere in which I was operating. I stressed that not publicly challenging the North Koreans on human rights did not reflect my lack of awareness but was simply a tactical decision for me to be able to continue to operate, which I felt remained a worthwhile endeavor on balance despite all the difficulties, even if it might have been more satisfying for some to publicly denounce the DPRK's human rights failures.

Instead, in my meetings, I spoke repeatedly about what I dubbed the "Three F's"—food, fuel, fertilizer—and how acute shortages of all of them were causing severe problems. Indeed, I judged that at present, these were the country's three greatest needs. When I spoke about the SDC's programs, and especially the Pyongyang Business School, my interlocutors were uniformly astonished. They found it hard to believe that the North Korea they knew of from a distance would ever tolerate a project involving so much contact with foreigners and exposure to outside ideas. But I used this example to stress my sense that, despite its human rights record and its combative response to those who raised the issue, the DPRK was gradually becoming both more used to and more open to dealing with the international community. This was an opportune moment, I argued, for more visits, and greater person-to-person contact to help demystify the country and its people.

I acknowledged that there would inevitably be differences and challenges, but my mantra was always "negotiate, negotiate, negotiate." As long as people outside the country were not fixated on a single, unchanging goal based on the way *they* did things, but were willing to listen and show some flexibility, I felt progress might well be possible. With the United States, however, flexibility remained a thorny problem, since Washington remained rigidly focused on denuclearization, while the DPRK was looking for better ties with the United States. For Kim Jong Il, the nuclear issue was just one item on the agenda—a bargaining chip to be used to extract concessions but also a tool to reorient the overall DRPK–United States relationship.

I repeated my message in favor of greater contact and exchange in meetings with people from a number of Washington and New York think tanks and research institutes, including the Center for Strategic and International Studies, the National Committee on North Korea, The Korea Society, and the EastWest Center. Conversations there covered possible new engagement strategies. I reiterated my sense that there were people in the DPRK who were eager to learn more about how the United States functioned and how Americans thought about politics, economics, culture, and so on, but that direct contact and access to information remained problematic for both the North Koreans and the Americans.

I arrived in New York just as an intense debate was underway at the United Nations about whether the UN Development Program should return to the DPRK. The program had suspended its operations in Pyongyang and withdrawn its staff under a cloud of allegations of financial and other malfeasance in 2007. In response to a stinging US Senate report in January 2008, the United Nations had set up its own independent review, headed by former Hungarian Prime Minister Miklós Németh. The three-member panel released its own 353-page report on May 31, 2008, emphasizing that no evidence had been found to substantiate the most serious allegations about illicit transfers of funds to the North Korean government, let alone that such funds had been siphoned off for use in the country's missile and nuclear programs. Acknowledging that the DPRK was a "difficult place in which to do business," the UNDP pledged to take a series of steps to address "any and all management and operational deficiencies."[12]

Beyond the specifics lay the broader question of whether cooperation on development—as opposed to purely humanitarian aid—was feasible in a country such as North Korea. My position remained strongly in favor of such cooperation. I felt the country needed both, and that humanitarian aid was not about just providing food; sectors such as health, water, and sanitation needed to be considered as well. I recognized that it was a learning process for both sides, and that for the DPRK, it was entirely new, but I was convinced that it was both doable and an important way to help put the country on a sounder economic footing. The debate over what the UNDP should do dominated my discussions not only with the UNDP but also with other UN officials, including those at the Executive Office of the Secretary-General, the Department of Political and Peacebuilding Affairs, and the Office for the Coordination of Humanitarian Affairs, as well as the UN envoys from Switzerland, North Korea, South Korea, the United States, Russia, Sweden, and Japan. Not surprisingly, the Americans and Japanese remained adamantly opposed to the UNDP's resuming operations, while North Korean Ambassador Sin Son Ho in a separate meeting urged me to push the Swiss government to support a resumption of the UNDP's work. My own view was that the benefits of the UNDP's returning outweighed whatever problems had previously existed, and when my opinion was sought, I made that point clear. It took another year, but I was pleased when in late spring of 2009, the UNDP finally reopened its office in Pyongyang.

As I returned to Pyongyang, the broader situation lurched back and forth between promise and peril. The United States, in response to the North's provision of a declaration of its nuclear capabilities, lifted restrictions that applied to the DPRK from the Trading with the Enemy Act of 1917 and initiated steps that could lead to Pyongyang's being taken off Washington's list of state sponsors of terrorism. But the six-party talks again stalled amid American complaints, driven by hard-liners in the Bush administration, Seoul, and Tokyo, that there was no satisfactory mechanism to verify the North's moves toward denuclearization. In response, Pyongyang threatened to restart operations at Yongbyon. Then, in mid-August 2008, sixty-six-year-old Kim Jong Il suffered a severe stroke. At the time, information remained sketchy, but when he failed to appear at a large parade to celebrate the establishment of the North Korean state on September 9, to which I and other members of the city's small foreign community had been invited, the rumors and speculation took on fresh intensity—as did the uncertainty about North Korea's future direction.

Meanwhile, the American presidential election was approaching, and in November 2008, Barack Obama was elected president. Although Obama declared a willingness to "extend a hand" to adversaries "willing to unclench [their] fist,"[13] the North Koreans, who had been observing an informal moratorium on missile tests throughout the ups and downs of the six-party process, showed their frustration at what they saw as American stalling, and also sought to send a signal that Kim Jong Il's 2008 stroke had not weakened the regime, by launching an Unha-2 rocket in April 2009. The launch triggered a series of new United States–supported UN sanctions, and effectively froze any possibility of serious negotiations between Washington and Pyongyang.

The situation was further complicated by the detention of two female American journalists on March 17, 2009. They had foolishly allowed their local Chinese guide to convince them to cross the narrow and ice-covered Tumen River separating the DPRK from China so they could claim to have stepped on North Korean soil. After a swift trial, the two were sentenced to twelve years in jail "for illegal entry into the country and for committing hostile acts." Their plight was much discussed in the Pyongyang foreign community, where the Swedish ambassador, who represented US consular interests in the DPRK, was allowed to make a few brief visits to them in detention.

We all speculated on how the North Koreans would utilize the two women to extract diplomatic concessions from Washington. It was evident that only a visit from a high-ranking American would secure their release. The North Koreans told the Obama administration that the envoy had to be former President Bill Clinton or the two would not be freed. Despite great reluctance on the part of the US administration, Clinton was duly dispatched to Pyongyang in early August 2009 to collect the two women. In a sign of how little interest Washington had in a thaw, however, the Bush administration gave the former president strict instructions to avoid, under any circumstances, smiling in the presence of Kim Jong Il or other North Korean officials during a meeting he had been granted.

However dramatic the international developments, once back in North Korea, I found they barely resonated among the North Korean people. For the average citizen, life went on. Living in Pyongyang, I was able to observe a certain rhythm to the daily existence of the people there—reflecting a combination of a regime determined to exert maximum political control and ordinary folk trying nonetheless to get on with their lives. As early as 5:30 a.m. on some days, cars mounted with speakers cruised through Pyongyang broadcasting key messages from the government, often accompanied by brass bands performing at full volume. On one occasion, it was to remind people of the birthday of Kim Il Sung. On another, it was to remember his death in 1994. In the spring of 2009, much of the activity was to generate enthusiasm for what the government called the 150-Day Battle. Inspired by the largely unsuccessful 200-Day Battle that Kim Jong Il had launched in 1998 to counter the worst effects of the famine, this new drive was intended to promote the construction of houses, revive farms, and expand the production of daily necessities.

Rodong Sinmun, the official newspaper of the ruling Korean Workers' Party, carried an editorial predicting "a shining victory in the 150-Day Battle."[14] For ordinary people, the campaign consisted of even more meetings and greater regimentation in their daily routine, with security units roaming the streets randomly stopping people to ask why they were not at work—all designed to boost output and further cement national unity. High school and university students, and even government officials, were sent to the countryside to work. I recall that one official explained his recent absence from meetings because of this policy. When I expressed skepticism, he took off his watch and said, "Look." While the rest of his arm had been turned brown by the sun, the skin protected by the watch was still white. He had indeed been deployed to the countryside and engaged in farming work.

I wondered how a population that often already seemed stretched to the breaking point would respond. In any event, apart from the broadcasts that woke me up early every day, and noticing even more propaganda posters mounted on the streets—some with slogans such as "Ride the Chollima horse to charge forward and storm our way through"—I saw little evidence that the battle was producing much progress. Indeed, my sense was that for most local people, it was just another burden, compounded by anxiety that another campaign would soon follow.

The dawn announcements often were mixed with other sounds, such as the footsteps of marching soldiers practicing parade formations for the many ceremonial rallies held in Kim Il Sung Square, or children rehearsing for the Arirang Mass Games. The synchronized spectacle of the games was the ultimate propaganda homage to the regime and the Kim family cult. It was a remarkable example of totalitarian regimentation, but to witness it was also fun, exciting, and uniquely North Korean—a spectacle I imagined no other nation would be able to pull off. Despite qualms over what must have gone into the preparations, almost every visitor wanted to go.

I did see evidence of fresh building work in the capital. For more than two decades, the unfinished skeleton of the Ryugyong Hotel, a pyramid-shaped 105-story building 330 meters in height that was originally supposed to be completed for an international youth festival in 1989, had loomed like an eyesore over the city. Problems with building methods and materials delayed it for years. Now, however, Orascom, an Egyptian private company, had agreed to invest in the structure. Work on the unfinished skyscraper was to restart, and the outer walls were to be covered with glass panels. Orascom planned to use the first few floors for offices and accommodations. It seemed possible that something that to me and many others had become a symbol of North Korea's failed ambitions on so many fronts might soon become operational.

One May weekend, I also noticed that many apartment block residents were suddenly on their balconies hammering away, removing all window frames—aluminum, plastic, or wooden—as well as glass and plastic sheeting covers. An order had been given for the beautification of all urban apartment buildings, especially those facing main roads. New flowerpots, usually five per window, some with real and some with plastic flowers, began to decorate balconies. Meanwhile, many buildings received a fresh coat of paint. According to the local rumor mill, Kim Jong Il, angered by descriptions in the international press of Pyongyang as a drab and colorless city, had ordered the facelift. Whatever the reason, word was that only at a later date would residents receive new windows and frames. Knowing the level of inefficiency so common in the country, I wondered whether the windows would be double glazed and come in time to keep out the cold before the bitter Korean winter arrived.

Despite the worst of the famine having ended nearly a decade ago, the picture was bleak outside Pyongyang. Although the bulk of my work now involved running the SDC's operations from the capital, I was able periodically to visit various projects, including some I had started while still at Caritas. It was clear that the food situation remained precarious. On any patch of lawn or grass, I saw teenagers, adults, and even the elderly picking grass, herbs, and roots. Unlike during the famine years, when it would have been for their own consumption—indeed, I was particularly struck that old folks still knew what to look for, a legacy of survival techniques going back to the Korean War—now it was probably to feed rabbits kept on their balconies.

Some streets were lined with wild apricot trees, and although the fruit was green and not yet ripe, people would still pluck some of it to take home. I noticed as well that every small strip of land was cultivated with vegetables—and guarded. Although fears persisted that small-plot farming might be prohibited, it remained an important source of food. The level of tolerance varied from area to area, but it appeared that the authorities generally recognized the importance of such private plots and, while not happy about it, allowed the practice to continue.

Tensions between humanitarian agencies and the government over food aid continued. The WFP had long applied the principle of "no access, no food," to ensure that its assistance reached those most in need. But the government abruptly turned the tables, insisting instead on "no food, no access." With hardly any food pledged by international donors, the WFP had to scale down its activities. Whereas the program once had operated in 131 counties, only fifty-nine outposts were open for food distribution by 2009, targeting the most vulnerable—children and pregnant women. The WFP's international staff had to be cut from fifty to fifteen. With more and more cases of malnourished children observed in hospitals and residential childcare centers, and the level of daily cereal rations provided for some reported to be only three hundred grams, or some thousand calories, per person, it was a bleak picture. The lack of fat, protein, vitamins, and minerals, as well as shortages of clean drinking water and inadequate health care, only added to the misery.

One remarkable midwinter train trip to Beijing gave me a particularly graphic picture of what life was like in the large swaths of countryside through which I passed. It was bitterly cold, with humanitarian workers across the country reporting acute shortages of electricity and heat. Indeed, the United Nations Population Fund (UNFPA) said that some of the medical injections they had supplied had frozen and had to be destroyed. As I watched from the train, which moved at a snail's pace, everything seemed dilapidated—shabby houses and unpainted tenements, many with only plastic- or cardboard-covered windows, despite the subzero temperatures. By the side of the tracks were numerous broken-down, rusting train wagons, some filled with timber or scrap metal. I saw people with shovels clearing the snow, while others were collecting snow in buckets to use for water at home. On frozen rivers, still others had cracked holes in the ice to collect water.

But it wasn't all depressing. I could see kids playing in the snow, and some skating on frozen ponds. And the landscape itself was breathtaking—flat fields with hills and mountains in the background. Not for the first time, I thought to myself that if one did not consider the poverty, North Korea was a beautiful country. I wasn't supposed to take pictures, but as I was alone in the compartment, with no North Korean traveling companion, I took as many photos as I could. My musings were cut short as the train pulled into a station near the Chinese border, where I saw piles of grain sacks, all heavily guarded—a sign of how desperate some people still were for food. It was disorienting to cross the bridge into China, with its shopping centers, nightclubs, restaurants, billboards, and neon lights.

While the authorities seemed willing to tolerate private plots, the expansion of markets remained a step too far. Moves to control market activity, and the economic liberalization it represented, became increasingly evident. Once the 150-Day Battle kicked into high gear in April 2009, Pyongyang's Tongil Market for a few weeks sharply reduced its operating hours, opening just from 4 p.m. to 7 p.m. Goods from South Korea disappeared from the shelves, and few items apart from food appeared to be available. At the same time, beginning in January 2009, the cabinet issued a decree saying that the farmers' markets, which had become crucial to the survival of people in the countryside, could again operate only every ten days—on the first, eleventh, and twenty-first day of each month.

Amidst these economic difficulties, on May 25, 2009, Kim Jong Il ordered the country's second nuclear test. Several missile tests followed. This led the United Nations Security Council to pass a new set of even tougher sanctions, further deepening the country's isolation.

Then, on November 30, 2009, Kim took the drastic step of ordering a revaluation of North Korea's currency. The government introduced a new version of its paper currency but allowed people to exchange only a certain amount of the old currency, at an exchange rate of one hundred old won for one new won. At a stroke, people's savings were wiped out. To many North Koreans who had stored cash to help tide them over during the lean winter and spring months, it was a devastating blow. Citizens were shocked, and whatever confidence the North Koreans had in their currency evaporated. It was the first time I had seen my North Korean acquaintances visibly angry. Panic buying swept Pyongyang, with people purchasing items they didn't need with the old currency they had rather than risk losing it all. The shelves in shops were quickly emptied. Restaurants closed for several weeks. Even foreigners were allowed to go to only one restaurant and one shop. The economy came to a virtual standstill. The few shops and individual traders who still had a few goods were not willing to sell anything, because nobody knew at what exchange rate deals should be made.

My notes for an excursion around Pyongyang on December 31, 2009, give a sense of the situation. "Afternoon shopping, empty shelves, even beer, flour and eggs were sold out, only goods left were those you don't really need or want, lollipops sold at an outrageous price, that's why they were still there. You can't live on salty potato chips. 2 kg of apples euro 7." With the start of the new year, eggs again became available at the diplomatic shop. But restaurants remained closed for all, locals and expats alike, with new prices not yet fixed and the new exchange rate not known.

The dramatic currency revaluation appeared designed to crush the markets and other unofficial economic activity, which Kim Jong Il may have seen as a threat to state authority, as well as to control inflation, weed out corruption, and target an emerging merchant class. It was, in effect, a way to confiscate the cash of those who had become relatively rich selling in the private markets. Instead, however, the revaluation provoked anger, as prices skyrocketed and shortages kicked in. There were reports of suicides, and even some almost-unprecedented public protests. The government was stung by the popular unrest. The chief of the party's finance department, Pak Nam Gi was blamed for the mess and reportedly executed in March 2010, and the government cautiously backtracked. By the spring of 2010, the markets had reopened.

CHAPTER SEVENTEEN

Black and White

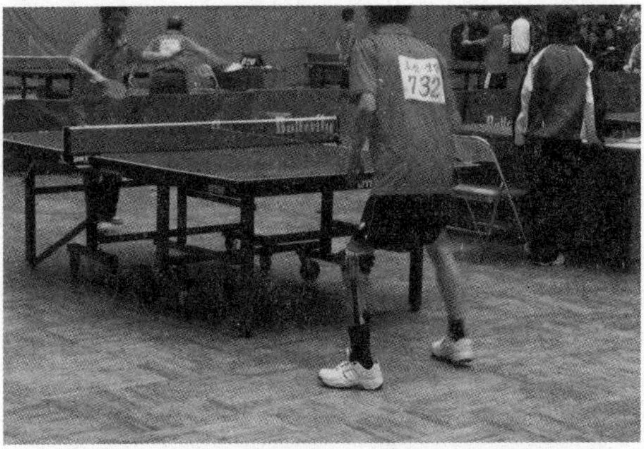

Some people with disabilities enjoyed the opportunity to engage in a small SDC-funded sports project.

One by one, the procession of people arrived at the gates of the old Bulgarian embassy, now home to Pyongyang's main foreign hangout, the RAC (Random Access Club). Dressed in wigs and other strange headgear, gloves, skintight pants, and a variety of other outlandish outfits, the crowd passed the puzzled and slightly alarmed North Korean security guards at the gate of the main diplomatic compound, who had no idea what was going on. It was the early summer of 2009, and Pyongyang's small foreign community was celebrating the life of pop icon Michael Jackson, who had passed away on June 25, with a costume party.

Wearing a curly black wig and long white gloves, as well as a black-and-white outfit, I had so changed my appearance that the bemused North

Korean guards at the exit of the SDC compound didn't recognize me. Other attendees were equally oddly dressed. I joked to the other attendees that "nothing is black or white in North Korea except for my outfit."

The party was the idea of the spouse of a World Food Program employee. A colleague who happened to have been in Beijing on a rest-and-recreation break was tasked with finding costumes and other props. A large cardboard coffin was constructed, decorated with Jackson's picture and plastic flowers, and placed in the center of the main RAC room. As his famous hits, such as "Black and White," "Billie Jean," and "Thriller," blared from loudspeakers, we danced the night away in a mood combining sadness and more than a little hysteria. For the small, usually overworked and overstressed international community, it was a welcome break from the day-to-day pressures of living and working in North Korea—a chance to let our hair down for an evening. No North Koreans attended, and there was no doubt that the North Korean security personnel at the compound gate thought we were more than a little crazy.

In fairness, though, by the late 2000s, expat life in North Korea was not nearly as grim as it had been a decade earlier. Once the fallout from the disastrous currency revaluation began to subside, restaurants started to reopen, and some goods were back on the shelves. Near the Ryugyong Hotel was a shop we had dubbed the "Blue Wonder," because it was a painted a garish shade of blue. Apparently, an Argentine businessman whose connections to North Korea were murky ran it; he stocked a variety of Argentinian goods, including a decent Argentinian Malbec wine—a pleasant surprise. I was even more surprised when I visited the Rakwon Department Store in the city center. Although it did not have many goods, I was astonished to find a bottle of 1997 Chateau Mouton Rothschild wine, with a label designed by the famous French American painter and sculptor Niki de Saint Phalle. The shop assistant was offering it for ten euros, but I knew it was something special and later learned that it was normally priced at $450. I could only assume that it had been a gift to a North Korean official or businessman, perhaps from a Chinese visitor, and, not aware of its value, the owner of the bottle was happy to get ten euros in cash from the store for trading it in. In any case, it was an enjoyable addition to my modest wine collection, and I still have the bottle today.

One popular gathering place was a new pizza restaurant. Rumor had it that the owner was a member of the Italian Communist Party. In any case, he had imported flour, cheese, and other ingredients, including salty, spicy anchovies, and brought experts from Italy to train the local chefs, who baked their pizzas in an authentic pizza oven. The atmosphere was always jolly, not least because the North Korean waitresses had been taught to sing Italian songs while serving. Their favorite was "O Sole Mio," which they sang over and over again. One evening, I treated the entire SDC team—all twenty of us, foreigners and North Koreans—to dinner there. The pizzas were a big hit. Everyone ate a lot, tasting every single pizza on the menu, but at the end, my North Korean colleagues asked, somewhat surprised and in anticipation, "Where is the main course?" No rice had been served, and although sophisticated and worldly by North Korean standards, they didn't believe a meal could conclude without rice being a central part of it.

Although golf is not usually associated with socialist austerity, there was even a golf course to which we expats had access. Called the Pyongyang Golf Club, it was located twenty-seven kilometers from the capital on the banks of Lake Taedong along the highway from Pyongyang to the port of Nampo. It had an eighteen-hole par-seventy-two course, a clubhouse, a pro shop, and a highly regarded restaurant. It was frequented mostly by foreigners, but occasionally we saw some North Koreans as well, presumably members of the elite.

The course was associated with one of the central myths of the Kim family, which was that in the early 1990s, Kim Jong Il in one game had scored five holes in one and finished thirty-eight under par. There was, of course, no way to confirm such an outlandish report, and it elicited more than a little derision. *The New York Times* quoted one analyst on the American Golf TV channel as saying, "Imagine the schedule he kept. Eight to 11—enrich uranium. One to four—destroy the world. Four to seven—play golf, shoot 11 holes-in-one and call it a night. I don't remember him popping up at the Masters."[15] But the Dear Leader's interest in sports was well-known. Indeed, when US Secretary of State Madeleine Albright visited Pyongyang in October 2000, among the gifts she brought was a basketball signed by Chicago Bulls star Michael Jordan.[16]

The scenery on the outskirts of Pyongyang was indeed lovely, as was much of the rest of the country, and it was possible to go for hikes and picnics. We often would come across North Korean families or groups of workers out for the day, making a barbecue and, invariably, singing and dancing. Meaningful conversations were never possible, but the people we met were always smiling and friendly and sometimes even invited us to join in. Their attitude and behavior were evidence that, even for people who didn't have very much, they were trying to make the best of things. It was an uplifting antidote to the tight controls and harsh rhetoric that usually surrounded us.

As an example of the tight controls, on one public holiday, the head of the WFP office and I took a walk along the Taedong River, which flows through central Pyongyang. We stopped to photograph some spring flowers, but suddenly a young official arrived, took us away into a guard hut, and forced us to delete the pictures. We must have inadvertently photographed something sensitive when shooting the flowers. Later, more senior officials came, but since the photos had been deleted, we had no way to prove that we had taken them, let alone that our intention had been to photograph only flowers.

Eventually, and with some difficulty, we managed to call the WFP's North Korean liaison officer, who rushed to the scene. As it was a holiday, he evidently had been drinking, and we noticed he seemed quite tipsy, but he managed to sort things out. We suspected he may have bribed the local officials with alcohol and cigarettes. In any case, it was a highly embarrassing experience. To have the heads of two major international organizations in the DPRK in such trouble was not a good look, even if our transgression, whatever it may have been, was done in all innocence.

More serious was when a group of NGO workers lost their way on a Sunday outing. Some foreigners working in the country could travel to certain areas without getting travel permission, so off they went—and by accident ended up stumbling into a military camp. The Ministry of Foreign Affairs eventually had to intervene in order to get them out.

That was hardly the only example of how what seemed like unexceptional aspects of daily life proved stressful. In the summer of 2009, we experienced nearly a month of nonstop electricity outages—sometimes as many as ten power cuts in three hours. The result was a shutdown of the stabilizer and the control panel that was programmed to automatically switch our emergency generator on. This caused serious problems for running and maintaining all of our electronic equipment, to the point that at times the office was no longer able to function. Indeed, one server was so severely damaged, it had to be replaced. We ordered a new one, and in addition we had to bring in technicians from Beijing to repair the stabilizer. It was only after a formal letter of complaint to the General Service Bureau for Diplomatic Missions that the situation began to return to normal.

For all the stresses, I do have many warm memories. Every autumn, we would have a "kimchi day" at the office. Making kimchi, the staple of the Korean diet and an important source of nutrition during the long winter, was an important ritual in every Korean family. I would gather all of the local and expatriate staff on our team, and together we prepared the two hundred kilograms of cabbage we had received for the office from the General Service Bureau. We would put that and the other essential ingredients into huge brown earthenware pots called *onggi*, and cover the pots with sturdy lids. We then buried the pots in the soil, where the cabbage would ferment and therefore keep for several months.

These kimchi days were always fun, filled with jokes, laughter, and camaraderie. I knew how close kimchi was to the heart of the Koreans, and felt this was a good bonding exercise that drew the team together. Other bonding activities including bowling—Pyongyang had a nice bowling alley—and, one Lunar New Year, to mark the arrival of the Year of the Pig, we had a dinner followed by a competition to see who could draw the nicest pig!

I also always made a point of holding a Christmas party every year and giving presents to the staff. One year, I gave a pregnant staffer a teddy bear. She spent the whole evening sitting on a chair and stroking the teddy. I could tell she was deeply moved. Another time, I showed the Rowan Atkinson comedy film *Merry Christmas, Mr. Bean*, which tells the story of the hapless Mr. Bean bumbling his way through Christmas shopping, gift-giving, and various celebrations in London. As the movie is highly visual and shows everything, the story is easy to understand regardless of the audience's level of English. Moreover, it was totally nonpolitical, so I thought it was a safe film to share with my North Korean colleagues—that they wouldn't get in trouble for having watched it. And that turned out to be the case. Indeed, I had never seen my team members laugh so hard.

I was not a particularly enthusiastic sports fan, but periodically I attended international football matches, which were a very big deal to the North Koreans. In April and June 2009, two important games took place, against teams from the United Arab Emirates and Iran, with qualification for the 2010 World Cup at stake. Switzerland had played a small role in helping the DPRK, offering training programs for North Korean football coaches, and in September 2008, the Swiss second-division team Concordia Basel signed the first-ever two North Korean football players to be hired by a European club.

A match I attended, against Iran—one of the world's better teams—in October 2008 was particularly intense. The stadium contained thirty thousand North Korean fans, along with about twenty Iranians who had made the journey from Tehran on one of the planes belonging to President Mahmoud Ahmadinejad to support their side. When the North Korean team scored a goal, the crowd went wild. When the Iranians did, there was absolute silence—except that the handful of Iranian fans had brought drums and trumpets, making much more noise than one would expect from their small number. The match ended in a 2–1 Iranian victory. Leaving the stadium, one of my North Korean colleagues, referring to the noise, declared, "Those were terrible football hooligans." I barely suppressed a laugh. In any case, in 2010 the DPRK qualified for the FIFA World Cup for the first time since 1966, a source of intense national pride.

But against the backdrop of the always interesting, often frustrating, and sometimes bizarre rhythm of daily life, the work continued. Apart from the SDC's large-scale projects—capacity development, agricultural programs, and so on—we supported a number of other initiatives. One of the most important was the SDC's contribution of a half million Swiss francs to the United Nations Population Fund (UNFPA) to conduct a census in late 2008. This was only the second census with international involvement that North Korea had ever carried out, the first one having taken place in 1993. It was somewhat surprising that such help was accepted, but presumably the DPRK leadership felt it was a price worth paying to get a better sense of the reality on the ground in order to develop the country's economy.

With the support of thirty teams from UNFPA, thirty-five thousand census takers fanned out across the country for fifteen days. They surveyed 5,587,767 households nationwide, soliciting answers to fifty-three questions about income, furniture, electronic home appliances, toilets, heating systems, tap water, and sewage facilities, as well as basic personal information such as age and gender.

In a nation known for its reluctance to share information, the published findings were fascinating. The total population was 24,052,000, up 2.84 million from 1993, a growth rate of 0.85 percent, suggesting that an uptick in births following the famine had compensated for the lives lost during that devastating time. The data also showed that North Koreans were getting older and less healthy than in 1993, with proportionately fewer children and more middle-aged and elderly people. Worryingly, the infant mortality rate climbed to 19.3 per 1,000 children in 2008 from 14.1 in 1993, the average life expectancy fell from 72.7 to 69.3 years, and women were living roughly seven years longer than men.

The census also provided other revealing glimpses into North Korean society. The country had 5.9 million households, with an average of 3.9 people in each. A female headed only one out of every ten households, evidence that the DPRK was still a male-dominated society, with few divorces and hardly any single mothers. About 85 percent of homes had access to running water, and about 58 percent had a flush toilet. In terms of work, farming provided employment to the single largest number of people, with 3.4 million people working the land. The second-biggest area of employment was the government, including the military, which employed 699,000 people. Interestingly, if that figure was reliable, it suggested that the size of the North Korean active-duty armed forces might be smaller than many Western analysts had long believed.

In negotiations with the government about the details of conducting the census before it got underway, I had pushed strongly for questions about disability to be included in the questionnaire. My interest in the plight of the disabled in North Korea dated back to my first trip in 1995, where I was, after some negotiations, allowed to visit a residential school for children with hearing problems. In a society so short of resources, I had long felt that disabled people were at the bottom of the priority list, often rejected or marginalized, with few support facilities, so I was always looking for opportunities to raise the issue or find ways to encourage the North Koreans to focus more attention on it. In the end, officials agreed to collect some data by asking individuals whether they had difficulty doing certain basic activities. Only a small proportion of the population reported any kind of disability: 2.5 percent acknowledged problems with mobility, and 2.4 percent said they had problems with their sight. The number of those willing to admit to hearing problems or mental handicaps was even smaller. More women than men said they faced difficulties of some kind. The data wasn't detailed, but I felt that anything that brought these issues to the attention of the authorities had the potential to do some good.

As always with North Korean statistics, it was hard to be sure about their accuracy. Nevertheless, from my perspective—even with the caveat that the data could be not totally reliable—a census with several dozen teams of international experts would provide important information for planning further humanitarian and development activities.

The SDC office had what was called a small projects fund—money that we could use at our discretion (in consultation with colleagues in Berne, of course) to support more modest initiatives beyond the large-scale projects that were our primary focus. Usually, we responded to requests or inquiries from the DPRK side rather than initiating anything ourselves. Even though it was a small amount of money compared with the other, more elaborate development projects the SDC was supporting, I thought these efforts were worthwhile, because they were addressing problems for which easily provided and non-bureaucratic assistance could play a positive role. Moreover, by getting involved with these other efforts, I was able to have contact with a wider range of people, see other parts of North Korean society, travel, and broaden my perspective and understanding.

I had been friendly with—and supportive of—the Korean Federation for the Protection of the Disabled (KFPD) for years, going back to its establishment in 1998 during my time at Caritas. Officials from the KFPD knew that I had returned to Pyongyang for the SDC, and we periodically kept in touch. One day, they came to me with a proposal—would we consider supporting an effort to provide recreational opportunities for disabled people, specifically to enable them to play sports? The idea was to stage a table tennis tournament. To me, it was a small sign of changing attitudes, in which welfare and rehabilitation centers for the disabled finally were receiving some official backing. The SDC agreed to pay for the equipment—table tennis paddles, balls, tables, and nets—as well as sports outfits, and I was an honored guest at the tournament.

The event was held in an auditorium, with several table tennis courts separated by green cloth dividers, a scorer's table, and players organized into teams. To see people wearing a prosthesis or struggling with other disabilities put their heart into the game was deeply moving, as was the sight of their families, who all had been invited, cheering in the stands. What struck me most was the sheer willpower of the participants, which came through in the intense way they played the games. At the time, the DPRK had not yet joined the Paralympics, but it did so in 2012. I like to think that the tournament we helped to sponsor may have played a role in creating an atmosphere in which the country felt eager to participate.

During my many years of working in North Korea, the lack of safe drinking water was a major problem throughout the country. Many people did not have working taps providing potable water at home and had to go to wells or rivers to get their drinking water. This was often contaminated and a source of disease, so when the head of the Save the Children Pyongyang office approached me with a request to support a clean drinking water initiative, we were pleased to help. The effort was focused on the city of Hamhung, where Save the Children had other projects as well. Hamhung was the second-largest city in the DPRK, located in the northeast, and had suffered badly during the famine years—its difficulties compounded by a lack of arable land—and, to some extent, was still just getting back on its feet.

The idea was to open a series of drinking water shops, managed by local people, where residents could get safe drinking water for a very modest fee. Although no one made any money from the payments, they helped keep the project afloat. And the small cost was outweighed not only by the benefit of having clean water, but by the fact that people no longer had to use precious coal or wood supplies to boil water acquired from other sources. On a trip to Hamhung, I visited two such water shops. The first, serving some twelve thousand people, was open from 5 a.m. to 9 p.m. On average, most families received ten liters of drinking water per day, and I watched citizens line up, carrying several big plastic containers, waiting for their turn. To encourage participation, the water was free for the first year; thereafter, people paid for five liters of water with a coupon that cost only one won. The second shop was located near the city's south gate. The locals had done all the work, including installing the pump, the tank, the pipes, and other fittings, while Save the Children and the SDC had paid for these materials.

The water quality was tested daily, and the initiative proved to be extremely popular. The two shops I visited were among nine that had been opened, with plans for six more. I not only was gratified to see the program's success but realized how much we in the developed world took things like drinking water for granted. In Hong Kong or Switzerland, we would not think twice about turning on the tap or about the quality of the water that came out. Getting safe drinking water was, although necessary, something of a luxury for all too many North Koreans.

But of all the small-scale projects, the one closest to my heart was the Hwangju Boarding School in North Hwanghae Province. This was one of about forty institutions around the country accommodating between eight thousand and ten thousand children, most of them orphans who had lost parents during the famine or other natural disasters, or from other causes. During my early Caritas visits, I did not know that such institutions even existed. It wasn't until my fifteenth trip that I began to get greater access. I found conditions at Hwangju to be pitiful, with the kids stunted or showing other signs of malnutrition, their unheated dormitories bitterly cold in winter, and hardly any school materials and toys. The hard-pressed staff were so overwhelmed with basic survival tasks that they were not really able to provide the children with much in the way of love, care, and concern. It was heartbreaking, described in my notes as a "cruel and terrible upbringing." So Caritas provided supplies of all kinds: canned fish, sugar, clothes, school materials, toys, soap, blankets, and more. But it often seemed that the staff, however dedicated, were so burdened by their work that a certain warmth was missing, and I always felt it would be so nice if we could bring kilos of cuddles as well.

I visited many times while working for Caritas, and felt deeply that I wanted to continue to support this boarding school. When I went there again after starting my SDC assignment and indicated that we might have some resources to continue to help, the staff received me like an old friend. I had built up a relationship of warmth and trust with the staff there, to the point that they often felt able to share concerns and feelings they would normally never acknowledge to a foreigner. I will never forget the harried and overstressed headmaster turning to me, sighing as he looked at the kids he was responsible for, and saying, in a pained voice, "I also have children." I could see that staff members were putting their hearts into their work here.

The stunting—a clear sign of chronic food deprivation, with an impact on physical health and possibly also on mental health—was particularly shocking. Fifteen-year-olds looked like eight- or ten-year-olds. The diet was insufficient, not only in terms of carbohydrates but even more so regarding proteins, fats, and micronutrients. The children ate a mixture of rice and maize, along with kimchi and soup. Meat or fish was available only on public holidays, and eggs also were a rare commodity. I was always stunned at how basic the kitchen was and what a hard job it was to prepare so many meals with so few ingredients. And such conditions were more or less the same in all the residential institutions.

In summer, children suffered from diarrhea and/or had skin problems. In winter, acute respiratory infections with symptoms of watery eyes, a runny nose, and a deep hacking cough were common. Heating was a big problem. After their lessons, fifty children often would stay in one room, huddled together to keep warm, with the proximity enhancing the risk of the spread of infections. Watching TV was virtually the only pastime and was done in shifts. A small room would be packed with children, glued to the TV. In summer, they could at least play outdoors.

Each dormitory room had space for four or more boys or girls. Each child had a small locker for his or her few personal belongings. As with the water project, I thought about the number of toys and variety of clothing many Western children had. School materials were also lacking. Books had to be handed down for many years, and two or three kids often had to share one book.

I became aware that our visits to these institutions also were providing the North Koreans with a window to the world. These children had never seen a foreigner before. I had learned to write the word "Switzerland" in Korean, and after my North Korean colleague had introduced me, I would write it on the blackboard as an icebreaker. The children would giggle, their amusement and curiosity further piqued because I am left-handed, something almost never seen in the DPRK. Such fleeting moments showed that even in this grim environment, there were traces of good humor and happiness.

And it was encouraging to see that the assistance provided was being put to good use. On one visit, staffers told me—and I saw for myself—that two hundred square meters of linoleum our assistance had helped them to purchase had led to resurfacing the rough floors in fourteen rooms, ten dormitories, and the clinic. And with the passage of time, the condition of most of the children gradually improved. We had subsidized the construction of a greenhouse at the Hwangju Boarding School, where cucumbers, tomatoes, mushrooms, lettuce, radishes, and cabbage had been planted. On one visit, I saw and estimated that about one-third of the roughly eight hundred kids were still somewhat malnourished or weak. In 2009, I was told that the nutritional status of 80 percent of the children had stabilized, although ten had been hospitalized for unspecified conditions. The food situation also was getting better slowly. In addition to rice and maize, the government had provided 300 kilograms of vegetable oil and one ton of soya beans, with the

SDC providing an additional 10,000 kilograms of vegetable oil. I was told that children were given 231 grams of rice, 103 grams of maize, and 25 grams of the SDC-provided vegetable oil each day.

The World Food Program also had been delivering assistance, but by 2010 its efforts had run into problems. During a June 2009 visit, I learned that the high-energy biscuits and vegetable oil the WFP had been supplying were about to run out, and nothing more was in the pipeline. I knew that the WFP had not been satisfied with monitoring arrangements. Given the relationship of trust I had developed, I bluntly told officials at the school that more openness and transparency were needed if they wanted additional assistance. We had difficult conversations. I stressed that being honest was important. The WFP staff were suspicions that the school had inflated the figures of what they needed to get more aid. I pushed on this point, warning that it could have serious consequences and that any further aid could lead to demands for stricter monitoring, but never got a clear answer. It was a sobering example of how, even in an institution run by compassionate and devoted staff trying to help the most disadvantaged, old habits persisted. Or perhaps the situations at the homes of the staff were equally dire, and that was why they wanted the additional supplies.

The uncertainty reflected a central fact about North Korea. Nothing was as black or white on the inside as outsiders often assumed. Beyond the apparent surface uniformity, there were layers of ambiguity and uncertainty, further blurred by a system where information was jealously guarded and suspicion of foreigners ran deep. For me, this less than clear-cut reality made trying to determine the right balance between the SDC's main mission—development cooperation—and a still-pressing need for humanitarian aid especially challenging. I was convinced that in the long run, focusing on development offered a better chance for people to improve their lives. But those who were still fighting for survival—a large proportion of the population—had little time or energy for development projects that would likely take months, if not years, to show results. Aid efforts, on the other hand, could often immediately improve dire conditions. Juggling these conflicting pressures on a daily basis, I found myself, for all the things that troubled me about the North Korean system, becoming less judgmental about what I was seeing. The frustrations continued, but I remained determined to do what I could to help.

CHAPTER EIGHTEEN

Women and the Five M's

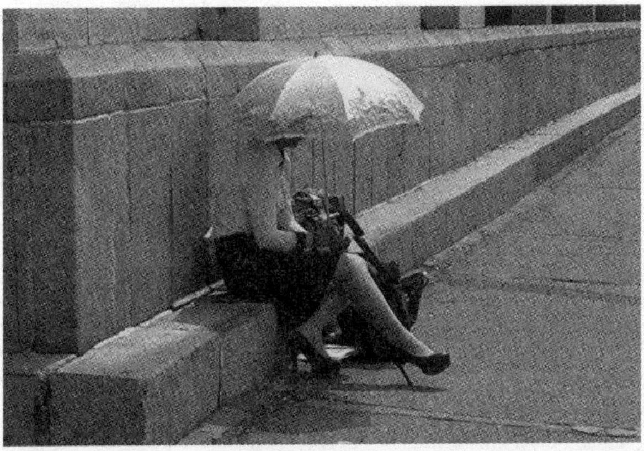

The growing popularity of high heels and parasols among women were signs of how a North Korean middle-class was emerging.

Over the years, I had many dealings with North Korean women—in schools, hospitals, nurseries, kindergartens, and farms, at the SDC, and elsewhere. For all the challenges they faced, I came away admiring—and deeply moved by—their strength, courage, and apparent refusal to give up as they carried multiple burdens under often difficult circumstances.

So I was heartened when, in 2010, during my fourth year in Pyongyang, North Korea passed a law on "the protection and promotion of the rights of women." The DPRK even submitted it to the UN Human Rights Commission, stating that it "comprehensively provides for...rights to social and political life, education, health care, work, personal inviolability and property, marriage, and family."[17]

It wasn't North Korea's first piece of legislation regarding women. Indeed, as far back as 1946, the government had adopted a law giving women equal rights to men. And DPRK propaganda long lauded women as the "flower of the household, society, and the state." Every year on March 8, International Women's Day, the government would stage a big celebration, to which I was usually invited. Officials would read long statements extolling the role of women, and then children would perform gymnastics, dance, and sing. At my office, my male colleagues would present me with a bouquet of flowers, and I would invite all female team members to my flat for a lunch that I would cook myself. For them, it was a rare opportunity to see how a foreigner lived, and they were curious about everything.

The few foreign women living in Pyongyang created the Pyongyang International Women's Association (PIWA). The group was quite active, arranging events such as bazaars and engaging in other charity activities to support needy North Korean children. My North Korean counterparts were somewhat surprised to see women from so many different countries working together so amicably and having so much fun in the process. I wondered what conclusions they drew from it.

As became evident on my many trips and in countless meetings over the years, the reality for women in North Korean society was rather different from the public stance. On numerous occasions, I would arrive at a meeting to discover that my half dozen or more interlocutors all were men. When I would ask, "Where are the women?" the response would be embarrassed laughter. Indeed, North Korea remained a deeply patriarchal society, shaped by centuries-old Confucian values in which women were expected to obey first their fathers and then their husbands. The vast majority of women faced intense pressure to prioritize family and domestic responsibilities over personal or professional ambitions—to serve the state by producing children to be loyal workers in the socialist system. Their professional work usually was limited to fields such as medicine, accounting, and teaching. Even there, traditional attitudes were deeply entrenched. At one meeting at the Ministry of Education, an all-male group of officials expressed concern that the educational system, with the predominance of female teachers, was becoming "too feminine."

The attitudes were not surprising, given that according to the 2008 census, only one out of every twelve women had completed a university education, as compared with seven out of twelve men. There were few women in high positions—the highest-ranking female official I ever met was a vice minister of agriculture—and many high-ranking women appeared to be relatives of senior leaders, as we see today with Kim Jong Un's sister Kim Yo Jong. The tradition of female subservience was strong enough that at one time, there was even a regulation barring women from riding bicycles—and subjecting them to a fine if they were to do so. Women also were discouraged from wearing trousers and speaking up in meetings. It was often a challenge, but in all the capacity development programs that the SDC sponsored—training, study tours, conference attendance—I always insisted, often in a humorous fashion to reduce the tension, that women be involved as a condition of moving forward.

The inequality was glaringly evident in farming. While the few men generally looked after machinery or sat on management committees, women did most of the heavy labor in the fields. I could see this on my travels throughout the country, and it was backed up by data from the 2008 census, which recorded that in agriculture, forestry, and fishing, a majority of the workers were women. Farming was tough, exhausting work. The hours were long, and many of the women suffered health problems, from diarrhea to malnutrition. Moreover, the government continually pressured farmers to increase production without providing additional agricultural machinery, and the women in the fields often were close to the breaking point already. No wonder that UNICEF data showed that 35 percent of women of childbearing age in North Korea suffered from anemia—twice as high in South Korea.

On top of this, they were still responsible for getting food on the table, keeping the house in good order, rearing children, growing food in their own kitchen gardens, and sometimes working in the unofficial economy. It was an enormous burden. During my earlier visits, in the mid-1990s, I'd often come across families with three or four children. But under the present circumstances, it was not surprising that many women now only wanted one child, or at the most, two children.

Ironically, it was the emergence of an unofficial, semiunderground economy during the famine—which then became somewhat legitimized with the profusion of markets—that triggered a dramatic change in the status of women, although the authorities did not sanction, and indeed only grudgingly tolerated, it. As I visited the large Tongil Market in Pyongyang, I was struck that almost all the vendors were women. They procured the goods, haggled over prices, and either kept the profits for themselves or shared them with loosely organized market cooperatives. Their presence was the result of a rigid, male-dominated structure in which men were assigned to ostensibly more respected and stable state-run workplaces—factories, workshops, the armed forces, and so on. The still-feeble economy meant that wages, food, and other state-provided benefits often arrived irregularly, if at all. And yet the men still had to clock in, even if all they did was spend their days in an idle factory. Monitored by a pervasive apparatus of control, many of these men were, in effect, stuck.

For women, as homemakers or agricultural workers or both, there was much less supervision and control, since they weren't required to show up at government jobs like men. And since the state often was unable to provide daily necessities, women had both an incentive and an opportunity to plunge into the unofficial economy to survive. Initially, it was often little more than trying to make ends meet by selling homemade baked goods, or vegetables and fruit when available, by the side of the road. The *jangmadang* (marketplaces) initially became the main source of survival for the vast majority of families in North Korea, and later, a source of regular income. As this process evolved, women increasingly emerged as the main breadwinners. It was hard work. With a lack of public transport, it was not uncommon to see women moving from home to market, or from market to market, carrying loads of thirty to fifty kilograms on their backs. Yet, judging from my own interactions and what I could see, North Korean women were tough and resourceful, and many appeared to thrive in this new and empowering environment.

Precisely how these markets worked—how and where the goods were procured, paid for, and transported—remained something of a mystery to us foreigners. The process apparently also involved smuggling, usually from China, using a network of middlemen who presumably would each receive a payoff. It had benefits, but it also exposed women to the danger of being left at the mercy of a world that operated on bribes and corruption. And the level of official tolerance often shifted from grudging acquiescence to periodic crackdowns. Indeed, I frequently heard the term "frog markets" used to refer to smaller, even less structured markets where the vendors would jump up, run, and disappear like frogs whenever the police showed up. These markets, I was told, were not only in many areas of Pyongyang but in the countryside too. They varied from small to quite big; usually sold foodstuffs, including homemade snacks; and often were open quite late in the evening. Whatever the case, it was clear that North Korean women were propelling the dynamic underpinning this quasi-underground business. In the process, they were learning all sorts of skills—networking, negotiating, monitoring price fluctuations, shipping, navigating the workings of the market—to which they otherwise never would have been exposed.

It was no surprise that the unofficial markets in the northeastern provinces near the Chinese border were livelier, better stocked, and more frequently patronized than those closer to Pyongyang. Interestingly, this dynamic also may explain why women comprised the vast majority of defectors from North Korea. This had always been the case, dating back to the end of the Korean War, but by the early to mid-2000s, the proportion of female defectors exceeded 80 percent.[18] Part of the explanation may have been a demand for labor in the booming Chinese economy; China was a way station for many refugees on the hoped-for eventual journey to South Korea. Certainly, the knowledge of the wider world acquired by being the leading force in North Korea's network of markets also played a considerable role in spurring women to choose to flee.

The growth of markets spread so widely that the government, although recognizing their crucial economic importance, sought to limit their impact. One way was to curtail the number of people involved by introducing a regulation in 2007 that only middle-aged women could work in the markets. This left many younger women in limbo, but the regulation seemed generally to be ignored. We also heard of more than a few cases in which younger women would pay bribes so the authorities would look the other way and allow them to join in the market activities.

The empowerment of women through their role in the markets changed the dynamic in many homes. Suddenly, women were earning more than men, so they had more clout in family decisions on a host of issues. One result was that the traditional Confucian preference for sons began to diminish, as parents saw daughters as being better able to take advantage of the benefits of an economy in which markets were playing an increasingly important role. Another consequence was that separation and divorce rates rose markedly, leading to a significant increase in the number of female-headed households. Indeed, women in the markets would joke, "If there is anyone who would buy my husband, I would be most happy to sell him—even at a discount!"

The market-activity space for women was hardly unlimited. As with everything else in North Korea, the government's political control, although manifested in different ways, extended throughout the society. For women, the state-run Korean Democratic Women's Union remained a powerful body. Although its influence diminished somewhat as the market economy grew, it was still crucially important in receiving and then transmitting orders or instructions from the top leadership down to the village level, and in ensuring that people obeyed the official guidance.

In June 2010, I received permission to visit Pujon County, in mountainous South Hamgyong Province, which largely had been off-limits to foreigners. The SDC was sponsoring an agricultural project in Pujon, which explains why I was allowed to go there. And I was able to meet with the chairwoman and vice chairwoman of the Pujon County Women's Union. It was the first time I had been given access to anyone from the union in the countryside. As befitting an organization whose main goal was to promote government policies—although achieving gender equality was another goal—the women told me that the union was, at that moment, focusing on motivating its members to work harder and increase agricultural productivity.

The two women from the union told me that most of their members were housewives, but membership also was open to single women. The group also organized training sessions on topics such as how to grow cash crops, such as sesame, and how to breed small animals. Indeed, I was asked if the SDC could supply some booklets about how to raise rabbits. The union also was in charge of nurseries and kindergartens, which were staffed mainly by volunteers, the women told me.

Another project in which women were involved was the construction of a small hydropower station—something that was badly needed, as highlighted by the erratic electricity supply in the guesthouse where I stayed. Touring the county, I was struck by the absence of young men. When I asked about it, my guide told me that most men between seventeen and thirty years old were in the army. Army work did not always mean purely military duties, as many men were involved in construction, road maintenance, and the like. Women and older men carried out most work in the fields.

Despite their hard agricultural work, women and their families still worried about food security. The World Food Program was providing blended food—with vitamins and minerals added—for young kids in nurseries in

Pujon, and enrollment was up because of this, the union officials told me. However difficult, the chairwoman told me, "malnutrition is no longer serious. We can cope." To me, that exemplified the kind of strong determination with which so many North Korean women I encountered confronted their circumstances.

My conversation with the two union heads was illuminating on other topics as well. They told me that the average age to get married was twenty-seven for women and thirty for men. They said arranged marriages still occurred, and the union itself often played the role of matchmaker. This did not altogether surprise me. One of the female team members in my office in Pyongyang told me her parents had given her six months to find a partner. Otherwise, they said, they would do so themselves. She was, of course, twenty-seven years old.

I had some additional dealings with the Korean Democratic Women's Union through Anita Fahrni, an exuberant and outgoing Swiss American who had been living in Switzerland since the 1970s. She had been deeply involved in working with women's groups there as well as in the developing world, and had a particularly long history of engagement with Mongolia, which she had been visiting for years and providing educational materials for its still-undeveloped educational system. She had first encountered officials from the Korean Democratic Women's Union in 2005 at a Beijing Plus Ten event, a follow-up to the well-known UN Fourth World Conference on Women held in the Chinese capital in 1995, and then had begun to bring groups of Swiss women to the DPRK. The union was her official host. Her delegations represented a wide mixture of Swiss women—politicians, businesswomen, farmers, members of the national women's federation Alliance F, and others.

As she had been doing in Mongolia, Anita also arranged to ship a twenty-foot container of books to Pyongyang. They included novels, school textbooks, even old issues of *National Geographic* magazine. The books were delivered to the Grand People's Study House—the national library—off Kim Il Sung Square. As the library stacks weren't open to foreigners, there was no way to know for sure whether anyone actually looked at them, but the North Koreans expressed gratitude for the donation.

I made a point to meet Anita and the groups she brought on visits, and occasionally accompanied them on field trips out of the capital. It was fascinating to sit in on the briefings the North Koreans provided. They insisted, for example, that there was no domestic violence and virtually no abortion in the country. Few details were provided, so there was no way to independently confirm these assertions—and defector accounts have repeatedly mentioned domestic violence and sexual abuse as a chronic problem—but the Women's Union members with whom we met were not prepared to discuss them.

Every so often, though, the encounters that arose from Anita's bringing her Swiss women's groups to the DPRK would produce a fascinating insight. On one occasion, I organized a picnic for her delegation and some North Korean colleagues. The discussion had turned to the question of imports and exports when, out of the blue, one of the North Koreans quietly said to Anita, "I wish they would export our entire leadership." It was a shockingly rare and exceptionally risky thing to say—something my North Korean contacts never would express in front of me. The conversation quickly shifted to other topics, but just for a moment, the mask had slipped off slightly. We wondered how many others privately shared the sentiment.

The opportunities I had to engage with Anita's groups, and what she told me about her experiences with the two delegations of North Korean women she'd brought to Switzerland, were revealing in other ways. It was clear there was a great hunger for more contact with and exposure to the outside world. This was a response similar to the one I had observed on the many visits abroad I had organized for various North Koreans over the years. Seeing how other societies operated usually was an eye-opening experience. Neither Anita nor I had any idea whether or how such exposure would have an impact back in the DPRK. But we knew that the North Koreans could not unsee what they had seen. I dared to hope that when the time was right, they might draw on these contacts with foreigners in ways that would make a difference at home.

It was in large part this mixture—of Confucian tradition, communist egalitarianism, Leninist political control, and unevenly emerging market forces—that made the situation for women in North Korea so interesting to me. As depressing as some of it was, I remained heartened by my personal encounters. However grim the circumstances, North Korean women were survivors.

Indeed, with a bit of cash in hand, some even began to display a fashion sense in their choice of shoes and handbags; some even wore a bit of make-up. I also was struck that, especially in Pyongyang, women began to walk around with little parasols, likely imported from China. Being suntanned was a sign one might have been working in the fields, and, whatever the talk about solidarity with the peasants, it was not an image that appealed to city residents.

More broadly, the base for discrimination in North Korea was changing from that of men versus women to that of the haves versus the have-nots. Money was increasingly what lubricated the society, determining who had access to education, health care, or other services—and even who was able to join the ruling Korean Workers' Party. It wasn't entirely healthy, but at least it meant that the rigid patriarchal structures that had been in place for so long were slowly beginning to crack a little.

Wrestling with how to characterize the changes I was witnessing, I created the term the "Five M's," referring to markets and money, which were playing a much bigger role in the daily lives of ordinary people; mobile phones, which had become a common form of communication; motorcars, whose presence was increasingly visible on the streets; and, most notably in Pyongyang, the emergence of a middle class.

The expansion of the unofficial but tolerated market economy underpinned the growth of this new, moneyed middle class, especially in the capital. There was even a Korean term for it: *donju*, loosely translated as "masters of money." Comprised of people who profited from the markets and trading and who often had access to foreign currency through their business ventures by working for international organizations or embassies, or through relatives working abroad—not to mention through corruption and high-level official connections—the *donju* group began to grow significantly in the late 2000s. In Pyongyang, so I heard, a *donju* was a person with the astronomical amount—for North Korea—of $100,000, while in the countryside, merely having $5,000 qualified a person to be considered a *donju*.

The signs of these changes in society were increasingly evident to me on the streets of Pyongyang. People patronized the growing number of restaurants, not just the Italian pizza place where I had taken my team but many others, including a Singaporean-run hamburger joint and a Viennese café where they could sip cappuccinos while admiring the broad vistas of Kim Il Sung Square, all the while paying with stacks of US dollars or euros. The women would make a point of displaying their jewelry in public, including fine gold chains or fashion from Beijing's Zara and H&M stores, while the men, often wearing Adidas or Nike sneakers, would smoke expensive imported cigarettes. I could see a growing number of cars on the roads as well as taxis—a half dozen new taxi companies were now operating—but still, the normal way of getting around was by bus, train, subway, bicycle, or what was known as "bus number eleven," the two ones in the number referring to people's two legs as they walked and walked and walked.

The members of the middle class were also able to purchase from a growing selection of consumer goods, from plasma TVs to squash racquets, many of them imported. There were increasing numbers of recreational and entertainment spots for them to enjoy as well, such as amusement parks, bowling alleys, other sports facilities, water parks, and aquariums. In the privacy of their homes, according to accounts from defectors, some people, using mostly smuggled DVD or MP3 players and USB devices, also had access to foreign entertainment. K-pop and dramas from South Korea were especially popular, but these forms of entertainment were extremely risky, and users could face harsh punishment if they were to be discovered by the authorities.

A central feature of the rapid change was the growing number of people using cell phones. The country's first cellular network was set up in late 2002. Operated by a Thai company called Loxley Pacific, it was confined to Pyongyang and to a special economic zone in the towns of Rajin and Sonbong near the Chinese border, although the latter effort ultimately failed. The network was based on a 2G system purchased from Hungary, and even with its high cost—750 euros to sign up and 300 euros for a phone—it quickly grew to have twenty thousand subscribers. But the government halted civilian use of the network for a period of time in the wake of the 2004 explosion at the train station in Ryongchon, near the Chinese border, shortly after a train carrying Kim Jong Il had passed through, amid rumors that it might have been an assassination attempt triggered by a remote-controlled wireless handset (although later, North Korea said the explosion had been an accident).

In 2008, however, the government revived mobile services and signed a deal with the Egyptian company Orascom to launch a 3G network. Orascom was no stranger to the DPRK. In 2008, it had signed a contract to refurbish Pyongyang's infamously decrepit 105-story Ryugyong Hotel. The nationwide cell phone service was called Koryolink, and Android phones rapidly became widely available. Soon it seemed that everyone was acquiring and using a mobile phone, attracted especially by the ease of calling or texting family and friends. Given the low incidence of landlines, with most available only for senior government officials, this was many people's first real opportunity to use a telephone, and they made the most of it. For young people and those in the growing merchant class, it became a daily necessity.

By the autumn of 2010, more than three hundred thousand North Koreans owned mobile phones. By the next year, 60 percent of Pyongyang's citizens between the ages of twenty and fifty had one, and by 2012, Koryolink reported over one million subscribers, with that number doubling in 2013.[19] I increasingly saw mobiles in the hands of not only the *donju* but of ordinary people, from teenagers to construction workers, and not only in Pyongyang but in other major cities and towns, not just for talking and texting but for taking pictures, listening to music, and playing games.

The cell phones were not cheap. The lowest-priced and most popular handset cost around $150. The majority of cell phones appeared to be Chinese models, most notably Huawei. There was a smaller market for smuggled South Korean Samsung handsets or even iPhones, which were considered much higher quality but risked being confiscated if discovered by the security police. In 2010, however, North Korea announced plans to manufacture its own device, to be called the Arirang, which would be cheaper and more accessible.

For a government that had long isolated people from one another as a tool of political control, it was a remarkable development. I was struck by the way people suddenly were able to communicate easily with relatives across the country, and by how quickly information could spread to remote cities, towns, and cooperative farms. Indeed, it became crucially important for traders, providing them with more efficient ways to exchange market information, including prices and exchange rates. The authorities evidently saw the growth of mobile communications as a symbol of modernity and a way to promote economic development, improve communications between Pyongyang and remote parts of the country, and increase productivity and efficiency. Moreover, Orascom's decision to create a joint venture with North Korea's Ministry of Posts and Telecommunications and invest $400 million could be used to show that the DPRK could be an attractive destination for foreign investment.

The criteria for owning a phone appeared not to be based on any kind of political litmus test, but rather on the ability of the individual to afford one. The authorities evidently believed that they had the surveillance capability to prevent cell phones from being used as a tool for dissent. North Korean users could not make or receive international calls, except occasionally by picking up a Chinese cell phone signal near the border with the People's Republic, and access to the internet was blocked, although the DPRK created its own intranet. While strictly censored, the intranet still made more information available than most North Koreans previously had had access to. One example: Portions of foreign books I had brought in, usually on business or technical topics, were made available on the domestic intranet. It occurred to me—and I told our North Korean partners—that if North Korea became more engaged internationally, this might become a copyright issue, but during my time there, it never did.

In addition, the government used its mobile network to spread official propaganda. The first Koryolink phone numbers began with the digits 1912, the year that Kim Il Sung was born. A service was introduced to allow the reading of *Rodong Sinmun*, the country's biggest state-run newspaper, on cell phones, and text messages were sent out covering other political topics the authorities wanted to highlight.

In contrast, the government set up an entirely separate system for the country's small international community, by which foreigners could call one another and others abroad, although they could not call local North Korean cell phone numbers. This was enormously important for foreign visitors trying to stay in touch with their home offices.

As the middle class grew, so too did the Kaesong Industrial Complex, just north of the Demilitarized Zone. I made several visits. It was striking to see over one hundred South Korean companies employing nearly fifty thousand North Korean workers, making everything from electronics and watches to shoes and household utensils. Most of the workers were women, with many having graduated only from high school. Although their working day was supposed to be eight hours, two-hour overtime periods and work on Sundays were frequently added.

Their wages were low—$60 a month. The state took most of that, amounting to nearly $4 million a month, while it compensated the workers with coupons for state stores and domestic currency. But the workers had decent dormitory housing and, at the complex's cafeterias, a reliable supply of food—for which they did not have to scrounge and scavenge—as well as access to childcare and medical services. In interviews, defectors from

North Korea regularly said that Kaesong was considered the best place in the country to work.[20]

On one trip, I visited a company that made cables for refrigerators and washing machines, as well as a textile plant making shoes and handbags. Although spartan by Western standards, the work environment was clean and bright, and the equipment modern, by North Korean standards. The workers, all dressed in factory uniforms, were generally friendly and smiling. Given conditions in their home villages or towns outside the complex, I could understand why they felt lucky to be there.

As one would expect, given the long-standing hostility and suspicion between North and South, the Kaesong project had its tensions. A key one revolved around North Korea's demand for a 400 percent wage increase in 2009. After fraught negotiations, Pyongyang agreed to a much more modest 5 percent. The North Koreans also rebuffed South Korean efforts to allow payments to go directly to workers, fueling a sense in Seoul that Pyongyang was exploiting both South Korean taxpayers and North Korean workers.

After my visits, I always felt that the fact that the North Koreans were being exposed to Western ways of operating, and to interaction with South Koreans, was a good thing and could contribute to the broader dynamic of change I was beginning to sense. Indeed, this prompted me to add a sixth "M" to my list: mindsets. Among the younger generation, especially in Pyongyang, people's thinking was slowly changing. These were young adults who had grown up in a time when the regime had stopped providing everything—food, clothing, and many daily necessities. Thus, they were not used to receiving government handouts, but instead were finding their own ways to make ends meet, developing a certain entrepreneurial spirit in the process. Women, of course, were very much a part of this new group. One reason may have been that whatever the other restrictions previously in place, few North Korean women (at least among the ones I met) were illiterate or had not gone to school. Moreover, they were clever, so it was not surprising that they made the most of opportunities.

But the dynamic underpinning these "Six M's" brought with it serious problems and questions. Chief among them was a growing gap between the predominantly urban haves and the overwhelmingly rural have-nots. While parts of Pyongyang increasingly resembled a modern twenty-first-century city similar to those found in many Asian nations, much of the countryside looked more like something from the early twentieth or even the nineteenth century—poor and backward; lacking power, transport, and infrastructure; life a daily fight for survival. Even with the rise of the *donju*, regular food supplies remained problematic in many areas.

My reports to the SDC from 2009 and 2010 give some sense of the situation.

November and December 2009: "There will be again a substantial cereal shortfall. During field trips it was noticeable how heavily guarded the rice and maize fields were. After the harvesting women, the elderly and children could be seen searching the fields for hours, collecting individual corn or rice kernels. Malnutrition rates remain high by WHO standards with some 37 percent of children under 5 stunted, 23 percent underweight and 7 percent wasted. With the continued food shortages, the legacy of hunger is passed on from one generation to another."

January to April 2010: "The pressure in the agricultural sector remains very high and returns from the hard work are not encouraging for the farmers. With farms having high quotas to fulfill and having to sell most of the harvest to the government for fixed (low) prices, recent observations are that even people on cooperative farms have not enough to eat."

May to August 2010: "For many ordinary North Korean people life remains tough, the food situation fragile, with pockets of poverty and only sporadic food rations from the government, if any at all. The lack of fertilizer, a delayed start of the agricultural season, and a short summer with much rain in the early fall will have an impact on this year's harvest."

September to December 2010: "Supply of staple food remained unstable causing see-sawing prices. The size of the rations allocated through the Public Distribution System varied, forcing more urban dwellers to purchase food from the markets."

As was the case in China and Vietnam—other socialist states that had embraced market-style reforms—there remained the possibility that, as the middle class grew and money began to trickle down through the system, this would be a temporary phase. As Deng Xiaoping, who had pioneered the reforms in China, once famously said, "Some people have to get rich before others." A more open, market-oriented economy might have been able to help lift out of poverty North Koreans who had so far not benefited from the changes. But the regime's ambiguous attitude during this period toward markets, trade, and investment with the outside world, as well as the existence of the *donju*, raised serious doubts about whether that could happen—although, as I was perhaps an incurable optimist, I certainly hoped it would.

With poverty no longer equally shared, there were sensitive political questions as well. As people began to support themselves and get what they needed outside the state economy, would they be less beholden to the authorities? Would a rising middle class in Pyongyang begin to demand political power commensurate with its economic clout? Would the endemic poverty that had scarred so much of the country lead to bottom-up pressure for change? How would the North Korean system respond to such challenges? Would the regime seek to co-opt the *donju* and enlist their newfound wealth to spur development, or seek to curb their influence? As the first decade of the twenty-first century came to an end, the honest response was that those of us following North Korea simply didn't know.

Not for the first time, North Korea posed multiple questions to those of us seeking to understand and interact with the society—without any clear-cut answers.

CHAPTER NINETEEN

Phase Out or Phase Down?

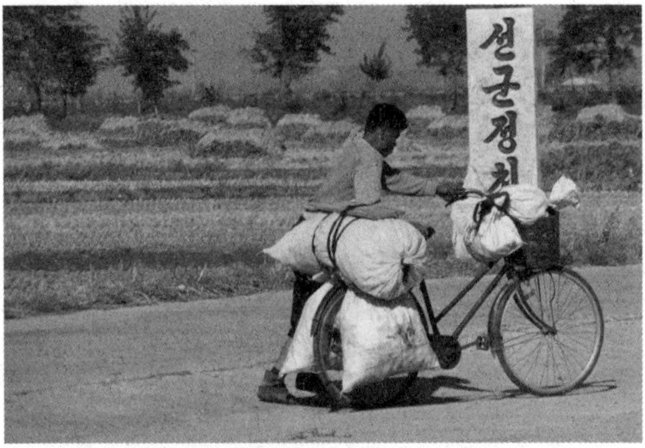

Economic problems persisted. Here, a farmer transports his rice crop on a bicycle.

I had arrived in Pyongyang for the SDC in late 2006, in the wake of the DPRK's first nuclear test on October 9. Because of the test and the country's generally poor international reputation, some conservative Swiss parliamentarians soon started calling for an end to the SDC's development cooperation in North Korea. And even some within the SDC doubted the value of this kind of involvement in the DPRK. Nonetheless, I had worked to build up our various projects and felt that, despite all the frustrations and obstacles, we were making some real progress in a country that was as important as it was difficult. But in the spring of 2008, the axe finally fell.

The Swiss Parliament ordered the SDC to halt its development program by the end of 2011.

The decision was part of a broader overhaul of the SDC's global efforts, triggered partly by budget concerns and partly by domestic political pressure to show progress that could be explained easily to the public and the Swiss political class. That overhaul led to the termination of SDC activities in Ecuador, Bhutan, Pakistan, and Peru as well as in North Korea. These sweeping cutbacks allowed the SDC to present its shutdown of the North Korea program not as specifically targeting the DPRK but as part of a broader recalibration of the SDC's approach. Yet, judging from the public criticism by politicians—most notably Gerhard Pfister, a leading figure in the powerful Christian Democratic People's Party and, from the beginning, the most vocal critic of engaging North Korea—as well as from private conversations with my colleagues at SDC headquarters, it was clear that the DPRK was seen as a special target. In the critics' minds, assisting North Korea in any way made it easier for the regime to devote more resources to its military and security forces, enabling it to continue imposing control over a population deprived of any liberty. As Pfister's motion in Parliament declared, the DPRK's "atomic weapon program violates international agreements. North Korea has shown itself to be utterly uncooperative, despite international efforts. It threatens to destabilize the region."

In an internal document providing staff members with guidance on how to explain the move to end our programs, the SDC asserted that "the potential for development partnerships is low in this country [North Korea], as the country does not have a strategy for reducing poverty—the hoped-for development progress has failed to materialize, partly because the political framework has not really improved. The chances of a real transformation are therefore slim."

Such negative views were hardly unique to Switzerland. Whether to engage or isolate the DPRK was a continuing topic of debate in Washington, DC. Different governments in South Korea also had veered from supplying aid and encouraging investment—most notably via the Kaesong Industrial Complex—to linking future aid with North Korean nuclear concessions. More broadly, UN agencies and NGOs had faced the problem of donor fatigue for years—to the point that by 2010, donors had provided the World Food Program with just 20 percent of its annual funding target for the DPRK.

Although bashing North Korea was quite popular among some Swiss politicians—and there was similar rhetoric in the United States, South Korea, and many other countries—the issue of whether the SDC should have a presence in the DPRK did not appear to resonate widely in the general Swiss populace. Apart from some desultory discussion in the Committee of Foreign Affairs, Swiss parliamentarians did not debate the issue in depth. This meant that the climate was not conducive to making the argument to the public and most politicians that changes indeed were afoot in the DPRK and that the SDC's activities were, in a quiet and nonthreatening way, a catalyst for further changes. Was there a way out? I pondered for hours.

Compounding my frustration was the slowness of official communication from Berne. Although I could see that the decision was coming, it was highly embarrassing for us in Pyongyang that the North Korean embassy in Berne, and thus the Ministry of Foreign Affairs in Pyongyang, knew before we did that the decision had been formally made. When I finally had a chance to discuss the matter with North Korean officials, they expressed regret, as they viewed the SDC as a pioneer in development cooperation, but accepted that this was Switzerland's sovereign right and thus respected the government's decision.

I felt sad, frustrated, and disappointed. I did not see the political sense in trying to further isolate an already isolated regime. Would it not be better to cooperate, or at least keep a line of communication open and try to contribute to solutions? In addition, I felt strongly that if Switzerland were to play a positive role in any moves toward a peace process on the Korean peninsula, it did not make sense to have an embassy in Seoul and Swiss military participation in the Neutral Nations Supervisory Commission—which nominally oversaw the armistice along the DMZ—but no on-the-ground representation in the North.

Yes, Switzerland had diplomatic relations with Pyongyang, but the Swiss ambassador to China, although accredited to the North, was based in Beijing and made only two or three visits to the DPRK each year. Moreover, in the wake of the famine, Switzerland had been one of the first countries, if not *the* first country, to offer humanitarian aid. The SDC had maintained an office in Pyongyang since 1997. And Switzerland was one of the few nations, if not the only nation, to gradually have turned humanitarian aid involvement into long-term development programs. These programs were aimed at improving the efficiency and sustainability of North Korean agriculture and—with capacity development programs such as the Pyongyang Business School and the many study tours, exchanges, and other trips we had organized—at helping the DPRK to forge greater connections with the international community.

All of this was now in jeopardy. But I did not give up trying to explain and generate support for what we were doing. One opportunity came with the visit of conservative Swiss parliamentarian Christoph Blocher not long after the SDC decided to end its North Korean development program. A right-wing billionaire industrialist and, from 2004 to 2007, a member of the Swiss Federal Council, he was a leader of the Swiss People's Party, which he had transformed into the country's largest political party. At one point, he had headed the Federal Department of Justice and Police. Blocher was a confrontational, flamboyant, and dominant personality. Some years later, Donald Trump's aide Steve Bannon would say that "Blocher was Trump before Trump."

Blocher had long been critical of SDC development work and indeed of our presence in the DPRK, but for reasons I was never clear about, he decided to visit with his family as a member of a tourist group. I was more than a little nervous about meeting him, but on October 21, 2009, I hosted him and his wife for dinner at my apartment. To make them feel at home, I prepared Swiss fondue, and we had a surprisingly good conversation. He was very interested in what the SDC was doing in North Korea, and despite his reputation, he listened very carefully. At the end of the evening, he wrote the following in my guest book, which translated from German reads:

> Despite well-known aversion regarding Switzerland's worldwide development cooperation, received very amicably by SDC in Pyongyang and with Swiss cuisine. To the Foreign Ministry in Berne: This humble development cooperation which is aiming at promotion of self-initiatives is to be continued! Ch. Blocher, former Federal Councilor.

In addition to Blocher's visit to North Korea, including his interaction with the SDC on the ground, which influenced his thinking, I met with another visiting Swiss parliamentarian, Christian Wasserfallen of the Free Democratic Party (FDP), which had merged with the Liberal Party in 2009. He had been a strong supporter of the SDC's work in the DPRK, and after returning to Switzerland, he and nine other members of Parliament issued a last-minute appeal to reverse the decision to terminate SDC's development projects there.

"SDC's targeted and pragmatic approaches are beneficial to the civilian population," the statement said. "Helping with soil erosion or pest control projects with the local population to develop the principles of successful agriculture increases the security of their own food supply. The programs are beginning to have an impact. The SDC knowledge transfer are important building blocks for future positive developments on the Korean Peninsula."

It came too late. The appeal was rebuffed. The shutdown of the development programs would proceed. In my discussions with colleagues, however, it became clear that there might be room to modify the SDC's involvement. Ambassador Blaise Godet suggested that my colleagues and I draft a concept paper making the argument that even if the development programs were ended, there would be value in the SDC's maintaining some kind of presence in Pyongyang. Making this case rested on two factors. The first was the SDC's own structure. The organization had two wings. One, with which I was associated, worked on development cooperation. The other, with its own staff and organization, concentrated on humanitarian aid. This, I thought, provided an opening, especially as the internal SDC document that had been so critical of the DPRK also noted, "The closure of the programs is not the same as the termination of any form of cooperation. The withdrawal means that this country is no longer a priority recipient of Swiss development aid. However, this is not the same as breaking off cooperation with a country without replacement."

After much consultation, debate, and discussion, we came up with a document entitled "Phasing Out and Exit Scenarios." In it, we again defended the projects currently underway, and offered a series of proposals about how to sustain an SDC presence after 2011. We laid out two key goals. One was to explore how to transfer to other international agencies—or, if possible, to the North Koreans themselves—programs that appeared to be working. But much more important was our strong belief that keeping a Swiss presence on the ground in Pyongyang, in some form, was absolutely crucial to maintain our influence in the volatile Korean peninsula. We warned of the danger that "first-hand information will no longer be forthcoming" and that there would be a "loss of visibility, influence, and trust with the DPRK," by which the annual bilateral political dialogue could be jeopardized, and therefore argued that "it is questionable whether a complete exit is the right step for Switzerland's external policy."

We proposed two alternatives to a complete exit. One was to continue financial support for select programs, focusing especially on food security, which could be managed by an SDC development attaché based in either Pyongyang or Beijing. The other, for which we had higher hopes, was to change the office in Pyongyang into one focusing on humanitarian aid, which remained a separate and distinct branch of the SDC. In either case, we stressed that, as we noted in bold lettering in our paper, an "in-country expatriate presence remains the prerequisite." It was, we contended, the only way to maintain working relationships with the North Koreans.

Godet backed our position and sent a cable to the foreign ministry in February 2009 noting that "Switzerland occupies a privileged position in North Korea. She is listened to and respected. This status has been earned over the years through patient work. The SDC's continued presence since 1995 has made a major contribution to this. Despite the very difficult environment in which they are conducted, SDC's programs make it possible to confront the North Koreans with other ideas and other development models. This long-term process requires perseverance and a difficult and constant dialogue with the authorities."

Godet even made his position public, telling Switzerland's leading newspaper, the *Neue Zürcher Zeitung*, that Switzerland had nurtured a consistent policy of engagement and political dialogue, adding that "we want to contribute to solutions."

With the help of supportive colleagues, I waged a low-key but persistent campaign to prevent a total Swiss pullout and build support for our alternative proposals. Early in 2009, I attended a meeting of Asia-based SDC staff and Swiss diplomats in Hanoi. The head of the Swiss foreign ministry's Asia department joined us. Regarding the DPRK, the discussion centered on whether to phase out or merely phase down our presence. Back in Switzerland for the foreign ministry's annual gathering of Swiss ambassadors from around the world in the resort town of Interlaken, the topic came up again. People repeatedly asked us about the effectiveness of the SDC's monitoring efforts and how sustainable our projects actually were.

The internal politics were complex. For one thing, some within the SDC were uneasy about how willing I had been to have contact with reporters, whom I saw as crucial to helping educate Swiss and international opinion about North Korea. This was contrary to the cautious way that the SDC generally dealt with the press. Indeed, one Swiss newspaper had complained that SDC staff in the field "had a mandate to say nothing."[21] Then there were the complex dynamics between the SDC and the Swiss Federal Department of Foreign Affairs, primarily because the SDC had a bigger budget than the ministry did. This was a source of some resentment, and helped explain why some ministry officials were pushing for the SDC to become less independent and more integrated into the ministry's activities.

I continued to argue that the SDC had been doing pioneering work in North Korea, and that we were playing a significant role in encouraging the country to gradually open up to more international contact. The DPRK government, I noted, repeatedly had expressed its appreciation for the development cooperation, as well as for the supplies of milk powder that Switzerland had donated almost annually to the World Food Program. Above all, I kept stressing the importance of being there. Even a small presence was better than no presence at all. Having people on the ground was, in my view, far more valuable than any amount of aid money.

In these constant rounds of meetings, emails, phone calls, and position papers, it became clear that there was a receptivity to trying to keep some of our development projects going as long as we could find other agencies to handle and finance them after the SDC's departure. The most promising post-SDC partner for the North Koreans appeared to be the Centre for Agriculture and Bioscience International (CABI). With offices in countries as varied as China, Brazil, and Ghana, CABI focuses on supporting agriculture in the developing world. The SDC already had partnered with CABI on our agricultural support programs, especially the Integrated Pest Management program, and CABI staff had developed good working relationships with their North Korean counterparts. Indeed, even as the SDC's time in the DPRK began to wind down, CABI helped to organize the first national workshop on integrated pest management. It attracted over eighty local and international participants, who shared research and compared notes. With the European Union willing to provide funding, CABI seemed well-placed to at least partly fill the void left by the closure of the SDC development program.

As for the Sloping Land Management program, no external organization was in a position to or wanted to replace the SDC. Yet it was my hope that, with the lessons learned through the SDC's assistance, the techniques being used in numerous localities would continue and perhaps expand. More broadly, as I noted in a report to headquarters, there was "a risk that without any further SDC involvement, achievements in food security [would] suffer a setback."

In terms of capacity-building, interest in programs such as the Pyongyang Business School remained high. Indeed, as word spread that the school would cease to exist after the end of 2011, the number of applicants for the few remaining courses soared. But without the SDC's backing, it was clear that this—perhaps the most innovative project of all, and certainly one of those closest to my heart—would have to cease operations. No longer would there be support for so many different training programs and study tours abroad either.

Even as we prepared for the end of the SDC's development program, I and my colleagues submitted a document to the foreign minister and, at that time, Swiss President, Micheline Calmy-Rey, making the case to authorize the establishment of a humanitarian aid office—and that a Swiss SDC official head it. After weeks of waiting, we received in early 2010 the news that Calmy-Rey had agreed. I was immensely relieved. While I was sorry to see so much of our good work come to an end, the decision meant that Switzerland would maintain what I had long advocated—a presence on the ground in Pyongyang. Moreover, the line between development projects and aid programs was blurry enough to hold out the prospect that some of what we had been doing that appeared to be facing the axe could, with a few tweaks or terminological changes, be salvaged. The sensation that so much of what I had poured my heart into for so many years was completely at risk slowly began to dissipate.

Meanwhile, the tentative thaw on the Korean peninsula began to fade. After the failure of a brief effort at diplomacy with the DPRK, the Obama administration adopted a policy described as "strategic patience"—declaring a willingness in principle to resume engagement but not aggressively pursuing it. Instead, the United States appeared willing to live with the status quo, while imposing sanctions on what Obama himself described as North Korean "bad behavior."[22]

It was difficult to judge how central a factor frustration with Washington was in what North Korea then proceeded to do. It may have gone ahead in any event, but starting in mid-2009 and continuing into 2010, the North undertook a series of what most in the international community saw as extremely provocative moves. These included resuming missile tests, announcing plans to manufacture a uranium-based nuclear bomb, and engaging in two violent incidents with South Korea. In March 2010, the South Korean naval vessel *Cheonan* was sunk, with the loss of forty-six lives, and Pyongyang was widely blamed. The North Koreans vehemently denied responsibility. Indeed, the foreign ministry called the heads of all foreign diplomatic missions, myself included, to a high-level meeting, where senior officials again insisted that the North had not been involved. Shortly thereafter, though, the DPRK shelled Yeongpyeong, a small South Korean–held island in the disputed waters of the Yellow Sea off the west coast of the peninsula.

It was against this increasingly tense backdrop that I waited one afternoon in November 2010 in the Koryo Hotel. I was due to have a drink with three members of a visiting delegation from Stanford University—John Lewis, Siegfried Hecker, and Robert Carlin. It would not be our first meeting. I had connected with Lewis, a distinguished sinologist and cofounder of Stanford's Center of East Asian Studies, some years before. He was a remarkable man—a veritable volcano of energy renowned for his formidable range of high-level contacts in Beijing, Moscow, Washington, and Pyongyang. He had been visiting the DPRK since the late 1980s, devoting his efforts to ways to improve mutual understanding and lower tensions. On several occasions during my time at the SDC, he had come to the North with Hecker, a professor of engineering.

A brilliant metallurgist, Hecker had previously been the director of the Los Alamos National Laboratory, best known for its role in helping develop the first atomic bomb as highlighted in the 2023 Oscar-winning film *Oppenheimer*, and had worked there to develop the US nuclear arsenal. Carlin, bearded and genial, was a visiting scholar at Stanford who previously for many years had been a North Korea analyst at the CIA and then the State Department's Bureau of Intelligence and Research.

Whenever these three men visited Pyongyang, we would meet for drinks or meals. On one occasion, I made them fondue in my apartment. Hecker and I discovered a particularly unusual connection. His parents were originally from Bosnia, but his father, conscripted into the German army, had died in World War Two. After the war, his mother settled in Austria, and in the early 1950s, under a program for underprivileged children—coincidentally run by Caritas, where I had worked for twenty-eight years—he had been able to spend three months in Switzerland and ended up in a village in the canton of Thurgau, which happened to be not far from my home village. It was a small world.

I suspect that, as I was a longtime foreign resident, Lewis, Hecker, and Carlin saw me as a resource to get a better handle on the domestic situation in the country. Although primarily focused on the broader geopolitics, they always emphasized their view, with which I heartily agreed, that North Korea was a three-dimensional place filled with real people, and to better understand it required getting beyond just discussing nukes and missiles, and acquiring a more nuanced and sensitive understanding of its culture and values. Meanwhile, they provided me with valuable insights about the nuclear issue, on which they had special expertise, having been given the unprecedented privilege on previous trips of visiting the Yongbyon nuclear complex and talking with North Korean nuclear engineers, as well as learning about the broader diplomatic situation. I also was able to assist them in making connections with Pyongyang's small diplomatic community and giving them brief character sketches of the ambassadors they were going to meet. We always had a fruitful and enjoyable exchange of views, and I was looking forward to another one on this crisp November 2010 day.

Yet the moment they entered the vast lobby of the Koryo Hotel, with its café/bar just to the left of the main door, I could sense something was different. All three looked tense and preoccupied. After a brief greeting, Hecker and Lewis apologized and said they had to go up to their rooms. Carlin suggested we go for a drink. Not surprisingly for someone with a background in the intelligence community, he was always somewhat reserved, but on this day, he was cautious to the point of awkwardness. He did say they had been taken again to Yongbyon, but it was clear that he was uncomfortable saying anything more. I did not push him.

Later, I learned what had happened. Earlier that afternoon, on what was their fourth visit to Yongbyon, the North Koreans had showed the three experts a vast new facility that had been secretly built to enrich uranium. Unlike so much in North Korea, which was shabby and run-down, the facility, as long as a football field, was gleaming, modern, and state of the art. Hecker calculated that it held around two thousand centrifuges. Although the facility technically was designed to produce low-enriched uranium (LEU), ostensibly for electricity, Hecker was certain it easily could be converted to make highly enriched uranium (HEU) fuel for nuclear bombs, raising the prospect of a dramatic expansion of Pyongyang's nuclear arsenal. No wonder all three men seemed preoccupied. In his hotel room, Hecker wrote up his notes before a dinner with senior North Korean officials, who indicated that the DPRK was still open to negotiations. Not surprisingly, the Obama administration was furious, denouncing the development as yet another provocation that showed just how dangerous the DPRK could be.

It seemed clear to me that the prospect of an expanded nuclear arsenal could only hurt the DPRK's struggling economy. As I noted in a 2010 year-end report to the SDC, "The leadership faces a dilemma: either maintain its nuclear program and therefore remain economically poor, or scrap its nuclear weapons and receive international assistance. At present, North Korean officials make little secret of their wish to be recognized as a nuclear-weapons power." Despite this worrying development, I remained convinced, as one American analyst put it, that "the only thing worse than negotiating with North Korea is not negotiating with North Korea." But for the moment, diplomacy seemed at a stalemate.

CHAPTER TWENTY

Farewell to the SDC

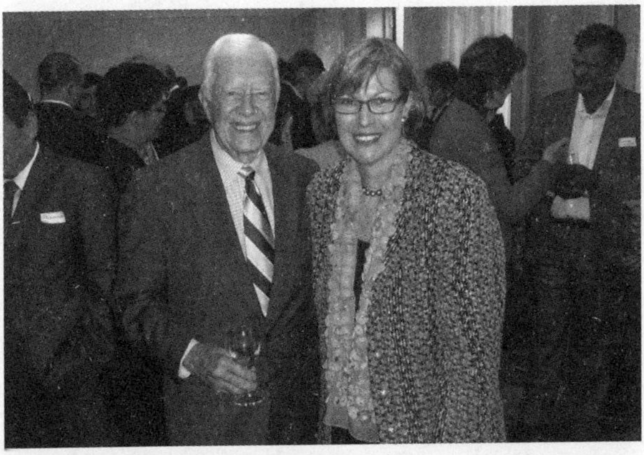

Spreading awareness of the problems through meetings with important visitors was also part of Kathi's job; here in 2011, with former US President Jimmy Carter, in Pyongyang.

The spring of 2011 was my fifth and last as a resident of Pyongyang. Springtime had become my favorite season in North Korea. As the days became longer, the air became fresher, and the trees began to blossom, the dark and freezing winter months faded into memory. It was as if life was beginning again. I watched as people cleaned their apartments, the streets were swept, and gardening and planting got underway. While young couples shyly embraced on their first spring walk, children played outside; roller-skating, skipping rope, and playing tug of war seemed to be their favorite pastimes. As old men played cards in the shade of a tree, other Pyongyang residents went out for strolls, many with cell phones pressed to their ears. I also came across grandfathers taking their granddaughters for walks along the Taedong river, the little girls so dressed up that they resembled dolls.

Some elderly men had stalls on the side of the road selling gas for lighters or offering to repair broken bicycles. Others sold drinks and snacks. I could also see women digging for roots, or collecting grass or leaves—but, unlike during the famine days, they were scrounging to feed not themselves but, in all probability, the rabbits they kept on their balconies at home. Occasionally a group of boisterous kids would follow me, eager to practice their English. The restaurants in the capital seemed full again. In one, I noticed a table of four young women having a good time, chatting and giggling—all well-dressed, with modern hairstyles, and all with mobile phones. Outside on the streets, I had made it a habit to observe women's shoe styles. They were becoming increasingly fashionable, often with heels that were so high, some women seemed to have difficulty walking, or platform shoes that would make them look five to ten centimeters taller. I wondered how many would twist their ankles on these rough roads while showing off the latest footwear.

It was a nice time of year. It was a moment too for one of my regular get-togethers with a man who had become a particularly useful contact: Guenter Unterbeck, a former East German diplomat who had been stationed in Pyongyang for years and spoke excellent Korean; after he'd ceased to have a country to represent, he stayed on and went into business. He had valuable insights, and I learned a great deal from him. East Germany had left behind a huge embassy compound in Pyongyang. Empty for a while, it had been turned into a so-called interest section for the German government before it became the full-fledged embassy of a unified Germany in 2001. In addition to housing both the chancery and the residence of the ambassador, it was so big that Sweden maintained its embassy office there as well, and the British had both its embassy premises and staff residences within the German embassy compound.

I regularly would treat this former East German diplomat to lunch at one of the best Pyongyang restaurants, the Arirang, where they served the most delicious *bibimbap*, my favorite Korean dish. He would always come with a rather big briefcase. The first time he did so, to my surprise, he pulled out not documents but two champagne glasses and a bottle of Rotkäppchen sparkling wine. Rotkäppchen is still famous throughout Germany, especially in the East, and the name is German for the fairy-tale character Little Red

Riding Hood. Sipping Rotkäppchen sparkling wine from champagne glasses in a Pyongyang restaurant was a slightly surreal experience—yet another example of the idiosyncrasies of living in North Korea.

And there were others. At the SDC compound, my assistant and I did a spring cleaning at our two big buildings, which felt like an endless task. One issue was that, as we had learned by now, North Koreans threw nothing away. Items that would go immediately into our trash bin were taken out elsewhere and used and reused. Occasionally, something we had thrown away two or even three times reappeared—almost anything was seen as a potential resource that might come in handy one day. I was quite certain that once the trash collection truck had left our compound, everything was sorted again and again. We also found among other stuff hidden in a cupboard around fifty cassette tapes of classical music I had given to the local staff two or three years before. I wondered whether they had been too afraid to take the cassettes home, let alone risk listening to Western music.

I also cleaned up files on my office computer. I thought I had discovered an interesting folder created by one of my predecessors. It was named "Innovative Ideas," but when I clicked to open it, it was empty. A cynic would say it was emblematic of things in the DPRK. I had a good laugh.

Later in the spring, we conducted a first aid training course for the SDC team with a UN doctor from the Philippines. This was a worldwide SDC requirement, and North Korea was no exception. Our Korean staff were very surprised, as they had never experienced such training. The doctor brought an inflatable doll with which to do various first aid exercises. It was serious but also fun, and there was a lot of laughter, as it was totally new for them. We had a safety training session as well, learning, for example, what to do if you have a fire in your hotel room. Even for me—an experienced traveler—it was interesting, helpful, and scary.

Despite the lighter mood in Pyongyang, the food situation around the country appeared to be getting worse again as I entered the final months of my tenure in Pyongyang. Heavy rains had caused serious damage, destroying homes and flooding farmland. Dozens of people had been killed, and many more were missing. A pumping station and treatment plant that supplied drinkable water to the 350,000 inhabitants of Sinuiju city was completely destroyed. Cross-border smuggling appeared to be increasing, while a UN Food and Agriculture Organization/World Food Program crop and food security assessment in late 2010 found that the country was facing a food deficit of 524,000 metric tons of grain. The assessment recommended providing some 305,000 metric tons of international food aid to the most vulnerable members of the population. Agriculture experts in South Korea, meanwhile, were predicting an even worse harvest for the early spring crop in 2011. The list of reasons was familiar: lack of fertilizers, pesticides, plastic sheeting, and diesel for the tractors, plus dilapidated machinery, soil depletion, and adverse weather conditions.

Despite all of our efforts and the undeniable—if often modest—success of some of our projects, as well as the visible improvement in the quality of life in Pyongyang, I began to feel that things were coming full circle, with a struggling agricultural sector and inefficient overall system creating more suffering for far too many ordinary North Koreans. This situation led the DPRK to ask again for international assistance and to push its diplomatic missions abroad to acquire food and send it back. There was even a barter deal under which China agreed to provide maize in return for North Korean coal.

The reports of renewed food shortages, along with heightened nuclear tension, led to the April 2011 arrival in Pyongyang of a group of distinguished global leaders called The Elders, established by the founding father of democratic South Africa, Nelson Mandela. They got me involved in helping them. The group consisted of former US President Jimmy Carter, former Finland President and Nobel Peace Prize winner Martti Ahtisaari, former Irish President Mary Robinson, and former Norwegian Prime Minister Gro Brundtland. Robinson, who had served as UN high commissioner for human rights from 1997 to 2002, and Brundtland were the first women to hold the top leadership positions in their countries. Brundtland also had served as the director-general of the World Health Organization.

After meeting senior Chinese officials in Beijing, including the foreign minister, the group began their DPRK visit by stressing their concern at the lack of bilateral dialogue between the North and South, as well as at the absence of broader multilateral talks on security and nuclear issues. Although their mission was wholly unofficial, the hope was, as had been the case in other crisis situations, that they might play a facilitating role in lowering tensions and generating both diplomatic progress and an uptick in humanitarian aid.

As I had missed the advance team for The Elders in Pyongyang because I was out of the country, I arranged a meeting with them while on a visit to Beijing en route back to the North Korean capital. Quite casually, I asked them who was going to host a reception for the foreign community in Pyongyang, where there was great interest in the visit. This was in large part because of Carter's historic trip there in June, 1994, when he met Kim Il Sung and brokered the resumption of United States–DPRK talks that led to the Agreed Framework deal later that year. Under that deal, North Korea agreed to freeze and eventually dismantle its plutonium-based nuclear program. In 2010, Carter had returned to Pyongyang and negotiated the release of an American teacher named Aijalon Gomes, who had been sentenced to eight years' hard labor after illegally entering the country from China.

Rather sheepishly, The Elders' advance team acknowledged they hadn't even thought about such a reception. So on the spur of the moment, I offered to host an event at the SDC compound—something they agreed was, in diplomatic terms, a bit unusual. Normally, the Swedish embassy represented US interests in the DPRK. Swedish diplomats, for example, were the foreigners usually allowed to visit detained Americans. So with a delegation headed by a former American president, there would have been a certain logic to the Swedes acting as reception hosts. But, for reasons I never figured out, they didn't, leaving the SDC and me to play this somewhat exalted diplomatic role.

The reception took place at the SDC compound on April 27, 2011, midway through the group's five-day visit. About seventy foreign diplomats, heads of UN agencies, and representatives of humanitarian organizations attended. Only three mission heads missed it. One of them was the ambassador of a Middle Eastern country. He apologized, explaining that he had a delegation arriving to negotiate a knotty problem: the North Koreans owed his country money and weren't paying. Instead, the North Korean government was sending workers to help repay the debt. It was a revealing insight into Pyongyang's often messy international relations.

I met all four of The Elders at the reception, although there was little time for substantive conversation, especially as I was busy supervising the event. It was clear that Carter was the person of greatest interest. It was a relatively relaxed occasion, but I also found it a bit curious. So few high-ranking Western politicians came to Pyongyang that to have not one but four figures of this stature was unquestionably an exciting development, especially for the foreign community. On the other hand, as one ambassador noted somewhat cynically, Carter was a "has-been accompanied by other has-beens." It remained unclear what the group might be able to achieve. Still, how Carter worked the room impressed me. As a good politician, he made sure to meet, shake hands, and engage in a few seconds of small talk with every single person in attendance.

During their stay in the country, the four held meetings with North Korea's foreign minister, chief nuclear negotiator, and titular head of state, Kim Yong Nam, as well as made a half-day trip outside Pyongyang. At the reception, Mary Robinson mentioned that they had visited a rural hospital with no running water in its operating room. In brief comments, Carter made no reference to the nuclear issue, but he did talk about the food situation, which was a key priority for the group. He had harsh words for South Korea and the United States for their failure, in his view, to provide sufficient food aid to address what was again becoming a critical situation.

In a report on their visit, The Elders noted that "recent assessments carried out jointly by the World Food Program (WFP), the Food & Agriculture Organization (FAO) and UNICEF…and, separately, by a group of US NGOs, concluded that a real crisis affecting up to a quarter of the entire population (six out of 24 million persons) was imminent." This was consistent with my own impression that a food crisis was looming. While the four VIPs acknowledged "legitimate concerns that the DPRK authorities may not be playing their full part in providing for the wellbeing of their own people, by not releasing food grains from strategic stock reserve," it was as clear to me, as it was to The Elders, that international aid again would become necessary to minimize the scale of the suffering.[23]

As I noted in a report to the SDC in May, "The food situation remains deplorable with rations, if any at all, as low as 200 grams per person per day (at times only 200 grams of potatoes and not 200 grams of grain). The consequences of not providing food aid are clear: stunted physical and mental growth of children; anemia in pregnant women, vitamin and iron deficiencies, increased risk of tuberculosis and other life-threatening diseases and probably countless preventable deaths." Whether, given North Korea's increasingly bad international reputation, sufficient help would be forthcoming was another question entirely.

There had been intense speculation that Carter, having met Kim Il Sung in 1994, would be granted an audience with Kim Jong Il, and the group's interest in such a meeting was palpable. But it didn't happen, just as Kim had failed to meet him during Carter's visit the previous year. The reason was unclear: an intentional snub to show deeper dissatisfaction with Washington's policies, a reflection of the North Korean leadership's perception of Carter as a has-been, the Dear Leader's poor health, or that the DPRK was dangling the prospect of such a meeting to lure Carter to make yet another visit at an unspecified future date. Officials, however, gave The Elders a letter from Kim Jong Il, in which he said he was ready to return to the six-party talks. Given South Korea's demand for unilateral denuclearization steps made by the DPRK before such talks could resume—and the Obama administration's support for Seoul—the prospects for a resumption of diplomacy seemed dim, and unlikely to improve because of The Elders' visit.

Still, it was an exciting moment for me to engage with these four renowned global figures, and I was as eager as the rest of the diplomatic community to glean whatever clues I could from them about the prospects for North-South or United States–DPRK relations. But they were cautious in their comments on these topics, and my excitement also was leavened by a dose of North Korean daily reality, which was reflected in my journal. "I met Jimmy Carter," I wrote, before adding the real highlight of the week: "We can now buy milk again." Key staples were so often in short supply that the prospect of purchasing milk again overshadowed my encounter with a former American president.

Meanwhile, for all the drama of high-level visits, and despite having to wind down the SDC's programs, my colleagues and I continued to work hard to keep the projects going until the last minute and, where possible, to ensure a smooth transition to those who would maintain and finance them after Swiss development cooperation ceased. We hosted several delegations from the SDC's humanitarian branch, and traveled with them to introduce them to both the country and the work we had been doing. For the Sloping Land Management project, we took them to various sites in which barren hills were clearly visible, highlighting the continuing need; fourteen new user groups with 108 new members had just been established. In addition, provincial and national workshops were held, an English-language forestry manual was translated into Korean, and a seven-person delegation from the North Korean Ministry of Land and Environmental Protection (MoLEP) visited Switzerland and saw agricultural schools as well as farms in the mountains there. When the North Koreans returned, some expressed surprise to me that Switzerland was as mountainous, if not more so, than the

DPRK—and that it was not cooperative farms but individual Swiss farmers who had to make a living off the often rugged land. At the same time, they came away deeply impressed with the modern tractors and other farm machinery they saw, as well as the nice houses and barns.

For all of our agricultural projects, the SDC had funded a collaboration between the North Korean Ministry of Agriculture, MoLEP, and the Centre for Development and Environment at the University of Berne. The focus was on developing the capacity to use geoinformation management for agriculture, which meant in part using electronic systems for mapping. The fact that more than one North Korean institution was involved in this work was itself something of an achievement, as communication and collaboration between different units were rare and often somewhat discouraged. The goal was to create a national geospatial database to contribute to better agricultural practices and improved management of agricultural resources, as well as build a curriculum of geoinformation technologies for future training. This would benefit many agricultural, forestry, and sloping land management programs, especially for strategic planning and monitoring. Despite the relatively short amount of time, the project, aided by a number of visits from consultants at the University of Berne, already had led to the completion of maps and models the North Koreans could use. I hoped a way could be found for this collaboration to continue.

With the capacity development programs set to shut down, a closing ceremony was held for the Pyongyang Business School in midsummer. Thirty people participated in the final round of classes. We also were able to fund two people from North Korea's Joint Venture and Investment Committee to attend a global conference on leadership of the next generation, supported by the Swiss bank UBS and held in Penglai, China. The 120 participants came from China, elsewhere in Asia, Europe, and Latin America. It was a good opportunity for the North Koreans to learn about investment policies and strategies—and problems—in other countries. A follow-up symposium was scheduled for the autumn in Switzerland, and the SDC agreed to cover the cost for the two North Koreans to attend.

In June, I made another trip to the United States, with seventeen meetings in Washington and fourteen in New York. Interest in the DPRK was generally very high, and I had good access to people both in and out of the American government, the United Nations, and various NGOs, as well as good turnouts at a number of functions where I spoke. But I found the mood to be darker than during my previous visit, with less receptivity to engagement and much deeper cynicism about any efforts to work with North Korea. Even on the subject of food aid, I found many of my interlocutors to be opposed, with some people calling the North "the worst regime in the world." American officials made clear that they would proceed only with the blessing of the South Korean government, whose president, Lee Myung-bak, was sticking to his long-standing hard line. I encountered that line when I met with the South Korean ambassador in Washington. We discussed conditions for a resumption of South Korean and/or US food aid, and of North-South relations. I explained the impact of chronic malnutrition and told him how we were trying to deal with poverty. Although the conversation was cordial, I felt that my presentation had little impact on his thinking.

My message was that it remained possible to work in North Korea and implement programs and projects successfully. I stressed that food aid was needed to help the most vulnerable, who bore no blame for the fact that they had been born in North Korea. I also argued that capacity development programs offered the possibility to plant the seeds of change, stressing what I called the need for the "Three F's"—food, fertilizer, and fuel—and offering my own observations about the growth of the "Five M's"—money, markets, mobiles, motorcars, and a middle class.

People I spoke with were surprised to learn that the North Koreans were thinking of starting joint ventures and two new economic zones. And I stressed as well that the impact of sanctions was only to heighten the already strong influence of Russia and China. I didn't find much agreement but was heartened that almost everyone I spoke with asked me to be sure to come back and meet with them on my next visit.

For the final Swiss National Day of my tenure, I arranged something special. Urs Buchmann, a Beijing-based Swiss businessman, was an old friend and an accomplished concert pianist who had started playing the piano at the age of five. I invited him to visit me and proposed that he perform a joint concert with a North Korean orchestra—something to which the North Koreans happily agreed. Indeed, as early as the spring of 2011, I brought the sheets of music Urs had given me in Beijing so the North Koreans could start rehearsing. The music was Piano Concerto No. 1 in B Minor composed by Sir Hamilton Harty, a brilliant pianist and conductor who also was the foremost Irish composer of the early twentieth century.

When Urs arrived a couple of days before National Day, we went to the Kim Won Gyun Conservatory—named after a famous North Korean composer—and met the head of the orchestra with whom he would be playing as well as the conductor, Ho Myong Gwon. Suddenly, in impeccable German, Ho asked if we spoke German. We said yes, that it was our mother tongue. He smiled and said, "In that case, we can speak German. I spent almost eight years in Vienna studying music." It was a total surprise. A North Korean conductor spending almost a decade in Vienna did not fit the notion of the DPRK as a society where no one had any exposure to the world beyond—and made Urs's collaboration that much more special.

National Day provided a unique opportunity for the SDC to invite its local partners as well as the members of the international community to a concert on August 1, 2011, at the Kim Won Gyun Conservatory; about 150 people attended. An SDC reception at the WFP compound followed, as the SDC did not have enough space indoors during the rainy season. Because the Swiss military attaché from Beijing was there, officials from the North Korean army attended as well. Although they were cordial, they were close-mouthed on any issues of substance. At the entrance, people put their name card or a piece of paper with their name on it into a box, and during the event there was a lucky draw with some ten prizes. It was great fun, and the prizes were a hit: a bottle of Swiss red wine, a Swiss Army knife, Swiss chocolates, and so on.

The North Koreans all wore their usual Kim Il Sung and Kim Jong Il badges, while we Swiss wore little Swiss flag pins. It made for quite a funny picture. We then hosted a lavish (by local standards) buffet dinner, where Swiss food, particularly sausages, cheese, and chocolates, were very popular. Having attended many such receptions during my years in Pyongyang, I always was struck by how much the North Koreans ate. It was as if even the more privileged officials—those allowed to go to diplomatic receptions—had such a meager or uninteresting diet that they came prepared to scarf down whatever food they could. One of my Swiss staff saw a local team member eating chocolate cake I had baked for the occasion, but, unfamiliar with Western eating habits, he had put ketchup on top of the cake as well.

As the most senior Swiss official in the DPRK, it fell to me to make some remarks. I talked about how the different people who comprised the Swiss population had "learned how to live together, to respect our differences, and resolve our problems peacefully in an open and democratic manner."

I summarized the range of the SDC's projects in the DPRK and stressed that "the bottom line is that Switzerland will continue to keep a presence in Pyongyang...albeit with a slightly different focus." I concluded with a heartfelt statement: "I have grown very fond of the people here in the DPRK. I wish them—and the country—prosperity, freedom, peace, and justice."

The concert generated a great deal of goodwill. Urs was thrilled with the opportunity to chat with young North Korean musicians, who were, not surprisingly, awed and slightly intimidated to meet a pianist of his stature. He was also the first foreigner they had ever encountered. But the goodwill—accentuated by the conductor's Vienna connection—was such that we came up with the idea of a small project using discretionary SDC funds to provide materials to overhaul the orchestra's musical instruments and provide some new ones. Although modest, the project was particularly satisfying.

Urs had another interesting encounter with North Korean culture. A passionate art collector, he had a large collection of paintings from all the countries he had visited, and was very eager to buy North Korean art. During my five years in Pyongyang, I had made many visits to art galleries and shops and had acquired a sizable collection of North Korean hand-painted propaganda posters. Indeed, it had become something of a hobby for me to wander through various galleries in the city on many Saturdays, inspecting the works on display and looking for posters, and I had become quite friendly with some of the young women who worked at these establishments. So I took Urs to the Korean Art Gallery on Kim Il Sung Square, a multistory building displaying traditional art, contemporary art, and socialist art, all very well presented in an attractive environment.

Urs was surprised by how nice the art shop was, and selected a socialist oil painting. The staff said they had to check to see if they had permission to sell it. Urs made a down payment, and I said I would pick it up the next time I was there and get it to him. Not long after Urs had gone back to Beijing, I returned to the shop. The assistants showed me a picture resembling the one that Urs had selected, but the colors were slightly different compared with the photo I had taken at the time of the deal. Somewhat embarrassed, they told me they were not allowed to sell the original but had asked an artist to make a copy, which they hoped would be OK. I contacted Urs, who said he wasn't interested. When I told the staff, they immediately gave me back the money. There was no ill will. But it was an interesting example of cultural differences. In the DPRK, as in China and other Asian countries, copying pictures is not viewed the same way we view it in the West. You often would find copies prominently displayed. Indeed, in North Korea, artists often expressed pride that they were considered good enough to be allowed to copy pictures of top artists. But Urs wanted an original, so the deal fell through.

I also took Urs and some other visitors to the circus, which I particularly enjoyed, because there was very little, if any, political propaganda—just an hour of amazing and, to me, often terrifyingly dangerous, exploits. Although I had been to the Pyongyang circus many times, I always froze in my chair watching the artists leap and twirl and take what I thought were shocking risks. I was continually amazed at their extremely high level of talent. There were two circuses in the capital—the city circus and the military circus. Both were equally good and had competed at the International Circus Festival in Monte Carlo, Monaco, where they had often won prizes. Some of the North Korean artists at one time even had toured with the most famous Swiss circus, Circus Knie. The performance was a welcome diversion from the usual stresses of Pyongyang.

For me, these final months were a frantic period. But the North Koreans' interest in our projects was there, and I was determined to squeeze everything I could out of the SDC programs while they were still operating. And, to be honest, I wanted to show the skeptics in Switzerland what could be done.

I still traveled out of Pyongyang whenever possible, but on more than one occasion, these trips became sad farewells to people with whom I had worked—in some cases, for years. In midsummer, I made another visit to the northeastern city of Hamhung and went to the Hamhung People's Committee, which I had visited a number of times over the years. A member of the committee whom I first had gotten to know while working for Caritas came to greet me, although he was preoccupied with damage from a recent storm that had caused severe landslides. Sadly, it seemed that nature rarely spared North Korea. When I left, it was an emotional farewell. He thanked me profusely for all the help provided, first during the Caritas years and now from the SDC. Gripping my hand, he asked me not to forget Hamhung, and declared that his great wish was that I should come back to the DPRK one day. I was deeply touched.

I also paid a last visit to the Hwangju Boarding School. I saw that the children were eating a mixture of maize and rice, a clear soup with a few mushroom slices, and kimchi. They were literally using iron rice bowls—a term used in many Asian countries to denote being supplied with enough to eat. Although I had witnessed such scenes before, I was again stunned by how often their heads seemed too big for their bodies—a result of the stunting caused by long-term malnutrition. The staff took me to the nearby mountains, where they now had a greenhouse, with people specially assigned to manage it. I gave the children sweets and some colorful balloons. We had a lot of fun blowing them up, although they always popped. I brought some footballs as well, which always were enthusiastically received. The children had made some paintings for me, one with the North Korean and Swiss flags. I got quite sentimental but tried not to show it. What would the future bring for those poor kids? I wondered if they would remember me, and if so, how? What would they make of this strange blonde woman dropping in from time to time and bringing goodies?

The city of Hamhung reflected the contradictions of North Korea. Despite the grim conditions at the cooperative farms and the boarding school, I was struck by the number of cars, trucks, and bicycles I saw on the roads, as well as by the large number of people using mobile phones. The streets of the city were full of people carrying jerricans to fetch water, while women were doing their laundry in the river as children enjoyed a swim. Yet at the Majon Hotel, which charged us an outrageous fifty-five euros a night, there was no running water, while hot water remained a dream. The contradictions were visible almost everywhere I looked. Despite the food shortages, further steps were being taken to reduce the country's isolation, with Air Koryo opening two regularly scheduled flights to Kuala Lumpur, Malaysia, as well as adding a weekly flight to Shanghai, China. And a month after The Elders left, the Pyongyang International Trade Fair took place, with the participation of 206 trading companies and groups from the DPRK, China, Germany, Malaysia, Mongolia, Syria, Singapore, the United Kingdom, Australia, Austria, Italy, Indonesia, France, Poland, and other countries. At the end of the fair, exhibitors usually would sell their items, mostly to locals with hard currency.

At the same time, however, tensions with South Korea rose. The South Korean military reportedly was using portraits of Kim Il Sung and Kim Jong Il for target practice, and North Korea seized over $300 million in South

Korean assets that had been invested to create a tourism center at scenic Mount Kumgang, just on the northern side of the DMZ. Yet in July, the United States and North Korea held talks. Separately, around the same time, Washington agreed to send $900,000 worth of emergency relief supplies following floods in the North. Meanwhile, in a sign of further economic malaise, the government announced that all universities in North Korea were going to be shut down for ten months so that the students could work in agriculture or industry. Some foreign observers speculated that another reason might be to preempt the admittedly remote possibility of campus protests.

The conflicting trends were reflected in my own shifting moods as I prepared to leave. There were days when things seemed bleak and depressing, and sometimes I wondered whether all my efforts over so many years really had made much difference. But when I took stock of everything, as I did in a predeparture memo to the SDC, it became clear that we had made a modest but real impact. While acknowledging the many setbacks and challenges, I stressed that our projects had helped to create better harvests, improve agricultural practices, transfer knowledge, provide valuable training sessions, and expand international contact and cooperation. I stressed the need for patience and perseverance, noting that "there is an enormous hunger for learning, for information…[but] sensitivity, creativity, negotiation skills and flexibility are needed in order to bring new ideas to people who have very little exposure to the rest of world." In conclusion, I noted, "The problem with North Korea will not go away quickly; with the political deadlock it will probably become even more complex and dangerous. We must move forward peacefully, not with aggression and confrontation, but with diplomacy and dialogue, with building bridges of understanding, respect and trust."

Two days before my scheduled departure, I visited the South Pyongyan Provincial Hospital in Pyongsong City about thirty-five kilometers north of Pyongyang. A Swiss friend in Hong Kong, Ruedi Bischof, had given me $10,000 and told me to do something useful with it. I got the idea of purchasing three thousand lenses for cataract operations. Working through my old contact Hugo Hörndli, who had been the intermediary for almost every item we'd purchased outside of North Korea during all my years of involvement there, we acquired lenses made in India. Provincial hospitals all had departments of ophthalmology, and the North Korean doctors were capable of conducting cataract operations. When I visited the hospital, they already had begun to do so, with great success. I suddenly realized how cost-effective this whole business was: For $10,000, three thousand people could have their sight restored or improved, with no additional medical training for the local doctors required. I stored this in the back of my mind, with the idea that I might be able to work with it in future. Indeed, although I didn't know it at the time, it would help provide an opening for me to return to North Korea and resume my humanitarian work.

Once I knew I would be leaving the DPRK, the question arose as to what I might do next. To my great delight, John Lewis—the distinguished Stanford University sinologist who also had made numerous trips to the DPRK, with whom I had become friends, and whom I had last seen feeling very shaken following a visit to the Yongbyon nuclear facility in late 2010—offered me a position as a fellow at the university's Shorenstein Asia-Pacific Research Center (APARC). I was absolutely thrilled at the opportunity to move to California. The team of Korea experts at Stanford was first-class, and many were good friends as well. Moreover, the program maintained cordial relations with the DPRK, which I thought might help keep the door open for me, as I definitely wanted to remain engaged and return periodically if I could. A university position would offer me a chance to decompress after so many intense years on the ground in the DPRK, and to try to pull together and further develop my own thinking and analysis about the country. And given the rigors of life in Pyongyang, a stint in the Bay Area was more than a little appealing. I accepted with alacrity.

Before I left, my SDC colleagues had a farewell party by the pool at the SDC compound, and the North Koreans gave me a "stone painting"—a piece of slate on which an image of my face had been created by grinding different stones to make colors. It was so lifelike, it resembled a photograph. This kind of stone artistry was a North Korean specialty, and I was deeply touched. They also gave me a set of twelve small kimchi pots, which today I use for all sorts of things. One has sugar in it, another holds flowers, and a third stores toothpicks. They are very practical and bring back good memories.

On September 30, I drove to the airport. I had made the trip hundreds of times, but this time it felt different. I was sad, knowing that I would never again see some of the North Koreans I had known, liked, and worked with. My local and Swiss colleagues came to see me off. They were visibly sad, but however emotional they felt, North Koreans never would allow themselves to be seen crying in front of a foreigner. As for me, the DPRK had been such a huge part of my life for so many years that this was like a leap into the unknown. I felt a mix of emotions—sadness, anxiety about the future, and the always present worries about the fate of the country and its people, plus concern about friends and unfinished work I was leaving behind. As the Air Koryo plane began to taxi down the runway, I shed a few tears.

CHAPTER TWENTY-ONE

Different Worlds

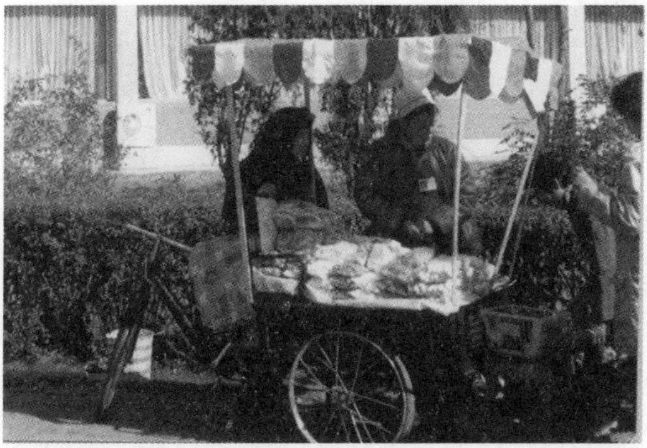

Gradually more goods were sold in small private stalls, but shopping in Pyongyang remained a challenge.

November 2011 marked a turning point in my life as I relocated from Pyongyang to Palo Alto, California, near Stanford University. It was, in some respects, a jarring adjustment, exemplified by a lunch I had with friends at a fancy hotel located not far from my new home. It had a view of the stunning Northern California scenery. I casually picked up a menu. It seemed oddly modest. A burger patty was ten dollars, salmon flakes were eight dollars, chicken was seven dollars, and steamed vegetables were five dollars. Then I did a double take. The menu listed a bowl of milk for three dollars, and homemade dog biscuits for five dollars. I hadn't noticed that at the top of the page was written "Furry Friends Menu." Here, in America, was a menu for dogs, while in North Korea, dogs were *on* the menu. Moreover, the canine treats on offer here made up a diet far healthier than that of the vast majority of North Koreans. My head was spinning. It was just one example of my disorientation as I struggled to adjust to the abundance of life in America after the harsh and shortage-filled existence that had characterized my five years in Pyongyang.

I began my tenure as a fellow at the Walter H. Shorenstein Asia-Pacific Research Center (APARC) at Stanford University in early November 2011, after a brief stop in Switzerland for final debriefings at the SDC. I was pleased that, despite the ugly politics that had forced the development cooperation programs to end, most of the colleagues to whom I was saying farewell were complimentary about what had been achieved during my tenure in the DPRK.

Arriving in Palo Alto, I rented a one-bedroom apartment in a three-story building. It cost half my income—the city is in Silicon Valley, one of the most expensive locations in the United States, but I had access to a swimming pool, which I used daily, a clubhouse, and tennis courts. And on the Stanford campus, about a half-hour's walk away on quiet back roads, I certainly enjoyed my newfound freedom and all the creature comforts, although it was so different from what I was used to that I sometimes felt like I was walking in my sleep. Going into lavishly stocked American supermarkets was an overwhelming experience. In Pyongyang, I had never taken a shopping list along, because I would never know what, if anything, might be available, and would feel lucky if I found a couple of items that I wanted to buy. Here, everything was to be found in abundance. I had a hard time choosing between twenty kinds of yogurts and dozens of kinds of milk. In Pyongyang, I had been happy to find any milk or yogurt on the often bare shelves. The cafés, restaurants, churches, art centers, fancy cars on the freeways, people going for bike rides at dawn, sense of wealth, and absence of the stressful issues that had made up my daily routine in the DPRK were, at first, bewildering. One thing that particularly struck me was the number of people wearing blue jeans, which were banned in North Korea. I had seen hardly anyone wearing jeans for five years. But I soon got used to the comforts of California and threw myself into my work.

My office at APARC was located in Encina Hall, the oldest building on campus. I found the university to be an inspiring place. It was created in 1891 by Jane and Leland Stanford in memory of their son, who had died of typhoid fever at the age of fifteen. They wanted to use their wealth to do something for other people's children. What a stark contrast to North Korea, a homogenous society in which the government created and controlled virtually everything. I often sat at outdoor cafés on the campus, soaking up the beautiful environment, full of greenery and lively young people of many ethnic and cultural backgrounds. I no longer had to think about what was allowed and what was not.

My new colleagues at Stanford were both welcoming and a colorful crew. Apart from John Lewis, Siegfried Hecker, and, on an occasional visiting basis, Bob Carlin, they included the director of the Shorenstein Center, a well-known South Korean scholar named Gi-Wook Shin. His deputy was David Straub, a soft-spoken, bespectacled former diplomat who had spent more than two decades in the US Foreign Service, much of that time dealing with Korea, both North and South. A fluent Korean speaker with a Korean wife, he had been the director of the State Department's Korea desk, had traveled to the DPRK several times, and participated in the six-party talks and other important diplomatic endeavors. We soon became good friends, and he took me under his wing, helping me not only to understand the center and the university better, but to get my bearings in a still-unfamiliar America. He took me to the surfing paradise of Half Moon Bay, south of San Francisco, to a local farmers' market, to his favorite German bakery. He and his wife generally helped me feel at home. The fact that he had some Swiss ancestry further strengthened our connection.

Other colleagues included Heather Ahn, the Korea Program manager at APARC, who particularly assisted me in adjusting to campus life; Tom Fingar, a China specialist who had served as director of the State Department's Bureau of Intelligence and Research; Karen Eggleston, a specialist on China and North Korea, with a particular interest in health issues in the DPRK; and Karl Eikenberry, a retired US Army lieutenant general with a background in China who also had served in South Korea and, from 2009 to 2011, as the US ambassador to Afghanistan.

Among its many other activities, the center had set up the Korea Policy Group, which I joined and where I was viewed as the person with boots-on-the-ground experience, as no one else there had ever lived as long in the DPRK or traveled there as much as I had. We held regular meetings, talks, and events. I presented to the group less than two weeks after arriving on campus. I found it a stimulating environment in which to think through my own views and experiences as I caught up on my reading and decompressed from life in Pyongyang.

On December 19, 2011, came the dramatic news that Kim Jong Il, who had been in poor health for several years, had died two days earlier. His son, Kim Jong Un, quickly emerged as the heir, taking the lead role in all the funeral ceremonies, which were broadcast on DPRK TV. I participated in a center-organized panel discussion titled "The Korean Peninsula After Kim Jong Il's Death." It was my first public appearance at Stanford. My presence at the university was not widely known at this point, so I was, to my relief, able to avoid doing media interviews, where I would have been pressed to spell out my views of what would happen next. I knew, perhaps better than most, how hard it was to predict events in the DPRK.

There was no doubt that a political transition, especially in a system as opaque as that of North Korea, would involve a degree of uncertainty. Yet I did not share the view, expressed by some so-called North Korea experts, that Kim Jong Un would prove a weak figure who would not last, or that the regime and the system were in jeopardy. Having seen the DPRK during its worst moments, I was convinced that, for all its idiosyncrasies and defects, it had an underlying resilience that would allow it to survive. More intriguing was the question of what kind of leader Kim Jong Un would turn out to be. He had, after all, been educated partly in Switzerland, and there were certainly hopes that, having been exposed to the outside world, he might continue or even accelerate the uneasy but clear process of change that I had witnessed during my years traveling and living in the country.

Indeed, in the first year or two of his rule, there were some intriguingly positive signs. These would include a more accessible leadership style than that of his father, who had been a distant and remote figure; some blunt talk about how the North Korean people would not always have to "tighten their belts"; and a purge of some members of the old guard. All this at first suggested that Kim Jong Un might indeed be an agent of change. Sadly, within a few years, those signs would disappear, and the hopes would be dashed—but in the early years of his leadership, I was not alone in my hopes.

As word of my presence spread, I began to receive invitations to give talks or join discussions, not only at Stanford but across the country. To me, it indicated a continuing strong curiosity among many Americans about the DPRK. In Los Angeles, I did a presentation on capacity development at an event hosted by the National Committee on North Korea, an NGO with a wide-ranging membership that worked to provide policymakers, the academic and think tank community, and the general public with credible information on the country. I spoke as well at the Council on Foreign Relations, the Asia Society, the Korea Society, and a variety of universities, including Harvard and the Johns Hopkins School of Advanced International Studies in Washington, DC.

It was a hectic but fulfilling time, and I was surprised and delighted when Stanford offered to extend my fellowship for a second academic year. One of the responsibilities that came with that extension was to teach a course, which I titled "An Insight into North Korean Society." I arranged for John Lewis, David Straub, and others with North Korea experience to talk to the class, and used my own experiences for much of the rest of the course content. Preparing the syllabus allowed me to review some of the most recent academic and journalistic work on the DPRK, and assembling a structure was helpful in sharpening my own analysis. I covered the history of North Korea, United States–DPRK relations, the North Korean military, the nuclear issue, everyday life, education, health care, the role of humanitarian assistance, human rights, and how the international media had been covering the country. When possible, I would bring things from North Korea to the class, such as copies of the *Pyongyang Times*, and the students were thrilled to be able to see and touch something from this place they saw as distant, strange, and mysterious.

I was impressed with those who took the course. I found them curious, eager to ask questions, and open to a less stereotypical and more nuanced view of the country. One of the things I liked about Stanford was its requirement that students had to take at least one course completely outside their major field, so I had people working toward philosophy, engineering, technology, and other degrees all flocking to learn about the DPRK. I framed their final term paper project as "not an academic research paper; the purpose is to provide students with an opportunity to present their views and opinions on issues facing North Korea, taking into account the class discussions and readings throughout the quarter." Their papers reflected the range of interests: "The US Approach to North Korea," "North Korean Refugees in China," "Entrepreneurship and the Black Market," "How the Attitude of Young Americans Towards North Korea Is Influenced by the Media," "The Korean War and How It Influences Chinese Attitudes Toward North Korea."

I found the teaching very satisfying, and at the end of the term, I took the entire class to my favorite Korean restaurant to celebrate.

The twelve months from October 2011 to October 2012 constituted the longest period that I had not visited North Korea since I'd first begun traveling there in 1995. But in the early autumn of 2012, I was thrilled when I was asked to join a delegation of mostly Swiss parliamentarians and their spouses who would be making a weeklong trip in October. This wasn't just a tourist group. The delegation would be holding a series of meetings with North Korean officials. The organizer of the trip knew from my media interviews that I had been dealing with the DPRK for many years. He asked if I could function as a kind of in-house expert, providing suggestions on where to go, and while in the DPRK, briefing them, sharing insights on different subjects to make their visit more meaningful and productive. Indeed, I would end up making some kind of presentation to the twenty-member delegation almost every evening.

Boarding the Air Koryo plane in Beijing for the flight to Pyongyang I had taken so many times previously, I had a strange sensation. Although obviously an outsider, I felt the kind of excitement one has when going home after a long time away. The sights, the sounds, the smells—all seemed so familiar. I was glad to be back. And because of the nature of the group and the kinds of meetings that were on the schedule, I knew I likely would be able to see many of my colleagues—who, not surprisingly, greeted me with open arms.

The itinerary included many of the standard experiences for visitors: a trip to pay respects to the embalmed bodies of Kim Il Sung and Kim Jong Il at Kumsusan Palace; a visit to the North Korean side of the Demilitarized Zone; a tour of the scenic Mount Kumgang area near the DMZ, where we all went hiking in the spectacular Nine Dragon Valley; a cruise on the Taedong River, which flows through Pyongyang; a visit to the circus. But there were many substantive meetings and visits as well. Through my connections, the group was taken to an SDC-funded Sloping Land Management project in North Hwanghae Province, which, I was gratified to see, was still going strong. We went as well to a WFP food factory in Pyongyang, where Swiss milk powder was being used to make blended food for children and mothers, and to a Swiss–North Korean joint venture that was producing simple medicines such as paracetamol. Some pharmacies recently had opened in the capital, and it was good to see some of their products on the shelves.

There also were high-level meetings with resident diplomats and aid workers, and with senior officials from the Korean Workers' Party, the People's Assembly, and the foreign ministry. A special treat was a session with my longtime acquaintance Ri Chol, who had been the North Korean ambassador in Switzerland for many years (where, unknown to me or almost anyone else at the time, he had supervised the young Kim Jong Un during his stint at Swiss schools). Now back in Pyongyang, Ri Chol was the head of a commission for joint ventures and foreign investment. I had known him for a dozen years, and he greeted me warmly. For all my skepticism about so much of the DPRK, I found it an encouraging sign that someone so senior, and with so much international experience, was in charge of an important part of what appeared to be a continuing effort to reach out and build connections to the rest of the world.

The emotional highlight for me, though, was a visit to the Hwangju Boarding School, whose work I had tried to support for many years through Caritas and the SDC. The staff were largely the same, and they welcomed me back, some with tears in their eyes, like I was a wayward family member returning home. I was delighted to see them, and deeply moved. The wives of some of the parliamentarians who accompanied me also cried—not because of the greeting I received, but because they were so shocked at the stunted kids, the decrepit facilities, and the overall grimness of an institution that, despite my many years of trying to help, still lacked so many basic facilities.

Nonetheless, as we prepared to leave the country after an exhausting week, I was heartened by the sense that the process of social change I had watched take hold during my SDC years—characterized by the "Five M's"—was still underway. Even in small village schools, English now was part of the curriculum. One of the North Korean TV channels provided English and Chinese language lessons regularly. When I walked into one hotel lobby, nobody was around. Everybody was in front of a TV concentrating on a Chinese language lesson. Moreover, the team members of the British Council were in high demand and were providing training-of-trainers programs. In smaller cities and villages, more low-level enterprises were being established. People knew not to count on the system to feed them anymore, and rules were bent so that they could fend for themselves. Coping strategies were growing in fits and starts, more in some areas than in others and still facing the looming presence of the state and its power to slow or reverse what was happening. I did feel that North Korean society was no longer static, that the dynamic of transformation was still alive.

Back in the United States, however, I found little receptivity for a more nuanced view of North Korea. This became evident when I participated as a panelist at a conference hosted by the Asia Society Northern California in San Francisco with the theme "North Korea: What Can the International Community Do?" The focus was mostly on North Korea's human rights situation. This was underscored by the presence of Michael Kirby, a former Australian High Court justice who was appointed by the United Nations Human Rights Council to lead an inquiry into human rights abuses in North Korea in 2013. Kirby participated in both panels at the conference, along with a young defector, Lee Seong Min, and Hannah Song, president and CEO of Liberty in North Korea (LiNK), a vociferous human rights lobbying group that—for understandable reasons—was sharply critical of the DPRK.

I found myself an isolated voice when I contended that simply condemning the North Korean regime did little to change the situation on the ground. Moreover, I voiced concern about certain activities of anti-DPRK activists, such as sending balloons with negative messages about the North Korean leadership, USB sticks with K-pop and South Korean dramas, and US dollar bills into North Korea across the DMZ from the South. North Korean officials had told me that ordinary citizens who picked up such messages were at great risk of getting into trouble with the state security apparatus. I argued that however satisfying the activists found these activities, and even if the chronicled abuses were true (and I had little doubt many of them were true), engagement, despite sometimes uncomfortable compromises, offered a better path to encourage real change in the North. I did not succeed in convincing many of the conference participants.

I returned to the DPRK in the summer of 2013 at the invitation of the Korean Federation for the Protection of the Disabled. I was able to see the process of change for myself. I had long been interested in the plight of the disabled in the DPRK, as mentioned. Indeed, on my first trip, in April 1995, I had been surprised to become one of the first foreigners allowed to see a residential school for deaf children. I had been told then that Kim Il Sung had, in 1993, started to pay greater attention to people with disabilities. I had forged a good working relationship with the KFPD during my years in Pyongyang, trying to support its efforts whenever possible, and in my initial application to become a fellow at Stanford, I had proposed writing a paper on the issue. As almost no material had been written about the subject, my new colleagues were enthusiastic.

My 2013 trip enabled me to gather considerable fresh on-the-ground information. In the process, I was able to get a sense of how much had begun to change. On a visit to Hamhung, I was taken to the Hamhung Orthopedic Hospital. Although built in 1954, it had recently undergone a significant expansion. Despite a leaking roof in one building, broken and outdated equipment, a lack of steady electricity in the winter, and a general shortage of medicine and medical supplies, the hospital was treating three thousand inpatients and over five thousand outpatients every year. Handicap International was providing some physiotherapy training. I took a photo of two patients sharing one bed. To outsiders, it might have seemed shocking, but given how many hospitals I had seen with empty beds—because there was no medicine, no food, and also insufficient personnel available to treat people, as staff would go to the mountains to collect herbs for traditional medicine—I actually found this encouraging.

Nearby is the Hamhung Orthopedic Factory, which manufactures prostheses and other orthopedic devices. As at the hospital, the facilities were dilapidated, with erratic supplies of water and electricity, but the factory was serving around a hundred patients a month. Here too collaboration had been established with Handicap International, which was helping to set up a more modern prosthetics and orthotics workshop and providing up-to-date training for the staff. Interestingly, the KPFD also had organized several mobile camps to support disabled people in remote regions, mostly mining areas, where accidents were common. Teams of eight to ten people, including technicians from the factory, physiotherapists, and KFPD experts, were sent to assist the disabled, repair old devices, and fit new ones.

And in Pyongyang, I visited the Korean Rehabilitation Center for Children with Disabilities, which opened in 2013 and was at that time integrated into a regular nursery. The manager and eleven staff members looked after twenty intellectually and physically challenged children—eight boys and twelve girls between the ages of four and seven. The children were in residence Mondays through Fridays and spent their weekends at home. Some activities, such as singing and dancing, were carried out with the other 130 kids at the nursery located in the same building, in keeping with the concept of trying to integrate the disabled children wherever possible. While

I could see the need for additional staff members, training programs, books, videos, and other material, it was striking here and at the other facilities I was shown how much more open the authorities were in acknowledging the existence of disability, and the need to do something about it. The change in attitude from my first trip was, I thought, highly encouraging.

That was the central theme of my paper, which I titled "People with Disabilities in a Changing North Korea." In the introduction, I wrote, "Though much more needs to be done, services for people with disabilities are increasing; public awareness of the needs and rights of the disabled is growing; and integration of the disabled into mainstream society is occurring, albeit gradually."[24] The paper summarized the evolution of North Korean attitudes toward the disabled, highlighting some of the major changes, both in terms of North Korean law and progress on the ground, and ended with a series of recommendations. These included calls for better training and research within the DPRK, especially within the KFPD. But I also argued for an expansion of collaboration with the outside world, which, I noted, would "provide opportunities for North Koreans working on behalf of the disabled, as well as for those with disabilities, to be exposed to international practices, ideas, expertise, and technologies. The exchange and sharing of information through a collaborative approach, by providing opportunities for study tours and training programs as well as by the simple act of donating professional books and subscriptions to disability-specific journals, will have a large impact on people with disabilities and those working in this field but will ultimately contribute to fostering improved relations between North Korea and the outside world."[25]

Yet calls for greater understanding always seemed to run up against the conventional view of the DPRK as reclusive, irrational, and dangerous, augmented by the grim picture painted in much of the media as well as in defector accounts of how daily life in the DPRK was dominated by a constant fear of arbitrary government punishment, imprisonment, or worse. Shortly after I finished writing my disability paper, a new rumor emerged that, if true, would personally affect me too. In November 2013, Kim Jong Un purged and executed his uncle, Jang Song Thaek. An official government statement said that Jang had engaged in "anti-party, counter-revolutionary factional acts." Many analysts believed that Jang had been becoming the center of a faction in the leadership with the potential to challenge Kim

Jong Un, and therefore had to be eliminated as a crucial step for Kim to consolidate absolute power.

Whatever the reason, Jang's downfall sparked a flurry of speculation about further upheaval in the regime. Japan's *Mainichi* newspaper then claimed that among the other victims of the fallout from Jang's execution was the former ambassador to Switzerland, Ri Chol, my acquaintance, who was reported in mid-December 2013 to have been put to death. The newspaper report had few details, other than to guess that Ri, who was widely believed to also have been managing the Kim family funds in Europe, including their Swiss bank accounts, may have had a falling out with Kim Jong Un over money.

Luckily, I was traveling when the news broke, so I was able to avoid the many media inquiries I received asking for comment. While I had no inside information, I was highly skeptical. Sensationalistic press reporting was a staple of the North Korea–watching world. Having seen Ri the previous year, I had detected no sign of stress, anxiety, or lack of loyalty to the new leader. But I was glad not to have to put my reputation on the line in public by either endorsing or dismissing the gruesome press accounts of Ri's alleged demise. Obviously, with no way to know for sure, I did wonder and, as I liked Ri, was somewhat concerned. But the whole saga seemed highly implausible.

Early the following year, in April 2014, Ri suddenly reemerged—not as a figure in disgrace, but as the DPRK's new foreign minister, and an active one at that, attending the UN General Assembly and taking on a high public profile. Privately, I felt not only relief but a sense of vindication. As I had suspected, the wild rumors turned out to be just that. It was a good lesson that, however strange North Korea seemed to outsiders, believing the many outlandish stories that made up the conventional view of the country was a mistake. As I noted in my paper on disability, "Many view the country and its people with preconceived notions. For a foreigner to obtain realistic information and develop an accurate understanding of the country and its people, long-term engagement, patience, and development of mutual trust are necessary."[26] I would be the first to acknowledge that this was much easier said than done—but the saga of Ri Chol's execution that didn't happen brought home to me the importance of continuing to try.

CHAPTER TWENTY-TWO

"Active and Positive Signals"

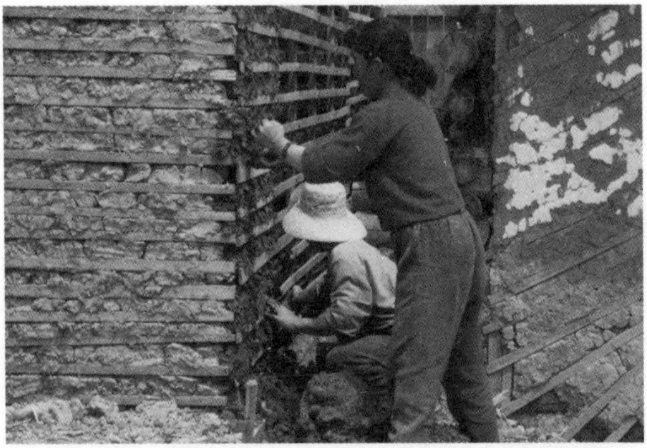

"Masikryong Speed," an expression used for jobs done quickly. Here, women are busy doing heavy construction.

It was the last thing I ever expected to see in North Korea, but the Masikryong Ski Resort took my breath away. Situated in a mountainous region a three-and-a-half-hour drive from Pyongyang, it features spectacular scenery, numerous chairlifts, and a luxury hotel—the nicest I ever stayed at in the DPRK—complete with a swimming pool, a sauna, and other facilities. Built by soldiers of the Korean People's Army in just ten months—so fast that North Koreans talked about conducting affairs at "Masikryong speed"—it was completed in 2014, twenty-one years after my first contact with North Korea. It was open to both locals and, significantly, foreign tourists and residents. The tour group I was accompanying was among the first visitors, and although it was summer, we were whisked up the mountain on the chairlift and had an enjoyable and scenic hike down.

Yet the backstory of the resort was—typical for North Korea—much murkier. The DPRK had placed a $7.5 million order for chairlifts with a Swiss company. The equipment already had been packed in crates when the Swiss government stopped the shipment, declaring the resort to be a "prestigious project for the North Korean regime"—meaning the shipment would have violated international sanctions imposed on North Korea that banned the sale of "infrastructure and equipment with a luxury character." But riding up the chairlift at Masikryong, I noticed "Ischgl" engraved on a metal plate on the side—the name of a famous ski resort in Austria. It turned out that the North Koreans had managed to procure the equipment secondhand, probably via China. It was another example of Pyongyang's resourcefulness in evading sanctions.

Various sanctions had been in place for years in response to the DPRK's nuclear tests of 2006, 2009, and 2013. They initially had been designed to block exports and imports of military supplies and technology to and from the North, but soon were expanded to cover coal, iron, crude oil, and luxury goods, and, more broadly, to shut the DPRK out of the international financial system. But the pressure did not produce any meaningful change in North Korean behavior, and the North soon proved itself adept at circumventing the restrictions. As one North Korean said to me, "We are not afraid of sanctions. The more the outside world reacts to our nuclear tests, the more our people think we need them to defend ourselves."

To me, the entire Masikryong venture was a symbol of North Korea at that period of time. On one hand, it was clear that Kim Jong Un had ambitious plans for further engagement with the rest of the world, and Masikryong was part of that. Tourism was being encouraged. On several of the more than two dozen trips I made from 2012 to 2019 following my departure from the SDC, I was a resource person for selected tour groups, which was how I was able to make two visits to Masikryong. More visitors were coming—not only from China but also from Europe. The number of flights in and out of Pyongyang's usually deserted airport was increasing, and the airport itself was getting a facelift. Aircraft now parked at new arrival docks, the arrival and departure halls resembled those of any small modern airport, and a new runway was in operation. Moreover, on the roof of the new airport buildings, the usually ubiquitous portraits of Kim Il Sung and Kim Jong Il were nowhere to be seen.

Overall, the situation for tourists appeared to be more relaxed. Taking pictures from a car was no longer forbidden, and tour guides seemed more accommodating in terms of special ad hoc requests. In 2014, a tourism college was established in Pyongyang, and there was even talk about developing ecotourism to take advantage of the country's spectacular scenery. Highlighting the changed atmosphere, a former North Korean SDC team member now working in the tourist industry informed me that there were currently fifteen local travel agencies in Pyongyang competing for business. Although some criticized tourism as supporting the regime, my own feeling was that it was helping to create a better understanding of North Korea and its people, shifting the focus away from politics and the nuclear and missile programs and toward ordinary life for citizens in the North. For all the limitations, I thought expanded tourism was a good thing, provided the groups were given good briefings.

But the sanctions also were a symbol that for much of the world, North Korea remained a pariah—characterized as a rogue state, seen as constantly flouting international rules, a country to be held at arm's length, pressured, and sanctioned. It was a paradox, because the reality was a combination of relaxation and tightening, engagement and confrontation, hope and fear—and it extended to much of what I saw and experienced in my dealings with the DPRK during those years.

Looking back now, I see that my existence during that time was a whirlwind of travel and meetings, all with a focus on North Korea; I crisscrossed the globe from Europe to the United States to Asia. Apart from my all-too-brief stays at my home village of Teufen, my time in Switzerland usually involved visits to Berne, Geneva, and Zurich for meetings with Swiss foreign ministry officials and politicians, senior officials from the SDC or other organizations, and North Korean diplomats stationed in the country. Some of the diplomats had been my translators ("guardian angels") on trips dating back to my Caritas days. I think many of them found their foreign postings to be stressful, difficult, and lonely, and I certainly got the impression they were delighted to see an "old friend" with whom they could speak and behave in a more relaxed manner. I was struck that at some of our meetings, they were dressed casually and weren't even wearing the obligatory Kim Il Sung or Kim Jong Il lapel pin, or even the pin featuring both.

In one case, a diplomat I had known for a decade was winding up a four-year tour in Berne, and we got together before his departure. He spoke fluent German and was accompanied by a newly arrived colleague whose only foreign language was English. Our conversation was candid, and when it turned to sensitive topics, we switched to German, which the junior North Korean diplomat did not understand, but he didn't seem to mind. I asked my friend whether the rumors in the South Korean press about the execution of Ri Chol were true. He vehemently denied them, said Ri was working on economic issues, and promised to convey my regards when he returned to Pyongyang. Of course, he was proved right when Ri Chol reemerged in public as the DPRK's foreign minister in 2014. My contact also told me he hoped I would continue to remain involved with North Korea, and expressed particular appreciation for the capacity development programs, like the Pyongyang Business School and the study tours abroad, that I had overseen during my time at the SDC.

But much of my time was spent outside Switzerland. After my Stanford APARC resident fellowship ended in 2013, I was invited to join the Center for International Security and Cooperation (CISAC), a group also based at Stanford's Freeman Spogli Institute for International Studies. The center's members met regularly to discuss North Korean and other security issues in East Asia, with a particular focus on concrete, doable steps toward future engagement with the country. I viewed the invitation to participate as a function of the eagerness displayed by many organizations and individuals to engage with someone with my extensive on-the-ground experience in the DPRK. CISAC attracted a fascinating range of people, not only Stanford professors and researchers but scholars from other institutions, lawyers, journalists, and more than a few current or former US government and military officials. Our discussions ranged widely, covering everything from the economy to sanctions to the nuclear issue and United States–DPRK relations. My role, as had been true at APARC, was largely to provide a sense of what it looked and felt like on the ground.

I also made a particular connection with a senior Pentagon official who focused on East Asia and was intimately familiar with military operational matters in the region. We became friends and initiated a dialogue on the DPRK that continued for several years. He confessed that he rarely thought about North Korea the way I did—as a living, breathing, complex society of twenty-four million individuals. Rather, to him, it was purely a strategic threat, a place to be monitored by satellite and targeted if conflict were to erupt. For me, it was an education to see how high-level people in the US military thought. For him, it was an opportunity to get a sense of how ordinary North Koreans—at least the ones I had encountered over so many years—thought and acted.

Our exchanges were fascinating. On one occasion, he mentioned that he believed there would be a massive flow of refugees from North Korea to China in the event of war. I replied that this might be the case but stressed my belief was that virtually nobody trying to flee would make it. For one thing, I said, it would take a drive of many hours to reach the border, on roads that were in terrible condition. Moreover, almost no North Koreans could drive or own cars, and public transport was terrible in the best of times, so one could only imagine how inadequate it would be in wartime, and in any case, North Korean security forces would probably shoot anyone trying to flee. At one point, my friend suggested that some North Koreans could perhaps look up possible escape routes on the internet. I pointed out that most North Koreans lacked computers and that the country had a limited intranet that was totally controlled by the government, so his idea was a nonstarter. For my friend, observations like these were a revelation, betraying the extraordinary lack of on-the-ground knowledge about the DPRK on the part of many top US officials. I like to think I may have helped inject a note of realism into his Pentagon deliberations.

On a separate occasion, I was introduced to another American with a military background. Some of my colleagues hinted that he also might have an affiliation with US intelligence. We chatted cordially enough until I asked him what he used to do during his military career. He said, "I flew B-52 bombers." That was enough to make me highly uncomfortable. I didn't have any further contact with him.

My credibility in these meetings and conversations—as well as during the many talks and briefings I gave to groups as varied as the Swiss Federal Institute of Technology, South Korean NGOs, Syracuse University, the Royal Asiatic Society in Hong Kong, and a cultural festival in the Czech Republic, among others—was based on my experiences in and access to North Korea. One of my tasks included preparing a short paper at the request of the Vatican's observer to the United Nations to serve as background information for Pope Francis, who was planning a visit to the United States in September 2015, with a scheduled address to the UN General Assembly.

Of particular interest were my exchanges with Chinese analysts. During this period, a host of different institutes and think tanks invited me to speak at or attend meetings in China. Given Beijing's close ties with Pyongyang, I had always assumed that Chinese experts got better access in North Korea than we Westerners. Yet I was surprised to discover in my many conversations that there was one constant refrain: a lack of access and on-the-ground information. The Chinese scholars often seemed just as frustrated as the many other North Korea watchers struggling to penetrate beneath the surface. My Chinese interlocutors were thus eager to hear of my experiences, as it turned out that I had seen much more of North Korea than they had. Still, given that institutions such as the China Institutes of Contemporary International Relations, the Shanghai Academy of Social Sciences, and the China Institute of International Studies all had close connections to the government, what I heard in my meetings provided intriguing clues to official Chinese thinking about the DPRK—summed up by one official as: "We won't let them starve, but they will not eat white rice."

As one example, in 2014, the deputy director of one institute implied that differences existed between the Chinese and North Korean governments. He said that Chinese leader Xi Jinping had his own ideas and was rethinking Chinese policy toward Pyongyang. He also noted that Beijing was concerned about the possible implications of Korean reunification, particularly the chaos that would likely accompany such a development. A common view was that the DPRK feared the United States and had—given the unhappy fates of Iraq's Saddam Hussein and Libya's Muammar Qaddafi, neither of whom had had nukes—concluded that having nuclear weapons was the only way to ensure its security. While acknowledging that China and the United States had a shared interest in preventing an expansion of Pyongyang's nuclear capabilities, the Chinese frequently stressed their view that Washington should make the first move to reduce tensions, possibly by issuing a declaration formally ending the Korean War. They also expressed concern about the emergence of a new cold war, with the United States, Japan, and South Korea on one side and China, North Korea, and Russia on the other. At the time, the fear seemed exaggerated. A decade later, sadly, it was close to reality.

In the middle of the decade, the polarization that would soon blight not just the Korean peninsula but much of the world was a distant prospect. For all of its idiosyncrasies, the DPRK was keeping its door at least somewhat open, and to my great delight, I was able to build on my previous experiences by continuing to travel there with almost as much frequency as I had done during my busiest years at Caritas.

One reason for my ability to return so often was the great variety of organizations who sought my expertise, ranging from NGOs to businesspeople to conventional tour groups. My earlier travels, however illuminating, had been focused largely on my role as a humanitarian worker. Now, this wide range of different organizations, all of whom had differing sponsoring bodies in North Korea, opened doors to parts of the North Korean system where I had had little contact, significantly boosting my understanding.

One of them was a Singapore-based nonprofit called Choson Exchange—"Choson" being an ancient term for the Korean peninsula. Founded by a young Singaporean entrepreneur named Geoffrey See, the group was running workshops to train North Koreans in the basics of business and commerce. To some extent, it felt like an effort to follow in the footsteps of the Pyongyang Business School, which had been forced to cease operation in 2011 when the SDC terminated its development cooperation programs. The group's courses focused on three themes: women in business, provincial development, and entrepreneurship among younger business leaders. Participants were chosen through an application process in collaboration with North Korean universities, and its official partner was the Committee for Cultural Relations with Foreign Countries, a body with which I had previously had limited dealings, and that turned out to be more open and flexible than many North Korean organizations. Choson Exchange was sending volunteers to North Korea and bringing North Koreans to Singapore. Beyond the specific content of the courses, the goal was to use the person-to-person connections forged to further encourage a gradual opening up of North Korean society.

Choson Exchange asked me to become an advisor, and invited me in August 2014 to observe one of its workshops in Pyongyang. Since the international political climate had led not only the SDC but other organizations to scale back or eliminate development cooperation, Choson Exchange was one of the few still operating, and I felt it was important that such an effort continue. The group's lectures certainly were of interest to the North Koreans, and I was struck by the need to take great care with translations, given North Korean sensitivity to terminology associated both with capitalism and South Korea. I also felt it would be a good idea for the foreign lecturers to be given a sheet of dos and don'ts to avoid embarrassing or awkward situations. Fundraising also remained a challenge. Better financial transparency—for example, by adding a financial statement to its annual report—might also be needed. Chosun Exchange also had received some criticism for maintaining a particularly high public profile, especially as their actual level of access to senior figures in North Korea seemed to be as limited as that of most other NGOs. I attributed this to the fact that the organization was staffed by young and perhaps excessively enthusiastic people. There was a risk that too much publicity might jeopardize their promising endeavor.

Assisting aid organizations was only one facet of what was turning into my traveling to North Korea every month or two. I was frequently asked to accompany foreign tourists. A unique one was Nicolas Berggruen, the son of a French mother and a German father, who had made a fortune trading stocks and buying and selling property in America. He had become known as the "homeless billionaire" because he lived out of luxury hotels and had no fixed abode, instead traveling the world on his private jet. Fascinated by philosophy, political theory, culture, and the arts, he founded a think tank, the Berggruen Institute, which publishes *Noema* (ancient Greek for "thinking"), a magazine reporting on politics, technology, climate change, culture, and much else. His wealth allows him to explore anything that captured his interest, and that included North Korea.

I had been introduced to Berggruen through a group linked to Eric Schmidt, the former CEO of Google, who, curious to learn how the internet worked in North Korea, visited there in early 2013. For someone as wealthy and influential as he is, I found Berggruen to be very easygoing and humble, not demanding in terms of accommodation and food, and interested in everything. He had wanted to fly to Pyongyang in his private jet, but I talked him out of it on the grounds that there wasn't enough time to go through the cumbersome bureaucratic process of getting permission. He may be a billionaire, but when we landed on the regular Air Koryo flight from Beijing, our hosts from the Korean International Travel Service (KITS) went out of their way to explain the three guidelines that all tourists—even VIP ones such as Berggruen—were required to follow: no taking photographs of the military; respectful handling of pictures of Kim Il Sung, Kim Jong Il, and Kim Jong Un; and not going alone for walks. Still, the KITS staff treated Berggruen with great respect, and one young fellow kept looking at him with great curiosity and suddenly blurted out, "So, I am meeting my first billionaire!" with a big grin on his face.

The North Koreans were eager to discuss investment opportunities, arranging meetings with the Investment and Development Office of the National Tourism Administration and the president of the International Economic Exchange Association. They explained the country's special economic zones and new tourist zones. These included the Rason Special Economic Zone, established near North Korea's border with China and Russia, which had so far largely unfulfilled hopes of becoming a manufacturing, tourism, and transportation hub. The North Koreans also were promoting the Wonsan-Kalma Coastal Tourist Area, a large-scale project to promote tourism on the eastern coast of North Korea. The centerpiece of the project was the redevelopment of the Wonsan-Kalma Airfield and Kalma Peninsula into a modern airport and a tourist area with multiple high- and low-rise buildings along a four-kilometer beach. Construction stopped during COVID but then resumed. Our hosts also took Berggruen and me to see new residential building projects, to visit the Tongil Market, and to have a meal at my favorite pizza restaurant.

In our conversations with North Korean investment promotion officials, Berggruen bluntly asked if the DPRK was going to follow the Chinese model of market-style economic reform. "We have our own style," was the answer. "We want to import successful models, not politics. We follow the motto of Kim Il Sung. 'Keep your feet in your own country and your eyes on the world.'" They explained that current economic priorities were in agriculture, consumer goods, retail services, education, telecommunications, the hotel industry, and mining, among other areas. It was such a sweeping range that it was hard to determine how much was simply ambition and rhetoric and how much might lead to practical results. Indeed, despite the long meetings, I was surprised that the North Koreans were not better prepared. They had brought no brochures or concrete proposals, and had no suggestions in terms of a visit to a special economic zone. Indeed, they didn't even have name cards, contact numbers, or email addresses. It seemed odd, given that this was an opportunity to pitch one of the world's wealthiest men, with lots of connections in the United States and Europe, on the value of investing in the country.

With the benefit of hindsight, I wondered whether the people from the investment office felt constrained because of internal developments about which we at the time—early November 2013—knew nothing. Yet barely a month later, in a shocking move, Kim Jong Un ordered the execution of his uncle, Jang Song Thaek, the husband of Kim Il Sung's only daughter. The charge was treason, and many analysts focused on speculation that Jang had sought not only to build up a rival power center but to push the DPRK closer to the Chinese model of reform and openness. It was a dramatic indication that the younger Kim, for all the signs that he too wanted to expand international contact and improve the economy, would act harshly to prevent any challenge to his own authority—and it was a sobering reminder of how deadly North Korean politics could be.

I continued to be in demand as a tour guide. In October 2015, Switzerland's largest newspaper, the *Tages-Anzeiger*, organized a trip in collaboration with a leading Swiss travel agency. Seventeen people registered, and I was asked to accompany them. Upon arrival, we were given a slight variation of the "three nos": no taking pictures of the military, no walks without a guide, and no distribution of sweets or other gifts to children. But our guides were friendly and helpful, and once they realized how well I knew the country, proved quite flexible in adjusting the itinerary to accommodate my requests—which included going to some of my favorite restaurants and visiting a cooperative farm. Moreover, as long as we avoided direct questions about the leadership, they were surprisingly open about political matters, including family reunions among relatives separated by the Korean War, a possible peace agreement, and the idea of reunification with South Korea. "We don't want to be reunified like Germany, which would mean being absorbed," one of our guides candidly acknowledged. "We want to do this in our own way and peacefully. We want one country and two systems, and to do this without foreign interference."

Upon arrival, I rented a mobile telephone for $24.50 and purchased a SIM card for $40. It was valid for seven days and enabled us to make international phone calls in case of emergencies. We stayed at the Yanggakdo Hotel, located on an island in the Taedong River, which flows through Pyongyang. To my surprise, the hotel TV was showing international news channels such as the BBC, Al Jazeera, and NHK, as well as several Chinese channels. The hotel was buzzing with official visitors and foreign journalists, all there to attend the seventieth-anniversary celebrations of the founding of the Korean Workers' Party on October 10. Tourists were not invited to the official ceremony, but our guides took us to the train station, where we watched the huge military parade among a crowd of thousands of ordinary North Koreans.

Later, we moved to a place where, after the official event in Kim Il Sung Square had concluded, many floats, including military ones, passed by. It was especially fascinating to observe the local people, both young and old, proudly cheering the military. We also were able to see other events connected to the anniversary, including impressive performances on a floating stage in the Taedong River, a torch march involving thousands of youngsters, and a huge fireworks display. To me, it all marked a forceful show of confidence by Kim Jong Un, despite the country's poverty and deep-seated problems. The tourists I was guiding were equally impressed, with many saying their sense of daily life in the DPRK was quite different from what they had been led to believe from reading media accounts in Switzerland.

In early 2016, the St. Gallen Foundation, an organization linked to the University of St. Gallen in Switzerland, approached me. St. Gallen is the nearest city to the village where I grew up, and I know it well. The university is recognized for what is generally considered one of the best business schools in Europe, and every spring hosts the St. Gallen Symposium—a weeklong gathering organized by the students in which global experts debate and discuss key economic, political, and social developments, with a special focus on enhancing dialogue across borders. Past participants have included UN Secretary-General Kofi Annan and International Monetary Fund Managing Director Christine Lagarde. Those who contacted me asked for my help in organizing a trip to learn more about the DPRK's educational system and explore whether the government might be willing to allow North Koreans to participate in the symposium.

As we held preparatory meetings for a visit planned for November, North Korea in September 2016 conducted its fifth nuclear test, the second of the year. The test triggered worldwide condemnation and a fresh set of international sanctions. To me, the expansion of Pyongyang's nuclear arsenal was extremely worrying, given the lack of evidence that sanctions would moderate the country's behavior. However, it only reinforced my belief that dialogue between the DPRK and the rest of the world was even more important to enhance understanding and reduce the chances that those weapons actually would ever be used. The St. Gallen group's visit, for which the North Koreans had given their approval, seemed to me to be a small step in that direction, so in November, I arrived in Pyongyang with two representatives from the St. Gallen Foundation. We had to collect our visas in Beijing, where we also met with Jean-Jacques de Dardel, the Swiss ambassador accredited to North Korea. Reflecting the prevailing international view, he seemed not very enthusiastic about our visit or hopes for engaging the DPRK.

Although I had had dealings over the years with a variety of North Korean educational institutions, my contact had been somewhat limited and almost always related to specific projects. We stepped out of the Air Koryo plane to be greeted by the Committee for Cultural Relations with Foreign Countries. This trip offered a rare opportunity for an in-depth look at higher education in the DPRK, with visits confirmed for three universities and one high school. Our trip got off to a sour start, however, when customs seized packets of business and travel books we had assembled as gifts for each educational institution. It took considerable time, explanation, and haggling before airport officials agreed to let us bring in the materials.

The visits to the Pyongyang University of Science and Technology, Kim Il Sung University, the Pyongyang University of Foreign Studies, and Pyongyang Secondary School Number One were illuminating, providing a glimpse of a side of North Korea even I had rarely seen. The routine at each place was the same—a greeting and an introduction from a senior university official, a tour, and then a visit to classrooms. The Pyongyang University of Science and Technology was new—established in 2010. Funded mostly by overseas Koreans and staffed by volunteer foreign professors, and with around six hundred students, it offered at that time undergraduate, master's and doctorate programs in information technology, life science/agriculture, international finance/management, and the medical field. The medical faculty was divided into dentistry, public health, and nursing. At the time we visited, the administration was building a research and development center for medical studies, and was especially proud of the cloud-computing lab, and the fact that it had sent some of the students to study abroad, in the United Kingdom, Brazil, and Sweden. We were pleased that Chancellor Chan-Mo Park expressed interest in nominating students to attend the St. Gallen Symposium.

The Pyongyang University of Foreign Studies is famous for training the interpreters who play such a crucial role in the DPRK's international dealings. A representative told us that they taught twenty-three languages. The key languages at the time were Russian, Chinese, and English, but the school was newly placing an emphasis on German. There also was an institute for simultaneous interpreters, although university representatives stressed that they lacked both teaching material and staff. That didn't dent the enthusiasm when we visited a German class and talked with the students in German.

We also saw an enthusiasm for German when we visited Kim Il Sung University, which was founded in 1946 and has more than ten thousand students. A representative took us to the Faculty of German Studies, and we had a chance to chat with six master's-level students. To our surprise, they asked us to speak in Swiss German; as we did, one student did an excellent job translating into High German. She was a charming young lady who was very likely the daughter of a diplomat who had been stationed at the North Korean embassy in Switzerland for several years.

Overall, we all felt the trip was positive, and the North Koreans appeared open to some kind of engagement with the St. Gallen Symposium. In our final report, we recommended remaining patient. Through our visit, we had sent what we described as "active and positive signals" regarding the symposium, and we planned to invite members of the North Korean embassy in Berne to attend the next year's symposium. The ball was now in Pyongyang's court.

CHAPTER TWENTY-THREE

An Endless Seesaw

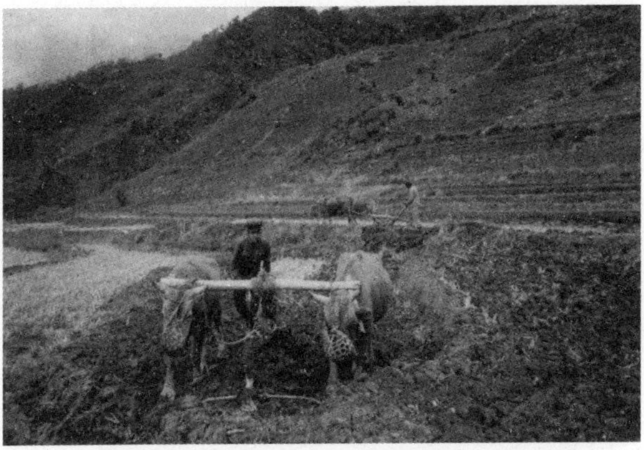

Despite some progress, the agricultural sector remained in desperate need of modernization.

My trips between 2012 and 2019 helped me assemble a kind of snapshot of the DPRK during the years immediately after Kim Jong Un became supreme leader and as he attempted to put his stamp on the country. As was so often the case in North Korea, the picture was full of contradictions and by no means the one-dimensional portrait that so many outside observers painted.

The "Six M's" I had identified some years before—the original five of money, markets, mobiles, motor cars, and a growing middle class plus the latest addition, changing mindsets—were still very much in evidence. The Kwangbok (Liberation) Department Store and Supermarket in Pyongyang's Mangyongdae District was as good a place as any to observe them. A fairly new three-story building, it was a joint venture with China that was considered the largest and most successful mall in Pyongyang. It was known as a place where one could change US dollars into North Korean won at the realistic—that is to say, black market—rate, rather than the absurd official rate offered at hotels. In August 2014, the official rate was 97 won to the dollar. At Kwangbok, the rate was 7,200 won to the dollar, and no one seemed to notice or care if foreigners crowded the counter to change money.

Many of the goods on sale were imports from China, although there were items from Indonesia, Thailand, Vietnam, and other countries as well. The first floor held stationery, cosmetics, and electronic goods, and had a large supermarket, including a fruit section, where I bought bunches of bananas to share with my North Korean colleagues. On the second floor, one could find locally made and imported clothing, as well as furniture in a store named Ikea. It offered Chinese and North Korean–made items and, apart from the borrowed name, for which I assumed no permission had been granted, had no relationship with its more famous Swedish counterpart. I was pleasantly surprised that the prices seemed relatively modest and that, unlike in so many shops in the DPRK, the shelves were always full. On the top floor was a food court where a beer cost one thousand won—at the black market rate, around twenty cents, probably the cheapest beer in the world—and at the entrance was an ice cream shop where a cone cost five thousand won. That was the same price as a bowl of Pyongyang's famous cold noodles. The mall was always packed on Sundays, when most North Koreans did not work. It was a common sight to witness families buying their excited kids ice cream at the front door or adults slurping down noodles. I visited often, as I found it one of the best spots in the city for people-watching.

Meanwhile, the Rakwon Department Store, which I had visited on my first trip in 1995, also was trying to change with the times. It now offered a loyalty card, which provided discounts, and had counters where customers could buy take-out food. The top floor had a microbrewery and restaurant run by Kenji Fujimoto, a Japanese man who had become known as Kim Jong Il's private sushi chef. The place had begun selling alcohol under the store's own brand: Rakwon beer and *makkoli*, the latter being a milky, off-white, and lightly sparkling rice wine. With an alcohol content higher than most beers, it packs a serious kick.

Strolling the streets, I noticed other signs of change. One store offered customers both a restaurant and a shop selling Dell and Lenovo computers. I learned of a half dozen shops that the Hwang Gum Bol (Yellow Gold Field) chain had opened. Open from 6 a.m. to midnight, the stores were not fancy, but they sold a variety of local brands and had become extremely popular. Choson Exchange had trained the people behind these and more than a few other businesses. A coffee culture also was beginning to emerge, with a café on the sixth floor of the Pyongyang Hotel at its center. In addition to beverages, it sold coffee mugs and small espresso cups with a cute picture of Pyongyang and the logo of the Pyongyang Café. With a cappuccino costing around six to seven dollars, however, business here was still limited largely to those at the wealthier end of the economic spectrum.

At the same time, I spotted many young women wearing quite short skirts and high heels. I noticed as well a growing number of mothers pushing babies in strollers, something I had never seen before, as North Korean mothers almost always carried their little children. Another interesting phenomenon was large numbers of people walking and reading at the same time, in the same way that so many people elsewhere in the world walk while glued to their smartphones. For the first time, I watched people using e-bikes, and one Pyongyang shop even sold such bikes. Equally striking was the number of stalls in the city's back alleys selling food and drinks. The willingness of people to spend money on such services and establishments was a sign that what the government was able to supply was decreasing, while the private and semiprivate sectors were growing.

For someone who had first visited the DPRK when the streets were virtually empty, I found Pyongyang's increasingly frequent—although minor to a Western eye—traffic jams nothing short of astonishing. Taxis, which had been almost impossible to find, were proliferating. Within a single district, a taxi ride cost sixteen thousand won (around two dollars at the black market rate); the meter kicked in when the taxi crossed into another district. There were days when only cars with even-numbered plates were allowed on the road, followed by days for only those with odd-numbered plates, although cars with foreign license plates (a different color) were exempt from this regulation. These rules were in addition to a long-standing rule prohibiting most driving on Sundays that had been implemented due to petrol shortages. The result was largely empty streets on those days.

Incidentally, I often thought that the photos that made their way to the West showing seemingly deserted streets may well have been taken on those empty Sundays. However, it turned out that controlling traffic apparently was not the only reason for the odd-even-day rule. It applied only to government cars, which had white-colored plates. These official cars often were used for personal reasons, and the restrictions were aimed at curbing this practice. But the fact that people were exploiting having an official vehicle for personal use was yet another sign of how residents would take advantage of opportunities to make their lives more comfortable.

One day, I bumped into a group of young medical students at the Grand People's Study House (the national library). Their teacher had gone for a cigarette and left the students free to chat. They had so many questions about life outside the DPRK—from what the medical services were like in Switzerland to how a credit card worked. It was nice to have an entirely relaxed and free conversation. I was continually struck by the difference between the younger and older generations. The usual manner of older people seemed to be to hold on to what was familiar, with the conversation full of the ritualistic praise for Kim Il Sung, Kim Jong Il, and Kim Jong Un, while younger people, often wearing more modern and stylish clothing, appeared eager to learn, move forward with new projects and ideas, and even, in subtle but unmistakable ways, signal a desire for change.

At the same time, Kim Jong Un had initiated a construction boom across the country, but especially in Pyongyang. Developers were building residential housing—the tallest structure being seventy stories—government buildings, business premises, gas stations, power plants, schools, amusement parks, and museums at a breakneck pace. There was a boom as well in the building of new greenhouses. Roads were being expanded and resurfaced. In Pyongyang, the buildings looked solid and modern. I also noticed that families with some money were able to purchase solar panels for their apartments—a good way to cope with still-frequent power outages. Some of the major hotels now provided saunas and swimming pools, and there was a period in the mid-2010s when CNN and BBC News were available on hotel room TVs, along with the Japanese network NHK and Russia's RT.

Yet, in contrast to the promise of cautious reform and gradual economic development (which DPRK officials still could not call "reform," instead using the term "policy improvements"), and the possibility that an emerging middle class with rising expectations might put pressure on the regime for further liberalization, I still witnessed overwhelming backwardness and poverty in so many places. Indeed, in my notebook, I compared the situation to a see-saw. Even in Pyongyang, fuel and electricity remained in short supply despite the increasing use of solar panels. In many apartment buildings, the water pumps were not working, and it was common to see people hauling buckets of water up many flights of stairs. Regular access to safe drinking water remained a problem. Still, Pyongyang remained a haven of wealth, comfort, and openness compared with the rest of the country. In one rural area, I saw women washing clothes in a river, where children were playing as well, while sewage was pouring into the water just a few meters away.

I traveled thousands of miles during my nearly two dozen visits between 2012 and 2019. Wherever I went, the roads were in terrible condition, worse than I remembered from my earlier times in the country. On many occasions, the minibus I was in had neither seat belts nor a first aid kit. I was not unhappy that these vehicles were generally old and not able to go very fast.

Food also remained a problem. Traveling around, I was struck that most rice and maize fields were heavily guarded, suggesting that the authorities were trying to prevent hungry people from seizing crops. Fieldwork still was done primarily by hand or with oxen, since hardly any agricultural machinery was available or still operational. In some cases, I observed older people scouring the fields for individual grains of rice or maize, a throwback to the famine days and a clear sign that the food situation remained difficult. I hardly ever saw a homeless person or a beggar, although I did see women by the side of the road selling agricultural products as well as mushrooms collected in the woods.

In 2014, the United Nations' Food and Agriculture Organization (FAO) estimated that the grain shortfall would be on the order of 340,000 metric tons, and noted that the average diet for most North Koreans lacked sufficient proteins, fats, and micronutrients. Yet donor fatigue, coupled with the DPRK's poor international reputation, meant that the supply of international aid was declining. Interestingly, the Russian Federation emerged at that time as the major food donor, providing 28,700 metric tons of wheat. This was an early sign of the steadily increasing closeness between Moscow and Pyongyang, which also included the creation of a business council to expand cooperation aimed at meeting a goal of $1 billion in bilateral trade by 2020. This closeness later would develop into a strategic partnership involving North Korea's providing troops to fight in Russia's war in Ukraine.

After Russia, China was also a major food donor, continuing to provide rice. Still, in 2014 and 2015, the food ration for the average North Korean fell to 250 grams of grain a day.

Recurring drought compounded the food problem. On a tourist trip in June 2015, I and three Swiss colleagues visited a cooperative farm in Kangwon Province, where the farm manager acknowledged water shortages. I was struck that the children at the farm, while appearing relatively healthy, looked scruffy and dirty and evidently had not been near water in a long time. That same month, the Ministry of Foreign Affairs called in UN agencies and the Swiss representative to tell them about the seriousness of the situation. Significantly, the Korean Central News Agency (KCNA) issued a report on the drought, confirming the scale of the problem. I was told that the groundwater levels were low and that, especially with the chronic electricity and gas shortages, many water pumps were not working. Riverbeds had dried up, and people were frantically digging new wells. Even in Pyongyang, I ran into tourists from Singapore who complained that water in their hotel was available only twice a day for brief periods.

As I traveled, I noticed that some rice plants had turned yellow and that the maize crop was stunted in many places. The soil was cracked, and people would carry buckets of water for long distances to use for irrigation. Although the DPRK often had suffered from floods, rain was desperately needed at this point. Otherwise, the main harvest would be in jeopardy. An increase in malnutrition cases was very likely. As always, the most vulnerable—children, pregnant and nursing women, the old, the sick, and the disabled—would be the hardest hit.

Conditions for international agency work varied widely during this period but, unfortunately, trended in the wrong direction. Budget cuts and North Korean recalcitrance had led to significant reductions in the number of foreign personnel on the ground. The situation was further complicated by a new mandate from the UN secretary-general calling on all agencies, offices, and funds to place "the protection of human rights…at the heart of UN strategies and operational activities."[27] On the surface, it was an absolutely legitimate aspiration, but North Korea was exceptionally sensitive to any criticism of its human rights record, so raising the topic was almost guaranteed to be counterproductive. In my view, a less political approach focusing, for example, on meeting basic human needs or on human rights education would have been a much better starting point for gradually working up to human rights talking points. For organizations struggling to maintain their position on the ground in the DPRK, it was an added burden. Those coming and going found the topic easier to address than did the foreigners living there.

Continuing sanctions made operational matters worse. When I was able to get to the interagency meeting held every Friday at the United Nations Development Program's Pyongyang office, the top question on everyone's mind was how to get money into the country. The main banking channel that the UN had been using to get funds in had become a casualty of the sanctions, making it exceptionally difficult to transfer money for daily operational costs or to pay local suppliers. The only route now was for remittances to go to Commerzbank in Germany, from where the funds were transferred to Commercial Bank Sputnik in Russia (which charged an astronomically high fee of 12 percent). Then the money, in rubles, was transferred to the DPRK's Foreign Trade Bank. Even for unsanctioned goods, it was becoming increasingly hard to find suppliers and forwarding agents, because they feared becoming a target of secondary sanctions. Efforts to get a special waiver for UN agencies were achieving uneven results, and often people had to carry in large amounts of cash, with no paper trail. Among other things, this created a lack of accountability, which I strongly suspected was leading to increased corruption. The sanctions also were further depressing what little enthusiasm existed among international donors to provide aid.

For North Korean organizations, the impact was even worse. Factories were running out of raw materials and had no hard currency or international transaction methods to purchase inputs or spare parts. The cost of almost everything inside the country was going up. A coupon for fifteen kilograms of gas now cost 29.4 euros, and a coupon for diesel was 25.5 euros. Bus and taxi fees also were skyrocketing. Fewer goods were available in the markets, prices were higher, and new fees and surcharges were imposed on many services. Even though medicine was supposed to be exempt from the sanctions, essential drugs were still in short supply in most North Korean hospitals. For example, sanctions banned the import of certain medical equipment containing even small metal components, which ostensibly also could be used in missile construction. I knew of one shipment of equipment to treat tuberculosis that was held up for months because it also contained nail clippers—which were of course made of metal. With the United Nations and NGOs facing ever-greater operational difficulties, further cuts, with a corresponding impact on medical services, were anticipated. One UN official gave an interview to the French news agency AFP, in which he said that UN assessments had found that some ten million people in the DPRK needed humanitarian aid, but because of the difficulties in getting resources into the country and raising funds from UN member countries, only 15 percent of them received help.[28]

As I wrote in my journal at the time, "The longer sanctions last, the greater the impact will be felt by ordinary citizens. It is a downward chain to the poor. Sanctions should not harm those who already have incredibly hard lives."

Compared with what I saw during my earliest visits in the mid- to late 1990s, however, North Korea unquestionably was showing signs of progress, although the tightening of sanctions and the still-grim economic situation in much of the country appeared to have unnerved the authorities. The result was that from the mid-2010s on, the government counterbalanced its moves toward relaxation—some of which continued—with steps to tighten control.

An outbreak of the Ebola virus in Africa in late 2014 and early 2015 gave the DPRK regime an excuse to impose tighter curbs on foreigners. For several months starting in October 2014, in an eerie precursor to how the government would behave during the COVID pandemic, the border was effectively closed and resident expatriates were ordered to quarantine in their homes. Everybody, even the envoys from Russia and China, was affected. Foreigners could not get appointments with the Ministry of Foreign Affairs and were treated like outcasts, with resident expats not allowed to meet their own staff even within their office premises. Since there was not a single case of Ebola on or anywhere close to the Korean peninsula, people debated whether this was a show of power or an attempt to intimidate the resident international community. The many weeks of border closings certainly had a negative impact. With no meetings or field trips possible, foreigners were tired of being forced to stay at home and not being able to work. Many started thinking of leaving their posts. Some organizations considered closing down their North Korea operations altogether. Just in the nick of time, the government reopened the borders in the spring of 2015.

In the meantime, several tighter regulations were put into place. One was a blanket ban on receiving information from the outside world. Suddenly, CNN and the BBC disappeared from televisions in the few major hotels where they had been available. The only international channels were China's CCTV, Russia's RT, and Japan's NHK. Hotel guests also discovered they no longer could make landline calls to resident foreigners, although cell phones still seemed to work. At the airport, customs officials became stricter, checking suitcases, hand luggage, computers, and other IT equipment for publications, photographs, and films. Nothing about Korea, North or South, including guidebooks, was allowed to enter the country. Increased controls were imposed on the use of electronic devices, with people now required to register with the authorities even printers they owned. I noticed more roadblocks, checkpoints, and controls over daily movements. In my own travels, we were stopped many times. Each time, officials checked the papers of my North Korean colleagues very carefully. At one stop, I observed how thoroughly an army vehicle was inspected. The driver not only had to show his papers but also get out of the car and open the trunk. Holding a flashlight, the security official then checked the contents and demanded that some items be unloaded.

The harsh new attitude also led in 2015 to the expulsion of the newly arrived head of the German NGO that had been working in the DPRK for a dozen years, Welthungerhilfe, whose name means "world hunger aid"; previously it had been known as German Agro Action. Without warning or explanation, the new country director, Regina Feindt, was ordered to leave, and a colleague of hers who had been in the country for twelve years left a month later. I learned that for days prior to Feindt's departure, North Korean security agents had followed her day and night, to the point where she no longer felt safe and briefly moved into the German embassy. In my two decades of working in or with the DPRK, I had never heard of such heavy-handed harassment. Speculation about the cause was rampant, with people wondering if it was an interview she had given to a German newspaper or tensions with her North Korean liaison officer. The true reason never emerged. The organization was allowed to keep a skeleton presence on the ground in Pyongyang.

Two developments in relation to South Korea, both of them negative, also occurred in 2015. One was that a big international NGO conference was planned for Seoul in early November. The Pyongyang authorities made clear to the resident international aid community that anyone who attended it would not be allowed back into the DPRK.

The second had to do with defectors. South Korea announced that as of January 1, 2015, a total of 27,518 defectors from the North were in the South, and that 90 percent of them had come after 2000. Another significant data point was that between 2008 and 2013, 2,400 to 2,900 North Koreans had made it to the South every year. In 2014, the number dropped to 1,396. And in the first six months of 2015, only 535 defectors had managed to get there—91 men and 443 women. It seemed clear that the tighter controls throughout the DPRK were making it increasingly difficult for people to escape. Looking at the figures, I was struck by the enormous disparity between the number of men and the number of women who got out. It occurred to me that this might be for the same reason women were so much more prevalent in the private economy. The vast majority of men were tied to work units, and even if they had little to do, they were monitored at their factory or workplace. Moreover, many young men had to serve in the military for up to ten years. Women, consigned much more to the role of housework and raising children, faced less supervision. So it made sense that it would be easier for women to slip away unnoticed and cross the border into China. In any case, though, the tough new measures meant that the path to escape was being shut down.

One day, I asked a North Korean colleague who had lived abroad working at a North Korean embassy what he missed most. He replied, "Freedom, internet access, and meeting foreigners."

Despite the heightened security, there was an enormous disconnect between what I heard on the BBC, Voice of America, or Deutsche Welle news, and what I saw and felt inside North Korea. Especially after Donald Trump became president in 2017, a war of words between the United States and North Korea suggested that an actual war might be looming. On most of my trips, when I greeted my North Korean colleagues every morning, irrespective of the nature of the particular visit I was on, they all wanted an update on the international situation. While people occasionally asked me who I thought would win such a war, my general sense was that it was very much business as usual in the North. However heated North Korean rhetoric sometimes got, and despite Trump's threats, there was no sense of crisis or military mobilization. Instead, the dynamic of loosening and tightening, loosening and tightening—something to which most people had adjusted—simply went on.

The restaurants, shops, and markets, especially in Pyongyang, still were full. The uniformity for which North Korea had been famous was now gone. The situation differed notably from place to place. Contrary to the conventional wisdom, there were now many new realities in the country. The door to the outside world, even if watched much more closely, had not closed entirely. As one example, six months after I had brought two members of the St. Gallen Symposium to the DPRK, I accompanied two members of the North's diplomatic mission in Switzerland to attend the annual symposium in the Swiss town. The theme of the symposium that year was, appropriately enough, "The Dilemma of Disruption." It was a small step, but amidst everything else going on, their attendance was a positive one—to me at least.

CHAPTER TWENTY-FOUR

KorAid

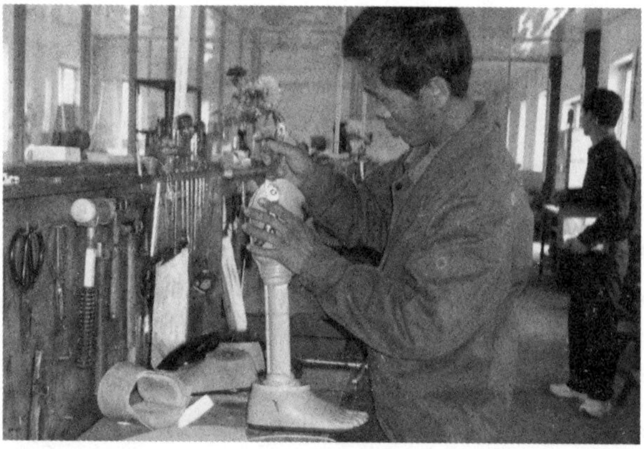

Help for the disabled was a KorAid priority, including support for the production of orthopedic devices in Hamhung city.

The South Pyongyan Provincial Hospital was a faded four-story building with grimy concrete steps leading to an entrance over which was draped a large propaganda banner. The white letters on a bright red backdrop read, "Let us health workers become the defenders of human life." The hospital was in Pyongsong, the capital of South Pyongyan Province. Located thirty-two kilometers northeast of Pyongyang, the city was, in better days, known for its automobile industry, as a center of science and technology, and as the home of several universities. On this day in December 2019, I was visiting the ophthalmology unit. There, I met a retired teacher who had just had a cataract operation. With a patch on one eye and tears in his other, he gripped my hand and thanked me over and over, in Korean and in halting English, for helping to restore his eyesight.

It was a moment that brought home to me the value of KorAid, an NGO I had established in Hong Kong in 2015. Among its projects was assistance for cataract operations in the DPRK. North Korean doctors knew how to do the relatively simple procedure but lacked the lenses and special eye medicine needed to carry it out. Once KorAid acquired these items abroad and shipped them, tens of thousands of North Koreans underwent the operation and got their sight back. To meet these patients was incredibly gratifying. It made worthwhile all the challenges and obstacles in setting up and operating a charity in the DPRK.

But it was still North Korea. When the grateful patient at the South Pyongyan Provincial Hospital announced that he wanted to invite me to his home for dinner to thank me, the officials in the room froze. I knew, as they did, that such a gesture, which would be unremarkable in so many other countries, would not be allowed in the DPRK. They got out of the potentially awkward situation when one of the doctors told the patient he would need to remain in the hospital for a few more days to reduce the risk of infection, and that I was visiting only on that day. All of us—including, I suspect, the patient—knew what was actually going on. But that was the way the system worked. Upon hearing this news, the patient gripped my arm even harder and kept saying, "Thank you." He was eager to pose for a photo.

As mentioned previously, I had been interested in the plight of people with disabilities since my first trip to North Korea in 1995. As my time at the SDC was running out, I had thought about trying to establish my own NGO to allow me to continue some kind of humanitarian work in the country. I felt I had the experience, the contacts, and the fundraising background to make it possible. I brainstormed with the people of the Korean Federation for the Protection of the Disabled, with whom I had long maintained a cordial relationship. I had found over the years that the KFPD, which I would call a semigovernmental organization, seemed to operate with slightly more freedom and flexibility than other institutions, and my exchanges with officials there often were more open than I had experienced elsewhere. It became clear that making cataract surgery available to the many people who needed it would be a worthwhile endeavor, so in 2010 and 2011, using my friend's donation, the KFPD conducted a trial run in Pyongsong, which was considered a great success.

I maintained my connection with the KPFD in the years immediately after my departure from the SDC in the autumn of 2011. That's when I also wrote my paper "People with Disabilities in a Changing North Korea," which Stanford University published in 2014—an experience that further heightened my desire to do something concrete to help this most marginalized section of the country's hard-pressed population. In 2013, the KPFD hosted me for two trips, taking me to a rehabilitation center in Hamhung that provided prosthetics for disabled people, an orthopedic hospital in the same location, as well as a center for Braille computer training for visually impaired children and adults, a school for kids with hearing problems, plus orphanages, baby homes, and boarding schools.

In 2014, I brought two experts on health and disability from Hong Kong to Pyongyang. We were taken to the Korean Rehabilitation Center for Children with Disabilities (KRCCD). The residential center now cared for around eighty physically and intellectually challenged children from the ages of four to ten. Many had been brought to the center by parents who felt unable to look after them properly. As was often the case in the DPRK, I found the facilities rather old but spotlessly clean, and the staff hardworking and dedicated. But the center lacked books, videos, and other material for assessing, training, and educating disabled children. We offered to do what we could to help.

My two colleagues from Hong Kong were warmly welcomed. They had brought written material on helping the disabled and gave a number of presentations. I found it interesting—and moving—to see that many parents were allowed to attend these sessions, obviously desperate for any advice to help them cope with the challenges of caring for a disabled child. They had many questions, and if the mother or father couldn't attend, a grandparent came instead. A few visits to existing health-care and rehabilitation facilities for children also were arranged. It was clear that the North Koreans did not have the basic tools to identify and assess special needs children, although historically the needs of visually and hearing-impaired children had been recognized.

At the end of our trip, the two experts and I prepared a detailed document full of specific ideas (including possible short-, medium-, and long-term objectives) for both the KFPD and the KRCCD. We offered to help with establishing a system for assessing each child and creating individual plans for following up. In addition, our report suggested setting up a resource center that parents and teachers alike could use to obtain more information, as well expanding teacher training. Finally, we proposed bringing a small number of KRCCD staff members to Hong Kong to observe the various systems there and for further training. All of these visits and activities generated enormous goodwill, regardless of the twists and turns in the broader diplomatic and security situation on the Korean peninsula, so by the time I began to set up my own NGO in early 2015, the KPFD and the KRCCD were eager to act as my North Korean partners.

Based on discussions with the North Koreans, my vision for KorAid—a project for which I enlisted my two Hong Kong colleagues as key volunteer advisors—initially had three main elements: to formalize and expand the cataract operation program by providing the lenses and special medicine to conduct at least three thousand surgeries a year; to support training programs for the staff, parents, and children at the KRCCD; and to fund the building of a greenhouse at an orphanage on the outskirts of Pyongyang so better nutrition for the approximately five hundred children institutionalized there could be provided—and hopefully serve as a model for other educational institutions to follow. It was clear that the North Koreans needed not just inputs but above all training, and my hope was to be able to provide this in a coherent, professional way. I asked friends and colleagues for suggestions about what to call my new organization. In the end, I decided on KorAid. It was short, snappy, and easy to remember.

I soon discovered, however, that creating an NGO to deal with North Korea was no simple task. I decided to base KorAid in Hong Kong. After so many years working there, I still had permanent resident status, the territory was a good base for traveling to the DPRK, and it had a reputation as a relatively easy place to do business. Moreover, attempts to raise funds in Switzerland had, apart from a few generous friends and family members, proved not very successful, and I thought I would have a better chance in Hong Kong. I found a friendly lawyer who was, like me, a member of the Hong Kong chapter of the International Women's Forum. She was willing to help me with the legal paperwork on a pro bono basis, but it turned out that the combination of international sanctions and tightening local regulations meant that getting set up wouldn't be so easy after all.

Indeed, many small businesses encouraged by InvestHK, the government's arm for businesses to get set up in Hong Kong, were complaining that opening a bank account locally had become a nightmare, largely because the territory's two biggest banks, Standard Chartered Bank and HSBC, had fallen afoul of US regulations in recent years. "Hong Kong is now the strictest and most difficult environment in the world to get a bank account," one of my colleagues warned me. Nonetheless, I assembled all the documents for registering KorAid Limited in Hong Kong, including the paperwork for creation of a three-person committee, since Hong Kong law did not allow for NGOs or companies to be officially run by just one person, and I had two expat friends who were willing to help. I submitted everything to the relevant government authorities, along with a letter requesting tax exemption. I was able to open an account at the Hong Kong branch of the Chinese bank ICBC, and by midsummer 2015, to my great relief, approval was finally granted.

My lawyer, in a formal document laying out KorAid's tax-deductible status as a charity, spelled out the organization's goals:

> To relieve poverty, suffering, hardship and distress of the needy people in…North Korea through donations, medical services and direct financial or material support…. For the prevention or relief of poverty, to create, promote, maintain, support and administer educational, health, welfare, training and other programs and activities for, and services to, underprivileged people with particular reference to people that are physically, mentally or intellectually disabled and children that are orphaned and deprived on a non-profit making basis.

In June 2015, the KFPD hosted me for the first time since the formal establishment of KorAid. In our conversations, I was struck by how much more engaged the North Koreans appeared to be on the broader issue of people with disabilities. I was told that the state—in a much more proactive way than previously—was encouraging the population to look after the disabled. Initiatives with a number of other foreign NGOs were moving ahead, including the provision of wheelchairs and the creation of vocational training programs. In addition, Handicap International, the Belgian-based

NGO that initially had been set up to help land mine victims in Cambodia in the early 1980s, was, at the time KorAid started, involved in occupational and physical therapy training programs at a home for the elderly and at some local clinics. The organization also was working on improving teaching skills for the blind.

I was pleased to learn as well that on North Korea's National Disability Day—June 18—the children from the KRCCD would, for the first time, participate. On their visit several months earlier, my two colleagues from Hong Kong had suggested such exposure. Moreover, with the assistance of the China Disabled Persons' Federation, a sports team of disabled people from the DPRK had arranged to go to China and train with Chinese teams. And a five-story building in the center of Pyongyang had been allocated for the Association for the Deaf.

After so much misery, it was heartening for once to be greeted with such encouraging news, and it was against this backdrop that I went with my KFPD colleagues to inspect the KorAid projects now getting underway.

The Mirim Orphanage, located on the outskirts of Pyongyang, housed at that time 550 children between the ages of seven and seventeen. All the kids were assembled to greet me. They looked generally healthy, but sadly, many were extremely stunted—a legacy of the famine years and the food deprivation that continued long after. In talking about the future of these children, I was told that a very few would go to university, about a dozen would join the army, and the rest were to be assigned jobs in factories or on farms. Two-thirds of the residents were boys. The explanation for the gender disparity was that in North Korea girls were adopted more often than boys. I asked staff members why, now that overall conditions in the country were better—it was almost twenty years since the famine—there still seemed to be so many orphans. They said that traffic and other accidents, as well as health issues, were still causing parent deaths. Moreover, if a widowed mother were to remarry, the new husband sometimes would not accept her children from a previous marriage.

The kids slept up to ten to a room. The electricity supply was not bad by North Korean standards, with power cuts lasting just two or three hours most days. The dining room was small, and meals were taken in shifts. I felt that the overall food situation now appeared stable, but the kids clearly needed a more diversified diet than one based largely on rice and maize. Moreover, vegetables were still in short supply, especially in winter. That's where the greenhouse that KorAid was proposing to support would come in. Not only would it help to provide better nutrition and act as a kind of insurance policy in case the food situation were to worsen again, but the children would learn how to grow vegetables—a valuable skill. More broadly, the greenhouse would serve as a model for other schools in the country, encouraging more educational institutions to be self-reliant.

I was then taken to Sariwon, the capital of North Hwanghae Province, about seventy kilometers southeast of Pyongyang, where I visited the 760-bed provincial hospital, which had been designated as one of the beneficiaries of KorAid's cataract program. I met two of the eight doctors working in the ophthalmology department. I found them open, relaxed, and easy to talk to. It was clear that the program would meet a major need. A KFPD survey showed that the blindness rate of people older than fifty in North Korea was 2.2 percent, and 50 percent of them needed cataract surgery. There were an estimated forty thousand to fifty thousand new cases per year nationwide, but only about ten thousand operations were being performed. The waiting lists were long.

As I explained the idea of KorAid's providing assistance, the doctors expressed great eagerness to collaborate. In the wards, I met several patients recovering from cataract operations, who were happy to chat. The doctors told me they conducted around seven hundred cataract surgeries a year but had a waiting list ten times as long—seven thousand patients. The lenses currently being used were produced at a factory attached to the Pyongyang Eye Hospital, but the doctors candidly acknowledged that they were of low quality, so the KorAid program would provide crucial assistance. I explained that my idea was to source better-quality lenses from a company in India, which had a good reputation for producing medical equipment, and have them shipped to the DPRK. We agreed that samples would first be sent from India to the KFPD, which, unfamiliar with the material, would conduct its own rigorous testing to make sure there were no problems. After that took place, KorAid would place an order. In early January 2016, the KFPD informed me that the first KorAid donation of three thousand cataract lenses and 1,500 vials of special eye medicine had arrived in Pyongyang and that distribution to three provincial hospitals was being organized. The KorAid team was thrilled.

I also met again with the head of the KRCCD. It was the morning after National Disability Day, and parents had taken their tired children, most of whom had participated in the event, home for the weekend. But Dr. Song Hyang Chun was eager to fill me in on the center's activities, and excited about future collaboration. She reiterated how valuable the input from the two Hong Kong experts I had brought with me on my previous visit had been, although she apologized that she had been too busy to follow up on a number of their suggestions, including displaying materials to update staff on trends in disability, and displaying the students' artwork. But she said that the KRCCD was carrying out a survey for the early detection of children with disabilities, and 320 kids had been identified. Dozens of parents had approached the center directly, and the waiting list was over 300. The demand exceeded the KRCCD's capabilities, so new admissions were limited, but staff were still making weekly home visits to some families to assist parents and caregivers.

I also had brought along a package containing toothbrushes and toothpaste; colored pencils, crayons, and pens for the children; and two books: *Recognizing and Planning for Special Needs in the Early Years* (which came with a CD), by Chris Dukes and Maggie Smith, and *More Play Helps: Play Ideas for Children with Special Needs*, by Roma Lear. The head of the KRCCD was very grateful but told me that equally valuable would be instruments for the children to play, especially those that didn't rely on electricity, as power supplies were so erratic. We also discussed the possibility of taking four staff members to Hong Kong for a study tour to see how disability issues were addressed there. She was enthusiastic, and we agreed to start the complex process of getting permission from the North Korean side and visas from the Hong Kong authorities.

I spent many months in 2015 and 2016 in Hong Kong. Much of that time was devoted to fundraising to get KorAid off the ground. I gave talks, attended meetings, and repeatedly made the point that even a small donation could have a large impact. The most graphic example: Each cataract surgery would cost about ten dollars. So I would tell prospective donors that for the price of a coffee and a pastry, they could give someone their sight back. The response was positive. As the funding began to come in, I was in touch with my North Korean colleagues about extending the program from three to six provincial hospitals, in the cities of Sariwon, Haeju, Sinujiu, Pyongsong, Wonsan, and Hamhung. In addition, there was talk of building a second greenhouse at another orphanage or boarding school.

Meanwhile, I ordered the material for building the Mirim Orphanage greenhouse from a Chinese company in the city of Dandong, just across the Yalu River from the DPRK. It was a slow and cumbersome process, with payment taking nearly six weeks to be processed. But once the money arrived, the items were shipped across the border, and greenhouse construction got underway. Luckily, this transaction took place before new sanctions came into effect prohibiting the delivery to the DPRK of any items containing metal.

On January 6, 2016, the DPRK conducted its fourth nuclear test, which the state-run media described as having been designed for self-defense against the United States. It was the country's first nuclear test in three years, and reflected both the continuing technical progress of North Korea's nuclear capabilities as well as Kim Jong Un's frustration with the Obama administration's policy of "strategic patience"—seeking to isolate and sanction North Korea and refusing to offer diplomatic rewards due to what the West saw as provocations. The UN Security Council quickly passed a tough new sanctions resolution. Nine months later, on September 9, 2016—the anniversary of the founding of the DPRK—came another nuclear test. In between, the North successfully launched a land-based medium-range Hwasong-10 missile capable of hitting the US territory of Guam and, according to some experts, possibly the continental United States.

The military moves completely overshadowed any efforts at humanitarian work. Moreover, they made the job of raising funds, purchasing materials, and shipping goods to North Korea much more difficult. Donors were becoming more reluctant to provide funds for projects in North Korea, making fundraising even more time-consuming and challenging. My colleagues at the KFPD also expressed concern about the sanctions. People frequently asked me if I had seen the list of all the items that the sanctions had mandated denying to North Korea.

Nonetheless, I remained convinced that despite the heightened tensions, the work of KorAid should continue. We were helping people in desperate need of assistance—powerless people who, I believed, didn't deserve to be deprived of care because of the actions of their government. Moreover, despite the bellicose behavior, my sense was that the North Korean regime was not completely pulling back from international engagement. I felt it was more important than ever to sustain humanitarian and people-to-people contact, however fragile, so long as even in a small way it had the potential to improve understanding and contribute to a lessening of tensions.

But it was getting increasingly difficult to settle bills for items ordered in China, where the logistics previously had been relatively straightforward, to be delivered to North Korea. Many Chinese banks, wary of being targeted by the United States, were refusing to accept payments for anything related to the DPRK. Humanitarian aid organizations, as well as diplomatic missions based in Pyongyang, started to carry cash, usually euros or US dollars, into the country through Beijing to cover operational costs and project expenditures. Legally, one was allowed to travel into or out of China with a maximum amount of ten thousand euros. Many organizations simply ignored this rule and carried in much larger amounts, but, afraid of getting into trouble, I scrupulously followed the regulation on each of my trips.

The headlines about nuclear and missile tests overshadowed what to me was a significant development. In the summer of 2016, the KFPD sent a seventeen-person delegation to the Special Olympics in Rio de Janeiro, Brazil, including two athletes who competed in different events. It was a small sign of Pyongyang's evident desire to remain at least somewhat internationally engaged and to give the plight of the disabled a higher profile.

Against this backdrop, I made two trips in 2016—one in the spring, one in autumn. The first focused almost entirely on the cataract operation project, and I visited four hospitals. The Red Cross Hospital in Pyongyang did four thousand cataract operations a year, all of them using locally produced lenses. Staff showed me their lens production facility, which consisted of two people in a small, dingy room using outdated equipment from Eastern Europe. They asked me not to take photos. The provincial hospital in Sariwon was one of those receiving lenses from KorAid. Staff told me that one thousand lenses and three hundred vials of eye medicine had arrived, with the remaining two hundred vials about to be sent on from Pyongyang. At the time of my visit, they had conducted 150 operations and said that all the lenses supplied by KorAid would be used by September. They told me that because of the lack of heat—it was March but still bitterly cold both outside and inside—they preferred to wait until late spring or summer to carry out the surgeries.

They introduced me to eleven patients—farmers, housewives, a seamstress, factory workers. It was easy to get detailed information about their backgrounds, experiences, and conditions. When my North Korean colleague told them that my friends in Hong Kong and Switzerland and I had donated the money for their lenses, they smiled broadly and effusively expressed thanks. The five-hundred-bed Wonsan Hospital also had received one thousand lenses and five hundred vials of eye medicine. I met thirteen patients, most of them elderly housewives but a couple of younger men as well. One, a forty-eight-year-old factory worker, told me he was overjoyed that he would be able to return to his job. One thousand lenses and five hundred vials of eye medicine also had been delivered to the South Pyongyan Provincial Hospital in Pyongsong.

At all the hospitals, I spoke with the most senior officials and doctors as my KFPD companion translated. They made a point of stressing how they were keeping detailed records of how the items that KorAid had donated were used. Once a month, they sent a list of beneficiaries to the KFPD. I was allowed to check their record books, which, as best I could tell, were in good order. There was no lack of transparency here. My interlocutors were extremely grateful for the lenses and eye medicine, but in a sign of how broken-down the medical system remained, they were not shy in spelling out the many other areas in which they desperately needed new and better equipment, including surgical instruments, scanning machines, even eyeglass frames. Unfortunately, that was beyond the ability and resources of my modest charity to provide. But I was heartened that the KorAid program was seen as so successful that plans were now being developed to add three more hospitals to the list of those receiving assistance.

In October 2016, I made my sixty-fifth visit to the DPRK. The response to the cataract program remained uniformly positive. It was agreed that for the next phase, six more provincial hospitals should become beneficiaries. KorAid was to provide six thousand lenses, three thousand vials of ophthalmic fluid, and six kits with surgery instruments and consumables. As on my previous trip, I visited numerous hospitals, and the experience of meeting beaming patients whose sight had been restored made me feel that all the hard work and frustration was worth it. In my notebook, I wrote, "The patients were all smiles, as the cataract operations make a huge difference in the quality of their lives."

Two of the hospitals I visited—in Hamhung on the east coast and Haeju on the west coast—also had dealt with an organization in Nepal called the Tilganga Institute of Ophthalmology, which ran a nonprofit, community-based NGO, the Nepal Eye Program. Its focus was on outreach, especially to rural areas, where medical care was limited. The program also offered training to doctors from other developing nations. Experts from Tilganga had spent several days at the hospital in Haeju conducting surgeries, and the chief ophthalmologist there had done a one-month training program in Nepal. At Hamhung, a team of eight doctors from Tilganga had visited twice, treating between six hundred and seven hundred patients. Back in Pyongyang, my KFPD colleagues and I discussed the idea of expanding training and collaboration with Tilganga. I was very supportive, and my North Korean colleagues were interested, especially in the idea of North Korean doctors receiving further training in Nepal or anywhere else.

At the Mirin Orphanage, the greenhouse material had finally arrived in July 2016, and construction had started immediately. Now the work was almost completed. In June, July, and August, several orphanage staff members had attended a ten-day training course at the Pyongyang Vegetable Science Institute, and they proudly showed me a short video of the training program. They told me that they would start planting in the greenhouse as soon as possible, beginning with cucumbers, tomatoes, leeks, spring onions, eggplant, spinach, watermelons, and other fruits and vegetables. A number of new buildings had been erected during the past year as well, and the capacity of the school was now 860 children. The number of teaching staff had been increased as well.

The biggest event for the staff and the children at Mirim had been a visit from their leader, Kim Jong Un, in July 2016. The staff told that me Kim, impressed by what he saw, said that the school was like a paradise. It was no surprise that a big slogan hanging from the main building read, "Let us become real sons and daughters of Marshal Kim Jong Un." My hope was that Kim's visit to an institution where KorAid was active would further legitimize our work in the eyes of the authorities, thus helping to overcome the bureaucratic difficulties that, given the nature of the North Korean system, even the most positive of projects periodically encountered.

During this trip, I also finalized plans for a four-member delegation from the KRCCD to make a ten-day trip to Hong Kong the following month. On November 29, 2016, the director of the KRCCD, who was a medical doctor, accompanied by a nurse, a teacher and an interpreter from the KFPD, arrived in the territory. I had met the director and one of the other delegation members in Pyongyang, although I did not know the other two. The director had impressed me. I felt that she really cared about the children at her center, and I was glad that, after we overcame a host of bureaucratic obstacles in both Pyongyang and Hong Kong, which already had produced a six-month delay, the trip was finally taking place.

For ten days, we kept up a furious pace, with two meetings or events each morning and two more in the afternoon. Altogether, the group visited nearly twenty institutions and centers working with or for intellectually challenged children, and met professionals in the health, social welfare, and education fields. My colleagues from Hong Kong and I took them to publicly funded health services and clinics as well as a number of NGOs. While we tried to expose them to a wide range of services for people with disabilities, their primary interest was on places focused on helping children with special needs. It was clear that the North Koreans lacked some of the basic tools to define and assess special needs, and I could sense a palpable urgency in their desire to learn as much as possible.

Wherever we went, the North Koreans received a warm reception and found their Hong Kong colleagues eager to be helpful. At one child assessment clinic, for example, they met with a doctor, a speech therapist, an occupational therapist, and a social worker. At the end, the staff said to them, "This is what we can do for you." I could see that the North Koreans were deeply moved. One NGO, called Heep Hong, had a display of handmade items—toys and tools and so on—for the children to use. The North Koreans were especially excited, because they could see how they could easily copy these items at home. An empty small plastic bottle filled with a few pebbles, for example, became a rattle.

Interestingly, in the view of my two Hong Kong colleagues—the ones I had brought to the DPRK and who were, along with me, acting as hosts—services in Hong Kong for intellectually challenged children in 2016 still were at a relatively rudimentary level. But for the North Koreans, what they were seeing was a revelation. The highlight of the visit was a training session done by one of my Hong Kong colleagues on how to assess intellectually challenged children. The North Koreans said they would begin to use those techniques, along with the assessment kits we provided them, as soon as they returned home.

Beyond imparting technical knowledge and skills, the visit also exposed the four North Korean women to life in bustling, freewheeling, exuberantly capitalist Hong Kong—a city about as different as possible from rigidly controlled, slow-moving Pyongyang. They said little to us about their feelings or reactions, even when we took them to meet our friends or for a meal at the Hong Kong Club, a posh relic of the territory's time as a British colony. But on many days, after I dropped them at the Caritas Guest House on teeming Nathan Road in the city's Kowloon District, I would wait discreetly across the street. Sure enough, after ten or fifteen minutes, I would see them emerge from the hotel and venture out into the crowded streets to explore on their own. How I would have loved to know what their conversations were like as they soaked up an experience unlike any to which they had ever been exposed.

CHAPTER TWENTY-FIVE

"I No Longer Feel Useless"

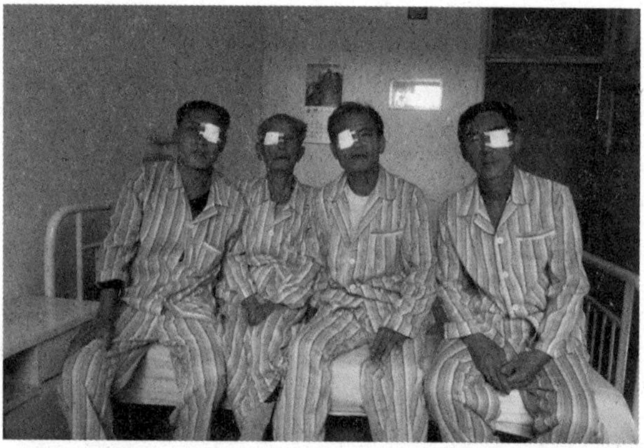

The provision of lenses and other medical supplies for cataract operations gave thousands of people their sight back, another KorAid project.

Whenever I happened to be in Pyongyang on a Friday, I made a point of attending the weekly interagency meeting, a gathering of international organization representatives usually held at the office of the United Nations Development Program (UNDP). This was an opportunity for diplomats and UN and NGO staffers to exchange notes and try to get a better sense of what was going on in the country and of how the North Koreans were dealing with the international community. The organizers always invited the North Koreans involved with these organizations, but they never attended. The meeting on September 15, 2017, however, was different—and more alarming—than any I previously had attended.

Tapan Mishra, a Columbia University–educated Indian with nearly two decades of UN experience, led the meeting. Since 2015, he had headed the UNDP's North Korea operation and was the senior UN official in the country. In a startling admission, Mishra told us that he had been in regular contact with his North Korean counterpart to discuss how foreign residents would be evacuated—or, if evacuation were not possible, provided with safe shelter—in the event of war.

The worrying discussion reflected the dramatic increase in tensions on the peninsula in the preceding months. Since Donald Trump had taken office in January 2017, he and Kim Jong Un regularly had been exchanging threats and insults. Throughout the spring and summer, the DPRK had conducted a series of missile tests, and press reports in Washington suggested that the North now had a miniaturized warhead that could be mounted on missiles capable of reaching the United States. In August, Trump had warned that the North Korean threat would be met with "fire, fury, and, frankly, power, the likes of which the world has never seen before."[29] In a defiant response, the DPRK conducted its sixth nuclear test on September 3.

No wonder the international community in Pyongyang was nervous. In my notebook, I wrote, "The mood at the inter-agency meeting was somber. The UN and the aid community were worrying how long they might be able to operate." I also observed that on the streets, "Talk of war seems to have increased." During my SDC years and thereafter, I had developed a hobby of collecting North Korean propaganda posters. The day after the interagency meeting, I saw some new ones. One had an image of a tank with the caption, "Nuclear Force Building." Another had the words "Answer of the DPRK—pre-emptive war."

Some North Koreans I spoke with were visibly nervous, asking me who I thought would win if war were to break out. That they raised this with me suggested that such a topic was on many people's minds and regularly being discussed within North Korean society. One expatriate friend encountered a North Korean who was more confident. "Let's get it done," the man declared. "We'll win," he added, in a revealing indication of what his real priority was, "so belt-tightening can come to an end."

Meanwhile, I noted that regular North Korean military exercises were underway, with some roads closed and camouflaged trucks visible. In

Pyongyang, people were darkening their homes and, as drills were conducted, filing into underground shelters. I was struck by how short the North Korean soldiers were.

There was, however, a strange disconnect between the alarming headlines, the anxiety within the international community and among some North Koreans allowed to interact with foreigners, and much of what else I observed on my regular visits. For the vast majority of North Koreans, the propaganda, however bellicose, was just routine background noise of the kind they had lived with for years. They appeared much more preoccupied with the daily struggle to survive or efforts to improve their lives than with Donald Trump or threats of war. Talk of "fire and fury" or additional nuclear tests seemed to be coming from another planet.

That certainly was the sense I got as I made regular trips to follow up on various KorAid projects, all of which, despite the geopolitical tension, were still moving ahead. For me, one of the most exciting ventures was taking place in Hamhung, the country's second-largest city and the capital of coastal South Hamgyong Province. Handicap International (HI) had approached KorAid for financial support to assist the Hamhung Physical Rehabilitation Center, with the funds going to help produce approximately one thousand orthopedic devices annually. Constrained by a lack of cash and the pressure of international sanctions, the center was unable to acquire the devices on its own. Interestingly, the orthopedic technicians had received three years of training in Cambodia, where loss of limbs due to land mines dating back to the Vietnam War remained a major problem.

HI had been the first organization to provide physiotherapy in the DPRK according to international standards. With the support of KorAid, which also had received a small contribution for this project from the SDC, HI ordered prosthetic and orthotic components from China, which reached Hamhung in the spring of 2018. None of the items could be produced locally. During that year, prostheses and orthoses were provided to support the needs of 990 people—894 adults and 96 children. After fabrication, all the devices were tailored to the needs of each individual. One doctor and one physiotherapist then provided rehabilitation services for each patient, including fitting the device and training the person on how to move with it.

Like virtually everything else in North Korea, the process was complicated by feeble infrastructure. The lack of electricity—the prosthesis workshop received only two hours of power in the morning and two in the evening—slowed progress. Indeed, on my first visit in early September 2018, there was no electricity, so we agreed to return a few days later in the hope of seeing the workshop in operation. A generator, funding for fuel, and new workshop tools were high on the wish list of the center's director. I also was not surprised to learn that even though meals were provided, food supplies for the forty or so patients in residence were, as I diplomatically put it in a KorAid report, "not quite sufficient." I even saw how maize had been planted in big flowerpots to add to the meager supply.

It was heartbreaking for me to see people, especially young people, who had lost one or both limbs in some freak industrial or car accident. But I was deeply moved by how determined the patients I met were to walk again and to resume as normal a life as possible. One twenty-two-year-old had lost both legs in a railway accident in January 2018. Just admitted to the Hamhung Physical Rehabilitation Center, he was very optimistic that with some practice using his new prostheses, he would be able to walk again. "My new legs are comfortable; I feel fine," he told me. "I can go to a factory and work there. I feel like flying when I stand up from the wheelchair. The prostheses are my wings."

A thirty-five-year-old miner had had his left leg amputated above the knee following a mine accident in 2017. I observed a therapist putting him through a range of motion exercises. "I can see the others can walk again. I am encouraged," he said with a broad smile. "Maybe I will also be able to walk again with orthotics and go home walking without crutches."

It was always heartening to visit a place like this. Not only were thousands of disabled people receiving treatment that would transform their lives, but the treatment—and the degree of independence it would afford the patients—would have an incalculable impact on their family members and friends as well. As far as I could tell, the center's and the KFPD's recordkeeping was clear and complete, and I was encouraged as I secured additional funding.

I also went back to the Mirim Orphanage, where a KorAid-supported greenhouse had produced its first harvest: eggplant, cabbage, spinach, and lettuce. Greenhouse farming was now included in the school's curriculum, thus combining gardening practice with classroom lessons. The topics included soil fertility, the selection and production of seedlings, watering needs, fertilizer selection, and general growing practices. The students had two lessons per week for practical work in the greenhouse and four lectures in horticulture. Each session lasted forty-five minutes and was offered to children between the ages of twelve and seventeen. In mid-2017, 280 children were participating. The teachers had a background in biology and were in close contact with the Pyongyang Vegetable Science Institute.

Staff told me that because of the greenhouse, children at the orphanage could now consume vegetables during the whole year. Some of the excess produce would be bartered for seeds. They also informed me that one of the big challenges now was watering the plants, as the orphanage lacked a drip watering system, which delivers water directly to the roots of plants using a network of pipes and tubes, preventing waste. I added that to my list of items to explore for potential KorAid help.

I also made several visits to the KRCCD. The staff told me that the team that had traveled to Hong Kong in 2016 was now applying what they had learned in assessing dozens of children, while also providing assessment training to other staff members. However, they had encountered problems with autistic children and those suffering from cerebral palsy, because different assessment protocols were needed for these cases, for which they had no experience. The center's head, Dr. Song, asked if we could arrange additional training and whether my colleagues from Hong Kong might be willing to return to Pyongyang. I was certainly happy to try to arrange another training visit, but the broader political climate created a more challenging atmosphere for raising funds from donors increasingly reluctant to support projects involving the DPRK, for finding experts willing to travel, and even for getting permission from the government in Pyongyang for them to come.

Still, progress was being made in other areas. An important positive step, which one of the Hong Kong experts had suggested, was that the KRCCD had started to keep a record book for each child. It included personal information, the diagnosis, a description of the first interaction with the child, weekly and monthly health and educational charts, a weekly rehabilitation overview (such as eating habits, toilet training, ability to clothe, communication, dancing, drawing, and playing), and observations by health and teaching staff. Having all the information easily accessible in one place made a big difference. The center also had created a "red book" that served as the communication means between the center and the parents. Recorded in this book were progress reports, discussions of problems, and tasks that needed to be done during the weekends when the child was at home.

It took months and months of planning, but by mid-2019, I finally arranged a follow-up visit for my two Hong Kong colleagues. It was their first time back in Pyongyang in five years—a sign of how slowly things were moving and how difficult it was to get things done in the DPRK. Three of the four KRCCD staff members who had visited Hong Kong in 2016 were still there and were delighted to see us. It was impressive that now, compared with 2014, the center was well-equipped with age-appropriate furniture, toys, exercise equipment, and teaching aids, both inside the building and outside in the play area, that Handicap International and other aid organizations had supplied.

The focus of this trip was very much on training, trying to provide as many tools as possible for our North Korean colleagues to assess and care for special needs children. One workshop concentrated specifically on autism and attention deficit hyperactivity disorder (ADHD). Using PowerPoint presentations and DVD reference materials, the two experts from Hong Kong discussed both theoretical and practical challenges in handling these difficult cases. I had, incidentally, told them before they left Hong Kong to print out their PowerPoint slides in the event of an electricity outage. They had looked at me in astonishment, but sure enough, in the middle of one presentation, the power did go off. The two women grinned at me as they were able to carry on.

In another session, they conducted demonstration assessments on three children to give attendees a hands-on explanation of the methodology and how to use the various assessment tools. This helped to determine the level of motor, language, emotional, social, and intellectual skills. My Hong Kong colleagues also provided assessment kits they had assembled to enable staff to better judge the strengths and weaknesses of the children. Personnel from several other institutions, including the State Education Commission, the Mansu Rehabilitation Clinic, the Okryu Children's Hospital—considered the best hospital for special needs children in North Korea—and Pyongyang Medical College, joined the sessions. Given how siloed the North Korean system usually is this was in itself something of an achievement.

Sessions also were conducted for the relatives of the children—usually parents or grandparents. Given the potential awkwardness of foreigners lecturing to a North Korean audience and the sensitivity of the issues, it was gratifying to see the large number of questions that came up, including on the use of oral medication such as Ritalin (which was then not available in the DPRK) and on how to handle the growing sexual awareness of teenagers. The Hong Kong experts stressed the importance of developing transition plans for adolescent and adult care.

By the end, the attendees had dubbed us the "three Hong Kong grannies," and the warmth they showed us was palpable. Our hosts took us on various sightseeing excursions, including to see the spectacle of the Arirang Mass Games, which my colleagues found impressive and enjoyable. Before departing, we came up with another detailed list of recommendations. This included developing a core team of KRCCD staff skilled in developmental assessment. The suggestion was for a staff of six, with three teams of two—for example, a doctor and a teacher, a nurse and a therapist, or a teacher and a therapist. We also urged the appointment of a designated care manager for each child, with a suggested ratio of one staff member to five children; regular case conferences by the treatment teams, with parents included; and reassessment every six to nine months to document progress. We also emphasized the importance of regular, structured communication within the rehabilitation teams (among the therapists, case managers, and teachers) and with the parents and the child. In addition, we suggested that targeted information about special needs children be made available to the general public, schools, and primary care doctors, possibly using app technology adapted to local mobile phones, to encourage greater awareness of the issue in North Korean society.

On my various trips, I continued to visit multiple hospitals to which KorAid was sending lenses, eye medicine, and other materials for cataract operations. At the Kangwon hospital in Wonsan, the KorAid goods had arrived just two days before I did. In my notebook, I wrote, "Watching the team of ophthalmologists and nurses opening the three big boxes was a humbling experience. Their clear joy of receiving the delivered goods was incredible, and they thanked KorAid profoundly for the organization's valuable assistance." I had a similar experience at the North Pyongan Provincial Hospital in Sinuiju, on the Chinese border, where the KorAid packages also had just arrived. The doctors told me there was a long waiting list for cataract procedures, and they had been using outdated, Soviet-era equipment, most of which simply did not work properly any longer. The staff were visibly excited. As I noted at the time, "It felt like Christmas as they opened the parcels."

During my hospital visits, I always was struck by how spartan and ill-equipped these facilities were. It meant that even the most modest additional equipment made a big difference. At the South Hwanghae Provincial Hospital in Haeju city, for example, which also was receiving lenses and eye medicine, I had brought a special battery for an ophthalmoscope. It had cost me thirty dollars in Switzerland. When I handed it over, the staff joyfully applauded. Still, the hospital lacked other equipment to do more precise assessments. When I asked about support from elsewhere, a staff member told me that, apart from what KorAid was supplying, nothing had been forthcoming for the past two years. Although locally produced painkillers were available, essential drugs were lacking, especially antibiotics and inputs for anesthesia. And hospitals still suffered from power cuts.

Still, I was impressed by the energy, commitment, and initiative of the medical staff. Starting in 2017, they began to organize mobile camps. Teams of three doctors went to county towns on nearly a dozen occasions, usually staying three or four days each time. North Hwanghae Province had twenty-two counties, and the aim was to visit ten to fifteen county-level hospitals annually. In the counties, two county-level doctors and three nurses assisted the Sariwon hospital teams. In addition to assessments, doctors performed twenty surgeries each day on average with equipment, lenses, and consumables they had brought with them. The patients greatly appreciated these mobile efforts, which freed them of the obligation to travel long distances to receive medical care.

At virtually all the hospitals I visited, I was able to meet and speak freely with patients who had undergone the cataract procedure. My KFPD colleagues would explain the reason for my visit, and the patients often would break out in cheers. This was an especially moving experience and gave me a sense of the individuals whose lives had been transformed by the efforts of KorAid. A few examples provide an idea of what the surgery meant to these patients: "My world was covered with fog," a seventy-year-old former tractor driver told me at the South Hamgyong Provincial People's Hospital in Hamhung. "I couldn't walk without the help of my son. You will never understand what I felt like. But now, the fog is gone, and the world has been given back to me."

A seventy-seven-year-old longtime farmer at the same hospital told me, "I lost my sight ten years ago. I could no longer do anything without the help of my family. I had to use walking sticks to go to the washroom. When others went to work, I was left at home and felt lonely. Sometimes I couldn't help crying. Right now, I can walk independently. I am really feeling happy. I really want to say thank you from the bottom of my heart to all of you, the organizers and the doctors who provided me with this operation."

In Chongin, at the North Hamgyong Provincial People's Hospital, I met a seventy-three-year-old woman. "I really wanted to see again," she said. "It was my greatest wish. Yesterday, when the plaster was removed, I couldn't help dancing around. I have two sons and two daughters. They are office workers. And now I can help them with cooking and cleaning. I no longer feel useless." As she spoke, she smiled broadly.

And as I was leaving the ward, an elderly woman from Myongchon County stopped us. Her feelings evident, she said, "I am from the mountains, and I got my eyesight back here. Next time, come and visit me at my home. I can make *bibimbap* for you. You stay healthy, and see you next year. I hope our friendship grows and you can provide more and more assistance to those who need help. Thank you."

For all the heartening signs of progress, I sometimes felt in my bleaker moments that our efforts remained inadequate. On one trip, I visited the Songchon Residential School for Children with Hearing Disabilities. Although it is not far from Pyongyang, it took us two hours to drive there, partly because of roadblocks due to military exercises and partly because, earlier in the day, civilians had been told to hide in shelters and were now walking back home along the roads. Security personnel frequently stopped our car and carefully checked our documents, especially the travel permits. Usually, after one quick look at me, the security personnel would wave us on.

The school in Songchon had a main building for classrooms and offices, and two others on the side for practical training, as well as dormitories, washing facilities, and toilets. The walls were cracked, and parts of the roof were leaking. In addition, with its broken boilers and rusty pipes, the heating system worked only sporadically. It was clear that major renovation was needed, but the principal told me no funds were available. Although the school had space for 240 children, it appeared that about 80—a third of the total—had returned home for the winter because of the poor living conditions, especially lack of heating. The principal seemed quite embarrassed and did not want to talk about the issue. However, a few classes were in session, and we had fun trying to teach the kids how to say "Switzerland" in sign language, and with me writing the word "Switzerland" in Korean on the blackboard. Still, as I observed in my notebook, "I felt very sorry for these disabled children having to spend their childhood at a school that was in such a poor state."

Another source of frustration was one hospital in Pyongyang where KorAid had supplied lenses. By 2018, three hundred lenses had been used in operations. But officials there appeared unenthusiastic about hosting training programs with participants from different ophthalmology departments or involving international experts, and were not eager to create a transparent reporting system. By the end of a daylong visit, I had concluded that it would not be worthwhile for KorAid to continue to offer support there.

And even in the hospitals where cooperation was proceeding smoothly, KorAid was now facing problems with our supplier in India because of the sanctions. He no longer was willing to send materials to the DPRK, forcing me and our regular supplier to make extra efforts to find a reliable source of lenses and eye medicine. Even though these items were supposed to be exempt from sanctions, the fear among so many companies and organizations about having anything to do with the DPRK was palpable, strangling efforts to provide even the most basic assistance.

Officials at the KFPD also showed a mixture of optimism and concern. They were elated when eight North Korean athletes competed at the 2018 Winter Paralympics held in South Korea. The exploits of the athletes received considerable coverage in the North Korean media, creating greater awareness of people with disabilities and their talents. In a reflection of the contradictory way things operated in the DPRK, the KFPD, displaying a surprising entrepreneurial spirit, had just launched its own taxi service despite government attempts to rein in market forces. The idea was to serve both people with disabilities and the general public. The cars had been leased from China, and any income initially would have to be sent to the Chinese vehicle owners. But the expectation was that as the business grew, it would generate funds for the KPFD. At the same time, though, officials acknowledged that their operations were being affected by the ever-stricter sanctions. While the organization still was allowed to import goods made with plastic, items containing metal parts were being blocked. It was part of a sweeping expansion of sanctions in 2016 and 2017 that included an embargo on fuel and all major imports and exports. Adding to their anxieties, KPFD officials said that they might need to return a plot of land that the government had allocated for the building of a rehabilitation center, as no donations for constructing the building had been forthcoming.

The frustrations indicated a broader trend: Despite the progress I was witnessing with the KorAid projects, things were tightening up, and the overall situation within North Korea seemed increasingly bleak. The chief of the EU's Food Security Office told me that there had been a significant decrease in market activity across the whole country, leading to job losses for many women and drops in family income. It was part of what appeared to be backtracking on the market-oriented changes that had begun to transform North Korean society. But it remained unclear whether this was part of a deliberate policy to severely curb private market activities—which, if expanded, would have the potential to create a broader political threat to the regime—or simply was meant to impose a greater degree of state control while still allowing the markets to exist.

Fuel shortages also remained a major problem. One consequence was that provinces producing a surplus of grain were facing difficulties transporting it to other, poorer locations. Moreover, organizations in the agricultural sector were having great problems importing items such as pumps, tractors, and spare parts for machinery as the sanctions grew tighter. Exemptions were offered to aid agencies only on a case-by-case basis, and in each instance, a written agreement from the UN Security Council was required.

Dramatic international developments intensified these internal tensions. In June 2018, Donald Trump and Kim Jong Un held a historic summit in Singapore. It was the first-ever meeting between the leaders of the two countries, and fueled hope that a broader breakthrough might lead to a sharp reduction in tension on the Korean peninsula. Eight months later, however, in February 2019, a two-day summit in Hanoi—which some had speculated could lead to a formal declaration ending the Korean War—collapsed in acrimony. Trump and Kim could not find common ground on the issue of the relaxation of sanctions or on how much of the North Korean nuclear program Kim would agree to give up. Trump abruptly ended the summit earlier than planned, abandoning a scheduled lunch and a joint signing ceremony. The dramatic rupture—which was not repaired despite a brief meeting between the two men at the Korean Demilitarized Zone in June 2019—had enormous consequences, generating a new spike in tensions and leading Kim Jong Un to conclude that seeking a fundamental improvement in relations with the United States was a dead-end street.

Adding to the dark mood, the Global Fund to Fight AIDS, Tuberculosis and Malaria announced that it was ending its activities in North Korea. The Global Fund had been operating in the DPRK since 2010 and had disbursed $69 million to tuberculosis projects and $34 million to malaria projects there, with the money handled by UNICEF and the World Health Organization. The TB program in particular was assisting some one hundred thousand adults and ten thousand children in North Korea. Without the Global Fund, the prospects for controlling the disease were bleak—120,000 cases of it had been reported in North Korea in 2016 alone—even though some NGOs, including the US–based Eugene Bell Foundation, which has an office in South Korea, and the American Christian Friends of Korea were also working on TB. A fund spokesman explained the reason for the cessation of its activities: "The unique operating environment in the DPRK prevents us from being able to provide our Board with the required level of assurance and risk management around the deployment of resources. We do independent checking in other countries in a way that is not fully possible in DPRK."[30]

I was deeply upset by the move, and by the vagueness of the Global Fund's explanation. The difficulties facing international organizations operating in North Korea were well-known but, as my own case showed, not insurmountable. The official statement said that no specific incident had triggered the decision but provided no other details. Given the lack of transparency, and the fact that Japan and the United States were among the fund's major donors and were outspoken critics of the DPRK, I wondered whether they had brought pressure on the fund to pull out. Whatever the reason, the move would have a terrible impact on the lives of tens of thousands of people at an already difficult time.

This was followed in 2019 by the decision of the Finnish Pentecostal charity Fida International, one of the few resident NGOs still operating in the DPRK and one of the largest overseas aid programs from Finland, to leave the country as well. Fida said the move was because sanctions had made it impossible to transfer any aid money. Funded in part by the Finnish foreign ministry, Fida had assisted since 2001 with the development of potato farming, a crop that provided additional food for rural communities while reducing malnutrition among children. In 2019, amid renewed shortages of food, the organization had also delivered over four hundred tons of emergency supplies of maize and soybeans, which helped sustain twelve thousand people. That aid would now cease.

The biggest shock came in late 2019, when Handicap International, which had been operating in the DPRK for twenty-one years and been a crucially important partner going back to my Caritas days, announced that it too was pulling out. I learned of the decision on my seventy-fifth trip, in December 2019, when I met the outgoing HI representative in Pyongyang. The official explanation was a combination of insufficient financial resources, problems finding good-quality local staff, and difficulties monitoring projects. These were the same factors that had played a role in the decisions of other humanitarian organizations to scale back or leave. The HI representative told me that as frustration within his organization had mounted, the move had been under consideration for some time. Although he provided no details, it was clear that there had been some tension with the North Koreans. As he candidly told me, "It was better to go now than later, when perhaps we would be told to leave."

For me, it was a particularly big blow. I had worked closely, and successfully, with HI for many years, and the staff had provided much practical assistance, including on occasion passing on messages from KorAid to the KPFD. I felt that the need for the services they offered to North Korea was more pressing than ever. Handicap International had been involved in many areas—disaster risk reduction projects, capacity-building programs, training in modern physiotherapy treatments (a first for the DPRK), and support for the KFPD—but I worried that the biggest gap would be in the area of rehabilitation, such as with the prosthesis project in Hamhung. I spoke with the SDC representative in Pyongyang about this, inquiring whether the SDC could help fill the gap, but was told that goodwill toward the DPRK was steadily shrinking in Switzerland too. Moreover, having provided support to the Hamhung venture once, the SDC could not do so again, as the organization had a rule not to fund the same project twice. I feared the people in Hamhung would be forced to go back to using the old methods, adding to the suffering of those in need of new limbs and other orthotic devices.

HI's impending departure cast a pall over my meetings with the KFPD. Even though HI was leaving all of its office equipment and two jeeps behind for the KFPD to use, I learned that the KFPD itself was facing a restructuring mandated by the government. The details were still unclear, but between the reorganization and HI's decision to pull out, I found my KFPD colleagues to be in a subdued and pessimistic mood. Other North Korean organizations dealing with the disabled, such as the Korean Rehabilitation Center for Children with Disabilities, were equally upset. People there also told me that the departure of HI would mean that contact with individuals and organizations in other countries would become more difficult.

The depressed atmosphere also was reflected in my discussions with people in the foreign community. Pyongyang seemed bleaker than usual, and in the Koryo Hotel, where I stayed, there were few tourists and even fewer businesspeople, although the hotel now offered Wi-Fi access at 13.8 euros per ten minutes. In general, people I knew seemed stressed and nervous. As I recorded in my notebook, "All the foreigners I met expressed that they felt they were facing many more challenges with their North Korean partners, along with increased demands and charges for every small service." The Ministry of Foreign Affairs was now screening resident organizations even more carefully and pushing for international staff to be reduced. Two European expatriates had received letters from the government stating that they had been in the country for too long and it was time for them to leave. A German diplomat informed me that a program to train DPRK medical doctors in Germany had been stopped. Organizing visits for foreigners also had become more challenging. In fact, he said, almost all engagement had been discontinued. The word "control" was used time and time again by locals and well as foreigners.

Diplomats also highlighted what they felt was a significant shift in tone in the DPRK's official media: While previous statements had talked of being prepared to defend the country, now there was talk of being ready for war. Indeed, two days before my arrival, the North Koreans had carried out another missile test, and during my visit, a North Korean foreign ministry official described negotiations with the United States as a "foolish trick" being played by Washington. Two days after my departure, there was another missile test. I was well aware that, while such tests unquestionably helped North Korea improve the technical capabilities of its arsenal, they were as much a political signal—a way to pressure the United States to offer better terms. But after the failure of the February 2019 Hanoi Summit, the Trump administration no longer seemed interested in negotiating.

Despite the gloomy atmosphere, I received no indication that KorAid projects were in jeopardy. Indeed, on the contrary, as I traveled the country that bitterly cold December, I saw visible progress. The first stop was a return visit the Songchon Residential School for Children with Hearing Disabilities, where KorAid had been supporting a major project to renovate the shabby and run-down facilities. We reached Songchon after a bumpy two-hour ride from Pyongyang in a dilapidated old minibus with no seat-belts and no heating. Luckily, I had brought a warm down jacket, and one of my KFPD colleagues, to my great relief, produced a hot water bottle and placed it in my lap every morning when we set off for our field trip.

Work on the dormitory had been completed, with new radiators promising some relief from the freezing winter temperatures. New doors had been installed for all the dormitory rooms, and the dining hall had new wooden tables and chairs. The school building also had received a new coat of paint, both outside and in. While the various materials had been purchased with a KorAid donation, the county had provided the construction workers and technical advice. When touring the premises, we saw that work was still continuing on the dining hall walls. In comparison with my previous visit, I was encouraged, because the school and dormitory buildings looked much better now.

The food situation seemed manageable. The government provided maize and rice regularly, with each child getting a ration of 450 grams per day. Fish was available once a month. The greenhouse that KorAid had supported was in good condition; mushroom cultivation had been added to the spinach, leeks, and lettuce being grown, and part of the greenhouse was being used to raise chickens, rabbits, and pigs. The vegetable and flower seeds I had brought from Switzerland were received with much appreciation.

From Songchon, I traveled to the South Pyongyan Provincial Hospital in Pyongsong, which I had not visited since 2016. By now, four KorAid deliveries of lenses and eye medicine had been received, although hospital officials said it had taken three months for North Korean customs to clear the most recent shipment. Further slowing things down, they said, were bureaucratic delays at the KPFD because of its government-mandated restructuring. Even so, the hospital was performing 1,500 cataract surgeries a year, and officials took me to a ward to meet and talk with patients. As a visit by a foreigner was still highly unusual, one of the doctors explained who I was and what KorAid had been doing. All six of the patients with whom I spoke through my interpreter expressed happiness and deep gratitude for getting their sight back. The head of the hospital expressed a desire for continued collaboration with KorAid.

The next morning, as Pyongyang received its first snow of the winter, I navigated the slippery streets to visit the Lions Hospital in the city's Raknang District. The name was the result of the hospital's being funded by the Lions Clubs International, especially the Seoul chapter. Its role, however, was not well-known and was kept very low-key, especially in Pyongyang. The hospital recently had been added to the list of KorAid cataract equipment recipients. I met ten patients, and the doctors were full of praise for the quality of the lenses and eye medicine they had received. They were eager to work further with KorAid, expressing hope that it might be possible to receive equipment such as ophthalmoscopes, slit lamps, and a portable biometry instrument in addition to the lenses and vials of eye medicine.

I had a similar experience at the North Hwanghae Provincial Hospital in Sariwon, sixty-seven kilometers from Pyongyang, which also had been using lenses and equipment donated by KorAid. Some of the instruments had been used so much during the previous two years that they no longer worked, and doctors asked if it was possible to get additional supplies. Here too, I was allowed to meet and talk with cataract patients. A retired teacher of Russian expressed delight that he could read books again, while an elderly cook said that one day she hoped she would be able to make a meal for me. Although always aware of the restrictions that existed governing the interactions of North Koreans and foreigners, I found these encounters to be deeply moving. They put a human face on all the paperwork, logistics, meetings, and frustration that managing KorAid involved. Altogether, KorAid had provided thirty-five thousand lenses for cataract operations. It was very satisfying to know that we had helped give tens of thousands of people their sight back.

On the day before my departure, I went to see the people at the KRCCD. I was touched that the director, Dr. Song, although battling breast cancer, insisted on leaving her hospital bed to come to the office to see me. I gave her three books on autism and ADHD. She was extremely grateful and told me that the assessment tools KorAid had provided were the ones they used most often. At the time of my visit, forty-two children were in residence. Six had recently graduated and were now attending a school run by the Deaf Association so that they could learn sign language. Newly admitted children had hearing problems, were autistic, or had Down syndrome. Hearing aids recently had been provided to twelve children.

We talked about plans for 2020, which, she told me, included auditory training and speech therapy programs. We also discussed developing an autism app. Dr. Song was interested in receiving more information, ideally on a memory stick and in English, about this possibility. She also asked if our Hong Kong specialists could provide more training programs, especially those involving the parents. She told me that my visiting the KRCCD the following June, as I had proposed, would be no problem. In fact, Dr. Song noted, that trip would be a milestone for me—the twenty-fifth anniversary of when I first had started working with the DPRK. When I returned, she said, we would celebrate the occasion together.

Dr. Song was one of the nicest, friendliest, and most competent people I had encountered in North Korea. There was no doubting her commitment and passion to helping the children in her care. I had come to respect her enormously. Even with the barriers that limited the interactions foreigners were allowed to have with North Koreans, I felt a genuine warmth and friendship, built around a shared desire to help kids who most needed it.

I got on the plane the next morning with a familiar jumble of emotions. There was always a certain relief to be leaving the bleakness, control, and aggravation that characterized so much of my dealings in the country, especially given the tightened controls that were becoming increasingly evident. But I was excited that, despite the overall atmosphere, KorAid's projects remained both well-received and, by any objective measure, relatively successful. After four years, I felt we were really accomplishing something, and I was looking forward to my return in 2020.

Less than a month later, a cluster of strange pneumonia-like illnesses was reported in Wuhan, China. The disease, called COVID-19, spread explosively across the globe. On January 22, 2020, North Korea closed its borders, cutting itself off from the outside world. In an instant, the work of KorAid came to a halt.

CHAPTER TWENTY-SIX

Quarantine

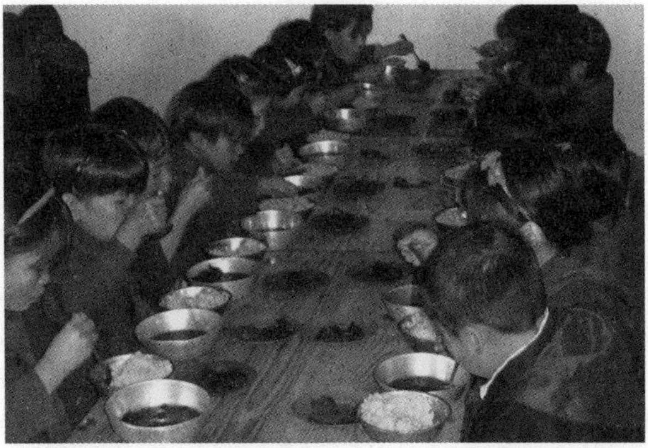

Difficult times again. The question remains whether such good meals will still be available to children like these?

Sitting in my home in Teufen in the winter of 2020, I watched COVID spread across the world. Like most other people, I had to stop traveling. I put off scheduled trips to Singapore, Hong Kong, New York, and Stanford, and canceled numerous planned face-to-face meetings. In early March, Switzerland recorded its first COVID death. Soon after, I received an email from a longtime North Korean contact—the representative in the northeastern Chinese city of Shenyang for the KFPD. He said that he was worried about me and asked for my mailing address, as he wanted to send me some face masks—in short supply in Europe during the early stages of the outbreak—from China. I was touched by his gesture. But it turned out to be the last communication I would have with a North Korean for many months.

In my nearly twenty-five years of dealing with the DPRK, I had never seen the country retreat into the kind of self-imposed isolation that the fear of COVID triggered. The borders were closed in late January 2020, with a shoot-to-kill order for anyone approaching the frontier without permission.[31] All flights in and out were stopped, followed by a cessation of ships from China. Schools and public sites were shuttered. Children and the elderly were instructed to stay home. The government launched a massive propaganda campaign to educate people on how to avoid this infection. Internal travel, limited to begin with, was severely curbed. There were even reports that soldiers had been ordered not to leave their bases.

Foreign trade plummeted. Markets, which had continued to flourish despite government pressure, began to wither. With few goods from China available for sale or barter—including food, over-the-counter medicines, and clothing—and even fewer opportunities for trade, ordinary people faced the loss of jobs and income, making it even harder to survive. Shelves in the shops of Pyongyang largely were bare. According to Chinese data, overall trade between China and the DPRK fell to its lowest level in decades, with a 78.5 percent drop recorded between February and July 2020 compared with the same period in 2019; imports were down 78 percent.[32] The delivery of raw materials for DPRK factories also came to a halt, as did deliveries of much-needed farming supplies, such as plastic sheeting, fertilizers, and pesticides.

The shortage of medicines seemed particularly serious. I heard reports that North Korean embassies in different countries were instructed to solicit for in-kind and cash donations to address this issue, but with all transport to the DPRK cut off, there was no way to get the goods into the country even if supplies could be found. Tourism also stopped. Although the scale was relatively modest, attractions including the Masikryong Ski Resort had brought in about $175 million in 2019, mostly from Chinese and Russian tourists. That revenue was now gone.

The small number of foreigners in North Korea when the epidemic broke out, mostly diplomats and a few aid workers, were placed under strict quarantine, confined to the foreign diplomatic quarter and denied any contact with North Koreans. There was no way to monitor ongoing projects, let alone get out of Pyongyang. With the borders closed and no banking channels working because of sanctions, many organizations were running out of money to cover basic operating costs. Under the circumstances, there seemed little point in remaining in the country. In early March, a special flight was allowed to leave with about eighty foreign residents aboard. The World Food Program, which for a long time had had the biggest international presence in the North, was forced to close all of its field offices. Not long after, a convoy of most of the few remaining foreigners was organized to travel by land to Sinuiju and then into China, where, after two weeks' quarantine, people were allowed to return to their home countries. Apart from a minuscule international presence, including skeleton staffing at the Chinese, Russian, Syrian, Cuban, and a few other like-minded embassies, the foreign community in Pyongyang basically disappeared.

As draconian as these measures appeared, I understood the reasons for Pyongyang's extreme response. A COVID outbreak in the DPRK would have been a catastrophe. Indeed, it would not be an exaggeration to say that an uncontrolled spreading of the virus could have threatened the country's very survival. However understandable, though, I felt that the restrictions were extreme, even by North Korean standards—not least because the DPRK was rejecting offers of help specifically to combat COVID. Following the email that the KPFD representative in Shenyang sent me, I sent a message to KPFD headquarters in Pyongyang offering to try to arrange a shipment of protective gear for the ten hospitals with which KorAid had been working. I never received a response. This appeared to be the result of a deliberate policy decision to further curtail contact with the outside world, even via email, snail mail, or telephone. I discovered that my effort would have been problematic even if the response had been positive, however. Unable to meet prospective donors face-to-face, I had thought of using the online fundraising platform GoFundMe. It became clear, however, that I would have had difficulties, because an NGO using the platform to generate financial support for anything to do with North Korea likely would have been viewed as a violation of sanctions.

The North also repeatedly delayed accepting a shipment of some 1.7 million doses of the AstraZeneca COVID vaccine from the international initiative COVAX. The main obstacles were the DPRK's concern about the safety and effectiveness of the vaccine, its reluctance to sign a liability waiver in case of side effects, and its refusal to allow international workers into the country to facilitate the shipment. In any case, the doses would have been sufficient to cover only around 850,000 people, or just over 3 percent of the North's total population. Other offers of vaccine assistance from the United States, South Korea, and even Russia also were rebuffed. The country's irregular electricity supply and lack of ultracold refrigerators and specialized delivery trucks for the vaccines, which needed to be preserved at specific temperatures, presented other obstacles. Médecins Sans Frontières (MSF) was granted an exemption from international sanctions and was able to ship some equipment, supplies for diagnostic purposes, and protective gear to the China–North Korea border, from where they were sent across. By the autumn of 2020, COVID aid from the International Federation of the Red Cross and Red Crescent Societies was allowed in, and India sent $1 million worth of desperately needed tuberculosis medicine. But no MSF or other foreign personnel were allowed in. And these episodes seemed to be the exception rather than the rule.

I was deeply concerned that the DPRK's approach to COVID would make the already hard lives of ordinary North Koreans even more difficult. With the closure of the Chinese border, critical imports such as rice, other grains, and key raw materials were suspended. As schools had closed, children no longer would be receiving the nutritional support they needed. I worried about what would happen to the most vulnerable: the ninety-five thousand acutely malnourished children, the over one hundred thousand nursery and kindergarten kids in need of fortified food, people with disabilities. There were reports from South Korea that even officers in the North Korean military were being given only ten days' worth of food rations per month, and that soldiers were being encouraged to breed rabbits for eating.

In a reflection of the grim situation, Kim Jong Un called on the country to prepare for another "arduous march"—the term the government had used to describe the famine years in the 1990s. Speaking to members of the ruling Korean Workers' Party, Kim referred to "many obstacles and difficulties ahead of us," although it remained unclear whether he meant specific food shortages or the broader economic difficulties that measures to prevent the spread of the virus were causing.[33] Underscoring the dire conditions, in April 2020 the United Nations released its annual *DPR Korea Needs and Priorities* document. It said that approximately 10.1 million North Koreans—about 40 per cent of the population—needed food assistance. The report called for the urgent provision of humanitarian assistance to the 5.5 million people it said were most in need.[34] Although I knew that the North Koreans were tough, hardworking, and more resilient than in the late 1990s, I wondered whether there were limits on how much more they could endure when facing new food, health, and economic crises.

Yet, by one critical measure at least, the draconian approach did appear to be working. The DPRK repeatedly declared that it had found no COVID cases among the population, and the regime seemed determined to keep it that way, regardless of the cost. There certainly was some skepticism outside the country about the claim, and it later emerged that there had been cases, but the North did appear to have avoided the large-scale spread of the virus that had devastated so many nations.

Sealing off the country was partially the reason for some significant internal political developments—among them the emergence of Kim Yo Jong, Kim Jong Un's sister, as an increasingly powerful hard-line figure. As a reflection of this new attitude, the North threatened action against the South in response to propaganda leaflets that defector groups had sent across the border. In addition, in June 2020, during the early days of the pandemic, the North blew up an inter-Korean liaison office that had been set up in Kaesong during an earlier period of rapprochement. Kim Jong Un himself was now describing Washington as the North's "principal enemy" and vowed to continue to develop the DPRK's long-range nuclear strike capability. It was a clear sign that in the wake of his failed summit with Donald Trump, Kim had changed his worldview. He no longer appeared interested in normalization with the United States or anyone allied with the United States. I worried that this also might mean a reluctance to further engage with NGOs that had a connection to the United States–led world, my own included.

These developments coincided with a growing closeness between Pyongyang and Moscow, triggered in part by the COVID pandemic and the different dynamics of China-DPRK and Russia-DPRK trade. Goods from China usually arrived in North Korea on trucks and trains that crossed the bridge over the Yalu River, linking the Chinese city of Dandong and the North Korean city of Sinuiju, both heavily populated, or were sent by ship to the North Korean port of Nampo. In contrast, trade from Russia crossed a bridge over the Tumen River to the sparsely populated town of Rason in the remote northeastern corner of the DPRK, while Russian shipping went to Rason port. Handling the trade in isolated areas involved much less human contact, thus, at least apparently in the eyes of the North Korean leadership, reducing the risk of spreading the virus. The upshot was that even as trade with China dropped precipitously, DPRK-Russia trade actually increased once the initial shock of the border closures wore off. It was one step in a burgeoning relationship that, with the easing of COVID, would lead to Russian leader Vladimir Putin's visiting Pyongyang in 2024, and Kim Jong Un's eventually agreeing to send North Korean soldiers to fight alongside Russian troops in Ukraine.

Meanwhile, I remained frozen out of the DPRK, and the activities of KorAid were at a standstill. Although communication with Pyongyang seemed almost impossible, I did maintain contact with North Korean diplomats I knew at missions in Switzerland, Hong Kong, Beijing, Shenyang, and Bangkok. It was fascinating to learn that they were finding that the information flow from their own foreign ministry had slowed to a trickle, and that communications with their head offices were often difficult and troublesome. Still, they remained under pressure to secure medical supplies to ward off COVID, as well as to get donations for the Pyongyang General Hospital, a large hospital under construction in the capital. The effort was complicated by the fact that, with the exception of medicine, sanctions still prohibited providing hospital equipment, which required special UN permission.

Most of my communications were by phone or email. Even in Switzerland, the DPRK ambassador initially was reluctant to meet in person—not least because, I had learned, most of the embassy staff did not have health insurance and could not risk falling ill. Eventually, however, to my surprise, he and one of his staff accepted my invitation to visit me at my home in Teufen. I had known him for a long time, and it was good to reconnect. He was not able to provide much news about what was going on inside the DPRK—he and his colleagues seemed almost as cut off as everyone else—but he did indicate that there still was a need for humanitarian help. The ambassador was now of retirement age, and he said he assumed that he would be called back to Pyongyang once travel restrictions were lifted. He said that after so many years abroad, he was looking forward to it.

Months went by with no communication from the KPFD in Pyongyang. I did hear periodically from KFPD staff in Shenyang, who asked if KorAid would be willing to support the KRCCD. The request was for help with training programs for physiotherapists, occupational therapists, and doctors; study abroad tours; and rehabilitation and education equipment. Although I was delighted to see that there was still interest, I made it clear that as long as the borders to China and North Korea were closed, KorAid could not help.

Then, on March 21, 2021, for the first time in fifteen months, I received an email from Pyongyang. It was written by a former KFPD staff member. She apologized for having been out of touch and indicated that because of COVID restrictions, even emailing foreign contacts had been banned, so this communication was a welcome surprise. She told me that her new organization lacked knowledge, experts, and inputs, and asked for support from KorAid. She promised to be back in touch with some ideas. Although we were both well aware that the borders had to open for visits and access to partners before any concrete progress could be made, I saw these messages as a positive signal. It was clear that my North Korean interlocutors were thinking ahead and retained at least some hope that a certain level of cooperation might be permitted again.

For the time being, however, despite the emails, the door to the DPRK remained closed.

Largely confined to Switzerland, I still had to manage the administration of KorAid. This included an annual audit, even though KorAid had organized no activities and spent no money. I also spent hours on the phone and participated in numerous conferences held via Zoom. It was a good way to keep in touch, but I found they were no substitute for face-to-face contact. It was difficult to establish personal relationships and build up trust on Zoom, and I found that many participants were cautious about discussing sensitive issues online. Still, the topics were often interesting, ranging from how the hard-liners were prevailing in Pyongyang to current US policy toward the DPRK, North-South relations, the plight of defectors in the South, human rights issues, the treatment of people with disabilities, and how diplomacy might be revived.

One Zoom conference, organized by the Washington, DC–based National Committee on North Korea and the East Asia Foundation, was called "How to Jumpstart and Sustain Diplomacy with North Korea." Participants included Moon Chung-in, an architect of the so-called Sunshine Policy—under which South Korea previously had sought to engage the North—and formerly a special advisor to liberal South Korean President Moon Jae-In, and Susan Thornton, a former US assistant secretary of state for East Asian affairs. As at many such events, though, the debate about the merits of concessions versus pressure—easing or tightening sanctions to get the North back to the negotiating table—ran up against a stark reality. President Joe Biden, who had succeeded Donald Trump in January 2021, appeared to see North Korea as a low priority, and Kim Jong Un seemed to have lost interest in making rapprochement with Washington a central policy goal. My general observation was that most experts were pessimistic about finding constructive solutions to North Korean issues. As one of the very few aid workers who seemed to get invited to participate, I tried at most of these events to offer a perspective focusing on the plight of ordinary people in the DPRK, which often seemed lost amidst the debates about high-level policy. I often felt frustrated that so few concrete actions would emerge from such gatherings.

In the meantime, I was pleasantly surprised to discover that in Switzerland, there was considerable interest in the large collection of North Korean propaganda posters I had accumulated during my many years working in the DPRK. The Swiss Federal Department of Defense, Civil Protection, and Sport was planning an exhibition at a library in Berne marking the seventieth anniversary of Switzerland's participation in the Neutral Nations Supervisory Commission (NNSC), an organization of observers who had been posted along the Korean Demilitarized Zone since the armistice of 1953. There was still a delegation of five Swiss military officers stationed at Panmunjom, on the southern side of the DMZ. The department staff asked if I would let them display some of my posters and if I would give a talk on the humanitarian situation in North Korea.

The Kunstmuseum in Berne, Switzerland's oldest fine arts museum, also approached me. The curator there asked if I could let them show some posters for a planned exhibition of North and South Korean art to be held in 2021. I initially deferred making a decision, out of concern that, given the state of inter-Korean relations, my participation might anger the North Korean authorities and jeopardize my future access, should they be upset at some of the South Korean art on display. But after extensive discussions about what would be the most appropriate posters—and how to ensure that the slogans would be translated accurately, since the Korean spoken in the North had evolved in a quite different way than that in the South over the decades of separation—I agreed to proceed, under the condition that the posters would have a separate room so they were not integrated into the rest of the exhibition. The posters were a big hit, and many visitors said that seeing them was the highlight of the exhibition.

As the COVID pandemic gradually subsided, I was able to resume some travel, although North Korea remained off limits. In the spring of 2022, I spent a month at Stanford, which provided a good opportunity to catch up and network. In New York, I met with UN staffers who had been dealing with North Korea, including Jerome Sauvage, the former head of the UNDP in Pyongyang. That September, I attended a conference on the prospects for peace hosted by Yonsei University in Seoul. I also met with officials from South Korea's Ministry of Unification and a number of NGOs, gave a talk to the Korean Coalition of Rehabilitation Therapists, and visited the Demilitarized Zone, where I was spoke with the Swiss members of the Neutral Nations Supervisory Commission. In November, I attended a conference in Kuala Lumpur, Malaysia, on mediating international conflicts.

Then I flew to Hong Kong, where I had a bad fall and broke my right arm in several places. It required surgery and a long period of rehabilitation, which put me out of action for several months. While still in Hong Kong, I was forced to cancel a planned meeting with staffers at the North Korean Consulate, and I phoned to explain why. Ten minutes later, they called back to say they were already making *bibimbap*, my favorite Korean dish, and that it would be delivered to my hotel shortly. What a nice gesture!

Back in Switzerland in the spring of 2023, as I labored through physiotherapy to strengthen my arm, I received a strange letter from the Hong Kong branch of the Industrial and Commercial Bank of China (ICBC). I had done my personal banking there for years, and it held the account created for KorAid in 2015. The letter said that both my personal account and the KorAid account were being closed. It gave no reason. I was shocked and disappointed. Given the sensitivity of any dealings with North Korea, I had gone out of my way to do everything by the book. The accounts were audited every year, with the paperwork submitted to the Hong Kong government to make sure everything was open and aboveboard. Inquiries by a lawyer in Hong Kong trying to understand the reason for the move produced no further clarification. Given China's own extensive dealings with—and political support for—the DPRK, it didn't seem to make sense that a Chinese bank would be so afraid of being sanctioned that it would act against an organization running such a small-scale and obviously humanitarian mission, or against the person who had created and was managing it. I was utterly perplexed.

I continued to make inquiries and spoke with a number of people familiar with the banking industry in Hong Kong and China. Eventually, a plausible explanation emerged. It had nothing to do with North Korea; instead, it likely was linked to the crackdown on NGOs and civil society that Chinese leader Xi Jinping had initiated. In the early and mid-2000s, China had seen a civil society emerge, with growing numbers of activists involved in labor issues, environmental protection, and promoting women's and LGBT rights; human rights lawyers; foundations started by entrepreneurs creating a new culture of philanthropy; and more. Now, as Xi was purging his rivals and concentrating more and more power in his own hands, the Communist Party had launched a sweeping crackdown to stifle this emerging civil society movement.

According to this analysis, with NGOs a key target of repression on the Chinese mainland and Hong Kong under a draconian new National Security Law that Beijing had imposed in 2020, major institutions in the territory, such as banks—especially Chinese banks—wanted nothing to do with any NGO, regardless of what it was involved in. There was no way to prove the correctness of this interpretation, but it made sense to me and helped explain why an organization providing humanitarian assistance to people in a country with close ties to Beijing would become a target. Given the work I had done in China dating back to the early 1980s, when I'd had my first contact with Deng Xiaoping's son and his organization that assisted people with disabilities in that country, it was ironic that the shadow of the Chinese Communist Party and its fear of any independent organization would lead to the dissolution of KorAid.

In any case, despite my still not fully healed arm, I flew to Hong Kong to ensure that I could at least retrieve the funds in the accounts before they were shut down. After exploring multiple options, eventually my colleagues and I at KorAid decided to donate the $34,432.32 remaining in the KorAid account to UNICEF, as its mission was in line with what KorAid had been doing and, even more so, because at this point UNICEF appeared to be the only UN agency managing to get goods into the DPRK. I initially approached the UNICEF office in Hong Kong, but they wanted nothing to do with North Korea. UNICEF headquarters in New York was more receptive. The money we sent, along with $50,000 I had in a Swiss bank account I was using for KorAid, was all used to procure micronutrient powder for children aged six months to twenty-three months. UNICEF procured 47,724 boxes, each with thirty sachets; 46,731 boxes were delivered to Pyongyang in July 2024, and the remaining packs arrived that November, just as KorAid was being legally dissolved as an organization in Hong Kong. The $50,000 was mostly small-scale donations from friends and family who were happy for me to send the money to UNICEF. I had also, however, received some larger donations from service clubs in Switzerland. When I contacted them about giving funds to a UN agency for work in the DPRK, they requested instead that I return the money so they could use it for other non-North Korea–related projects.

It was a bittersweet moment. Given the stress and anxiety the ICBC's decision had caused, I was immensely relieved to have been able to get hold of the funds and gratified that UNICEF had been able to use the money to purchase badly needed supplies that would help deprived North Korean children. This was very much in keeping with my own values and priorities. Given how much time, energy, and emotion I had invested to create and build up KorAid, however, and given the promise so many of our programs had shown, it was crushing to see the organization disappear—and with it, my hopes of further humanitarian engagement with the country that had played such a big role in my life for so many years. However, I was encouraged that, when I told my North Korean contacts abroad what had happened with KorAid, they said I would still be welcome with or without a supporting organization, and they expressed the hope that I still would be able to provide much-needed support.

Conclusion

In 1995, at the end of my first trip to North Korea, I concluded my report for Caritas–Hong Kong with the following, written as I left Pyongyang: "Many thoughts crossed my mind: People functioning like robots, the reality of brainwashing, the uniformity, the wretched lifestyle, the isolation, even George Orwell's concept of thought-crime. Comparing China to North Korea, China appears to be a free country."

As I write this thirty years later, there's no question that North Korea leaves such an impression, especially to a first-time visitor. But after my seventy-five trips, five years in residence, and decades of intimate involvement, it is equally clear to me that this description is incomplete. With patience, determination, good humor, flexibility, and a willingness to try to understand the world as North Koreans saw it, I encountered variety, complexity, nuance, commitment, conflict, compassion, love, hatred, ambition, despair—the full range of emotions and experiences that reflect the human condition.

While I had no choice but to deal with the system as it was, with all of its oppressiveness and idiosyncrasies—and no question, the system imposed severe constraints on foreigners—my ongoing involvement, which included visiting every province as well as many places other outsiders were not allowed to go, gave me a sense of North Korea as a living, breathing society of twenty-four million individual people, each with his or her own hopes, fears, and aspirations. Amid all the discussion of nuclear weapons, missile tests, sanctions, summits, and talk of war and peace, I always felt that the emphasis needed to be on ordinary citizens. These people did not choose to be born North Korean but were struggling to make their way as best as their circumstances would allow.

Those circumstances, particularly the broader geopolitics, are very different now than when I made my first visit—and indeed when I made, for now, at least, my last one in December 2019. For almost thirty years, beginning in 1990, successive North Korean leaders—Kim Il Sung, Kim Jong Il, and Kim Jong Un—pursued a policy of seeking better relations with the United States as a counterweight to China and Russia. It was in this context that the DPRK asked for foreign help during the period of the famine, implemented or at least tolerated a certain degree of economic reform in the years afterward, allowed a surprisingly large number of Western NGOs and UN and other international agencies to be based in the country, and sought to learn more about how the rest of the world worked. That was the climate in which I began my work in North Korea with Caritas, was later based in Pyongyang for the Swiss government, and subsequently pursued projects with KorAid.

At the same time, however, North Korea's leaders kept the nuclear option as a fallback in case a rapprochement with Washington—which would end what they saw as the US threat to the survival of the DPRK—could not be achieved. There is a clear link between the ups and downs of Pyongyang's diplomatic dealings with the United States and the watershed moments in the DPRK's development of its nuclear weapons. But the failure of the 2019 Trump-Kim summit in Hanoi led to a profound strategic shift in Kim Jong Un's approach. He abandoned hopes for normalization with the United States; turned away from engagement with the West; gave up on progress with South Korea, which he declared to be an enemy state before taking the idea of peaceful negotiated unification off the table; steadily expanded his nuclear arsenal, which some experts believe now numbers between fifty and sixty warheads; and aligned himself with Moscow in a deeper—and from a Western perspective, more problematic—way. This has been underscored by the deployment of thousands of North Korean soldiers to fight with Russian forces in Ukraine.

The return of Donald Trump to the US presidency in January, 2025 fueled speculation of a new American outreach to Kim Jong Un. Even if Kim were to agree to renewed diplomacy, however, the dynamic would be very different from the previous Trump-Kim summit. The US would find Kim in a much stronger position than in 2018 and 2019, having further consolidated his power at home, strengthened his military capabilities, and solidified key alliances. Normalization with the United States is no longer the North Korean priority it once was. If Trump were prepared to offer meaningful concessions, such as US diplomatic recognition or a significant easing of sanctions, Kim might at best agree to a kind of arms control accord that would maintain North Korea as a nuclear state.

That raises the difficult question of what this might mean for those, including myself, who long have supported engagement with the DPRK. The total closure of the country because of COVID ended in 2023, and Pyongyang since has reopened the border to some trade and official delegations, including welcoming a small number of foreigners, mainly Russians and Chinese. Nonetheless, as of the time of writing, the international community in Pyongyang remains tiny, and most of the aid agencies who had operations in the years before COVID are no longer there. And given the country's diplomatic reorientation toward Moscow and Beijing, which has led to a hardening of attitudes toward the DPRK in many countries around the world, including Switzerland, it is legitimate to ask whether this may remain the case for some time to come.

Nevertheless, one of my conclusions from years of dealing with the DPRK is that, for all their ideological posturing, North Koreans are at heart pragmatic. Moreover, Kim Jong Un must know that in the end, given his many public pledges to improve the lives of the population, including a reference to "no more belt-tightening," he does have to do something for the North Korean people. If indeed he feels more confident domestically, it is possible that at some future point he will feel more confident about opening up the country again to the international community, and especially to the UN and NGO agencies that previously had been so deeply involved in the DPRK. With the passage of time, the conviction that foreign aid is "sugar with poison," as one North Korean official voiced to me, might conceivably fade.

Adding to the likelihood of such developments, a large number of North Koreans, many of them now middle- or high-ranking officials, were exposed to how education, health, trade, markets, agriculture, and diplomacy operated in the rest of the world over the two decades prior to COVID. This happened through the programs that I and many other humanitarian and development agencies helped to arrange. Even if the domestic political climate requires these people to remain passive or silent at the moment, they cannot unsee what they saw or unlearn what they absorbed on visits to Vietnam, Cuba, Hong Kong, China, and Europe, or in projects like the Pyongyang Business School and initiatives that required them to make decisions at the local level rather than just follow orders from the center. At some point, if the atmosphere changes, they well could become a catalyst for revived change. Even though the DPRK often seems static and unchanging from the outside, one of the things I have learned is that the on-the-ground reality is much more fluid than it may appear. So, notwithstanding the current grim climate, I remain hopeful.

Indeed, despite an incredibly rigid political system deeply suspicious of outsiders, I found that it was possible to do more than I ever imagined. The tens of thousands of North Koreans who survived the famine because of international aid, and the thirty thousand people whose sight was restored through the help of KorAid, show that it is possible to get things done, to help those who need it the most, even under the most difficult of circumstances. It is possible to live up to the slogan I saw at the Caritas office in Switzerland when I first joined the organization in 1978. "A world where one person suffers less," it declared, "is a better world."

Notes

1 Elisabeth Rosenthal, "In North Korean Hunger, Legacy Is Stunted Children," *New York Times*, December 10, 1998; https://archive.nytimes.com/www.nytimes.com/library/world/asia/121098nkorea-food.html.

2 Kim Jong Il, "The 21st Century is a Century of Great Change and Creation," *Rodong* Sinmun, January 4, 2001.

3 Swiss Federal Department of Foreign Affairs, "Switzerland Condemns Nuclear Test by North Korea," press release, October 9, 2006, https://www.swissinfo.ch/eng/swiss-politics/switzerland-condemns-north-korea-nuclear-test/5493268.

4 Permanent Subcommittee on Investigations, *United Nations Development Program: A Case Study of North Korea*, staff report, January 24, 2008, p. 2; https://www.hsgac.senate.gov/subcommittees/investigations/hearings/united-nations-development-program-a-case-study-of-north-korea/.

5 Ibid, p. 1.

6 *Letter from the Permanent Representative of the DPRK to the United Nations Secretary-General*, March 13, 2007; available at: https://digitallibrary.un.org › record › 595019 › files › A_61_800-EN.pdf.

7 Bo Lager, "Agroforestry Is Taking Root in North Korea, Swedish International Agricultural Network Initiative, blog post, March 15, 2015, https://www.siani.se/blog/agroforestry-taking-root-north-korea/.

8 World Agroforestry Centre (ICRAF), "North Korea Opens its Doors to Agroforestry," *Science Daily*, August 27, 2010; https://www.sciencedaily.com/releases/2010/08/100827082328.htm.

9 The information on Capacity Building, Sloping Land Management, Maize and Cabbage (IPM) in this chapter comes from my own recollections, as well as copies of an *Asia Brief* that SDC's East Asia Division and its agricultural experts published regularly, and to which I also contributed. In particular, I relied on the following:

"Cabbage for All in DPR Korea," *Asia Brief*, October 2007.

"Under Biological Control—Enhancing Maize Production in DPR Korea, *Asia Brief*, December 2009; https://www.eda.admin.ch/dam/deza/en/documents/publikationen/briefing-papers/asia-brief-2a-2010_EN.pdf.

"Food from the Hills—Sloping Land Management in DPR Korea," *Asia Brief*, August 2010; https://www.eda.admin.ch/dam/deza/en/documents/publikationen/briefing-papers/asia-brief-2a-2010_EN.pdf.

"Catching Up on Capacity in DPR Korea Partnership Results," *Asia Brief*, January 2011; https://www.eda.admin.ch/dam/deza/en/documents/publikationen/briefing-papers/asia-brief-1-2011_EN.pdf.

10 George Packer, "The Quiet German," *New Yorker*, November 24, 2014.

11 "DPRK Foreign Ministry Spokesman Blasts Anti-DPRK 'Resolution,'" Korean Central News Agency, March 29, 2008; available at: https://www.globalsecurity.org/wmd/library/news/dprk/2008/dprk-080331-kcna03.htm.

12 United Nations Development Programme, "Statement on Senate Investigation into UNDP Operations in DPRK," January 23, 2008; available at: https://reliefweb.int/report/democratic-peoples-republic-korea/undp-statement-senate-investigation-undp-operations-dprk.

13 Barack Obama, "Inaugural Address" (speech, Washington, DC, January 20, 2009), US Government Publishing Office; https://www.govinfo.gov/content/pkg/DCPD-200900001/pdf/DCPD-200900001.pdf.

14 "Let Us All Become Speed-Campaign Heroes in the 150-Day Battle to Win a Shining Victory in the Grand Construction of a Prosperous and Powerful Nation," editorial, *Rodong Sinmun,* September 23, 2009.

15 Jere Longman, "Kim Jong Il, The Sportsman," *New York Times*, December 20, 2011; https://www.nytimes.com/2011/12/21/sports/remembering-kim-jong-ils-ventures-into-the-sporting-world.html.

16 Massimo Calabrese, "The Strange World of N. Korea's 'Great Leader,'" *Time,* October 28, 2000; https://time.com/archive/6928154/the-strange-world-of-n-koreas-great-leader/.

17 Cited in Jina Yang, "Women's Rights in the DPRK: Discrepancies Between International and Domestic Legal Instruments in Promoting Women's Rights and the Reality Reflected by North Korean Defectors," p. 223; available at: https://ww3.lawschool.cornell.edu/research/ILJ/upload/Yang-final.pdf.

18 Thomas Maresca, "Why the Overwhelming Majority of North Korean Defectors are Women, *USA Today,* updated December 10, 2017; https://www.usatoday.com/story/news/world/2017/12/10/most-defectors-north-korea-women/923072001/.

19 Citations in Wikipedia and Yonho Kim, "Cell Phones in North Korea," US-Korea Institute, SAIS, 2014; https://www.38north.org/wp-content/uploads/2014/03/Kim-Yonho-Cell-Phones-in-North-Korea.pdf.

20 Christopher Green and Yongseok Shin, "The Kaesong Industrial Complex: Setting the Stage for a Successful Second Act," 38 North, June 27, 2019; https://www.38north.org/2019/06/cgreenyshin062719/.

[21] Urs Schoettli, "Der Fall Nordkorea: Ein Mandat zum Schweigen?" [*The Case of North Korea: A Mandate to Say Nothing?], Neue Zürcher Zeitung,* February 15, 2008.

[22] Barack Obama, "Remarks by President Obama and President Lee of the Republic of Korea in Joint Press Availability," press conference, White House Office of the Press Secretary, Washington, DC, June 16, 2009; https://obamawhitehouse.archives.gov/the-press-office/remarks-president-obama-and-president-lee-republic-korea-joint-press-availability.

[23] "The Elders' Visit to the Korean Peninsula and China, April 2011," The Elders; https://theelders.org/news/report-elders-visit-korean-peninsula-and-china-april-2011.

[24] Katharina Zellweger, "People with Disabilities in a Changing North Korea," Shorenstein Asia-Pacific Research Center, Stanford University, March 1, 2014, p. 2; https://aparc.fsi.stanford.edu/publications/people_with_disabilities_in_a_changing_north_korea.

[25] Ibid, p. 45.

[26] Ibid. p. 2.

[27] António Guterres, *The Highest Aspiration: A Call to Action for Human Rights* (New York: United Nations, 2020); https://www.un.org/sg/sites/default/files/atoms/files/The_Highest_Asperation_A_Call_To_Action_For_Human_Right_English.pdf.

[28] Mythili Sampathkumar, "United Nations' Own Sanctions Hinder its Humanitarian Aid Efforts in North Korea," *Independent,* April 12, 2018; https://www.independent.co.uk/news/world/north-korea-nuclear-weapons-humanitarian-aid-united-nations-a8302181.html.

Robert R. King, "Humanitarian Engagement with North Korea—Great Need but Increasingly Difficult," Center for Strategic and International Studies, September 4, 2018; https://www.csis.org/analysis/humanitarian-engagement-north-korea-great-need-increasingly-difficult.

[29] Donald J. Trump, "Remarks by President Trump Before a Briefing on the Opioid Crisis," (speech, Bedminster, NJ, August 8, 2017), White House archives; https://trumpwhitehouse.archives.gov/briefings-statements/remarks-president-trump-briefing-opioid-crisis/.

[30] Talha Burki, "North Korea and the Global Fund," *The Lancet Infectious Diseases,* vol. 18, May 2018; available at: https://www.thelancet.com/journals/laninf/article/PIIS1473-3099(18)30238-X/abstract.

[31] Byungjin Park and Joonmo Cho, "North Korea's COVID-19 Policy Dilemma: Epidemic Prevention Conflicting with Trade," *Globalization and Health,* January 16, 2024; available at: https://pmc.ncbi.nlm.nih.gov/articles/PMC10790389/.

[32] Ibid.

[33] Olivia Enos, "Critical Signs to Watch for Famine in North Korea," *The National Interest,* June 29, 2021; https://nationalinterest.org/blog/korea-watch/critical-signs-watch-famine-north-korea-188838/.

[34] *DPR Korea Needs and Priorities 2020,* United Nations Humanitarian Programme Cycle, April 2020; https://dprkorea.un.org/sites/default/files/2020-04/2020_DPRK_Needs_and-Priorities_Plan.pdf.

Index

B

C

K

R

Acknowledgments

Deepest gratitude to the people of North Korea—ordinary citizens and government officials—who, in a largely closed society with a long history of suspicion of foreigners, opened themselves and shared information, access, and details of their often challenging lives in ways this book has sought to convey. For understandable reasons, we cannot name them.

Particular thanks for the access I was given over so many years to nurseries, kindergartens, schools, baby homes, orphanages, boarding schools, hospitals, cooperative farms, factories, universities, other institutes of learning, and the many individual families I met.

Many North Korean organizations facilitated my visits and work over the years. Special thanks to the North Korean Flood Damage Rehabilitation Committee (FDRC), the Korean Federation for the Protection of the Disabled (KFPD), the Korean Rehabilitation Center for Children with Disabilities (KRCCD), the Korean Democratic Women's Union, the Korean Catholic Association, the Education Commission, the staff at the Kaesong Industrial Complex, the Korean European Coordination Agency (KECCA), the North Korean Ministry of Health, the Ministry of Agriculture, the Ministry of Land and Environmental Protection, the Ministry of Labor, the Ministry of Foreign Trade, and others. We are particularly grateful to the Ministry of Foreign Affairs, which, often in record time and almost always without problems, granted visas to me for seventy-five trips as well as permission to live in Pyongyang for five years, in addition to giving Mike visas for his seventeen trips to the DPRK. The North Korean embassies in Switzerland and Beijing and the North Korean Consulate General in Hong Kong also were very welcoming and helpful.

Special thanks are due to all those who, particularly during the worst of the famine years, provided financial and other support to the relief effort, especially the Catholic Church in South Korea and many other organizations there—in particular, Caritas in South Korea and the Catholic Priests' Association for Justice. At an international level, thanks to the Canadian Foodgrains Bank and the Mennonite Central Committee, as well as to all members of the worldwide Caritas family and other donors big and small.

Caritas Switzerland hired and sent me to Hong Kong. Then, in 1995, Caritas Internationalis entrusted me with the often delicate and challenging responsibility of managing its programs in North Korea. Caritas–Hong Kong, Caritas Switzerland, and Caritas Korea all also played crucial roles. I am especially grateful to two men who served at different times as secretary general of Caritas Internationalis, Gerhard Meier and Duncan MacLaren. Without their backing, and that of all other Caritas colleagues, the work conducted in the DPRK would have been impossible. Special thanks as well to the Vatican for its support.

The Swiss Agency for Development and Cooperation (SDC) appointed me to head its office in Pyongyang in 2006 for five years, an experience for which I am deeply grateful. Special thanks to my SDC colleagues—both international and North Korean, as well as the many visiting consultants—who shared work experiences, enjoyable camaraderie, and many memorable occasions. These efforts were supported by the Swiss government's Federal Department of Foreign Affairs, particularly the Swiss embassy in Beijing, especially Ambassador Blaise Godet and Berne-based desk officer Andreas Gerrits. The Swiss embassy in Washington, DC, and the Permanent Mission of Switzerland to the United Nations in New York also provided valuable assistance.

Beyond the SDC, I extend warmest thanks to friends and colleagues in the international community in Pyongyang: the World Food Program, the World Health Organization, the UNDP, the FAO, the UNFPA, UNICEF, the Federation for the Red Cross and Red Crescent Societies, the International Committee of the Red Cross, Handicap International, and members of the diplomatic community in Pyongyang, as well as the staff at the EU office there and all resident and nonresident NGOs.

Other organizations who played important roles in my work over the years, and to whom I offer deepest thanks, include the Central European University in Budapest, which accepted North Koreans for training programs in economics as early as the late 1990s; and the Geneva Centre for Applied Studies in International Negotiations (CASIN), the University of Basel's Institute for Global European Studies, and the Institute of Federalism at the University of Fribourg, which also all were open to receiving and training people from

North Korea. In addition, special thanks to the Centre for Agriculture and Bioscience International (CABI), based in Delémont, Switzerland; the office of the International Center for Research in Agriculture (ICRAF) and the Kunming Institute of Botany in China; the China Disabled Persons' Federation, which was started by Deng Pufang, the disabled son of longtime senior leader Deng Xiaoping; and a number of Chinese institutions and think tanks focusing on North Korea with whom I had the opportunity to exchange views. The Hong Kong Management Association (HKMA) and its capable staff played a crucial role in the success of the Pyongyang Business School.

I am also particularly grateful for other support from Hong Kong, including donors who helped to fund my work. In addition, special thanks to the two Hong Kong–based experts in health and disability who traveled with me to North Korea and did presentations and training programs, as well as all staff at institutions working with intellectually challenged children in Hong Kong who received a delegation from Pyongyang with open arms. Thanks as well to Geoffrey See and his colleagues at Choson Exchange, and also to the two members of the KorAid committee.

The many journalists who interviewed me over the years (including Mike, when he was a CNN correspondent) deserve special acknowledgement. I am especially grateful to CNN anchor Patricia Chew, who guided me through a nerve-racking first TV interview! That and other coverage was crucial in bringing news of the suffering in North Korea to the rest of the world.

The authors want to single out a number of other individuals as well.

Leon Sigal and Robert Carlin read every single page of multiple drafts of the book, and offered crucially important criticism, corrections, and advice. John Delury, Barbara Demick, Eason Jordan, Philip Revzin, Siegfried Hecker, Jean Lee, Anna Fifield, and Jerome Sauvage also read the full manuscript. Their feedback has made this a much better book, and we are profoundly grateful. Others who read specific chapters and offered comments include Monsignor Celestino Migliore, Father Gerard Hammond, as well as Mike's sister, Clara, and sons Dan and Ben.

Our agent, Marc Mikulich, is one of a kind. He believed in this project from the moment we contacted him, never got discouraged, and expended tremendous effort to find a home for it. We are profoundly grateful for his wise counsel and assistance.

At Post Hill Press, special thanks to Debra Englander, Lexi Vanatta, Elena Vega, John Mitchell and their colleagues for their help and support.

Several Stanford University North Korea experts befriended both Mike and me over the years. John Lewis, Siegfried Hecker, and Robert Carlin helped deepen our understanding of the DPRK and also played a crucial role in shaping my professional future after I left Pyongyang, by inviting me to join the university's Walter H. Shorenstein Asia-Pacific Research Center (APARC). Gi-Wook Shin and his team at APARC—David Straub, Heather Ahn, Karen Eggleston, Karl Eikenberry, and Tom Fingar—offered me a new and supportive base to continue to follow developments in North Korea, as did Stanford's Center for International Security and Cooperation (CISAC), which invited me to join their group on North Korea and other security issues in East Asia.

We also would like to thank the following individuals:

Felix Abt, former Finnish President Martti Ahtisaari, Ruedi Bischof, former Norwegian Prime Minister Gro Brundtland, Urs Buchmann, former US President Jimmy Carter, Mayling Chan, Roberto Christen, Simone Dellemagne, Anita Fahrni, Louis de Saint-Gall, Monsignor Paul Richard Gallagher, Umberto Greco, Mary Healy, Stephan Herzog, Thomas Hoerz, Hugo Hörndli, Merete Johansson, Tapan Mishra, Monsignor Luis Mariano Montemayor, Park Kyung-seo, former Irish President Mary Robinson, Kim Robinson, Hans Roth, Abu Salim, Adrian Schlaepfer, Erwin Schurtenberger, Wilhelm Strohe, Helen Tinsley, Amy Tso, Christian Wasserfallen, Erich Weingartner, Thomas Wettstein, and Xu Jianchu.

Finally, special thanks to friends and family.

For Mike: his wife, Inez; sister, Clara, sons Dan and Ben; and cousin, the writer John Krich; as well as Woodrow and Unit Two, provided crucial intellectual and emotional support.

For me: Winnie Kan, my long-time assistant at Caritas, who kept my office running smoothly during all my travels; Guido Furrer, Michelle Garnaut, Ornella Julita, Jean Lee, Ildiko Moran, Elaine Pickering, Joan Polinsky, Hanspeter Spörri, and so many others helped with brainstorming a title of the book and gave other valuable input. Thanks to siblings Frieda, Gret, Hans, and their spouses as well as cousin Hansruedi for their patience when I often would say that I had no time for anything else because I was busy with the book. A special thanks also to my sister Heidi, who came to see me in Pyongyang, and also other friends and colleagues who were eager to visit and learn more about life in North Korea.

Apologies if people have been omitted, for mistakes in the text, or important issues neglected.

Deepest gratitude on my part goes to Mike Chinoy, who came up with the brilliant idea of writing this book. Without him, this book would not exist.

About the Authors

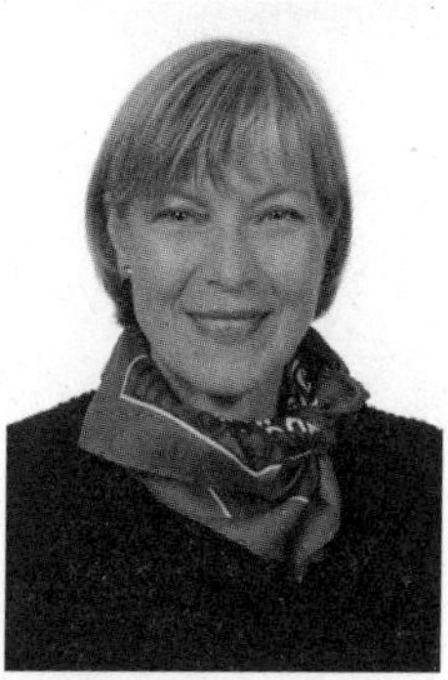

Kathi Zellweger is a senior aid manager with over thirty years of field experience in Hong Kong, China, and North Korea. She was based in Pyongyang for five years (2006–2011) as the North Korea country director for the Swiss Agency for Development and Cooperation (SDC), an office of the Swiss Federal Department of Foreign Affairs. Before joining SDC, from 1978 to 2006, Zellweger worked in a senior post for the Catholic Agency Caritas in Hong Kong, where she played a key role in pioneering Caritas's involvement in China and North Korea.

She also managed the Hong Kong–based KorAid Limited, a nonprofit she established in 2015 to focus on serving children in institutions and people with disabilities in North Korea. Zellweger is affiliated with the Center for International Security and Cooperation (CISAC) at Stanford University in California. She holds a master's degree in international administration from the School for International Training in Brattleboro, Vermont.

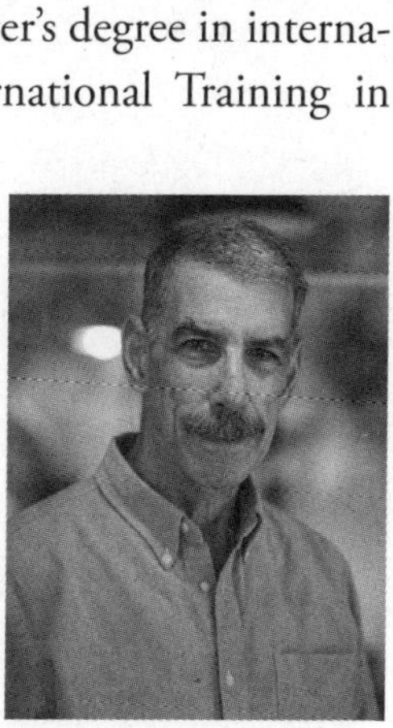

Mike Chinoy is a nonresidentscholar at the 21st Century China Center at the University of California, San Diego. Previously, he was a nonresident senior fellow at the University of Southern California's US-China Institute. Before joining USC, he spent twenty-four years as a foreign correspondent for CNN. He was the network's first bureau chief in Beijing, bureau chief in Hong Kong, and senior Asia correspondent. He also worked for CBS News and NBC News in Hong Kong.

Chinoy won Emmy, DuPont, Peabody, and ACE awards for his coverage of China, and also made seventeen trips to North Korea. After leaving CNN, he was a senior fellow at the Los Angeles–based Pacific Council on International Policy, focusing on security issues in North Korea, China, and Northeast Asia before joining the USC US-China Institute. He is the author of five other books. He has an MS degree from Columbia and a BA from Yale.